EXERCISE ELECTROCARDIOGRAPHY:
Practical Approach

Publications by Edward K. Chung, M.D.

(Williams & Wilkins Co.)

Digitalis Intoxication, 1969.

Cardiac Arrhythmias: Management (Tape Series), 1973.

Principles of Cardiac Arrhythmias, Second Edition, 1977.

Cardiac Arrhythmias: Self Assessment, 1977.

Artificial Cardiac Pacing: Practical Approach, 1979.

Exercise Electrocardiography: Practical Approach, 1979.

EXERCISE ELECTROCARDIOGRAPHY: Practical Approach

Edited by Edward K. Chung, M.D., F.A.C.P., F.A.C.C.

Professor of Medicine
Jefferson Medical College of
Thomas Jefferson University and
Director of the Heart Station and
Attending Physician (Cardiologist)
Thomas Jefferson University Hospital
Philadelphia, PA. 19107

Fellow, American College of Cardiology
Former Governor for West Virginia, American College of Cardiology
Fellow, American College of Physicians
Honorary Fellow, Philippine College of Cardiology and
    Philippine Heart Association
Member, American Federation for Clinical Research
Member, American Heart Association
Member, American Medical Association

Editorial Board Member for the Cardiology,
The Journal of Electrocardiology, Heart and
Lung, Drug Therapy, Primary Cardiology,
Hospital Physician and Current Prescribing

THE WILLIAMS & WILKINS COMPANY
Baltimore

Copyright ©, 1979
The Williams & Wilkins Company
428 E. Preston Street
Baltimore, Md. 21202, U.S.A.

Made in the United States of America

Library of Congress Cataloging in Publication Data

Main entry under title:

Exercise electrocardiography.

Includes index.
1. Electrocardiography. 2. Exercise tests. 3. Heart function tests. I. Chung, Edward
K. RC683.5.E5E95   616.1'2'0754   78-15889 ISBN 0-683-01569-9

Composed and printed at the
Waverly Press, Inc.
Mt. Royal and Guilford Aves.
Baltimore, Md. 21202, U.S.A.

To My Wife, Lisa
and
To My Children,
Linda and Christopher

Preface

Exercise electrocardiography (the exercise ECG test or the stress ECG test) is clearly one of the most important and the most popular non-invasive diagnostic tests in the field of cardiovascular disease.

The primary purpose of exercise electrocardiography is to determine the nature and the etiology of chest pain. By doing so, the early diagnosis of coronary heart disease can be made by the exercise ECG test.

In addition, the efficacy of medical as well as surgical therapy for the cardiac patient can be assessed. Furthermore, the functional capacity of the cardiac patients can be evaluated by the exercise ECG test.

The aim of this book is to provide useful information regarding exercise electrocardiography for the diagnosis and management of cardiac patients. This book presents 17 Chapters including Introductory Remarks on Exercise Electrocardiography, Master's Two-Step Test, Preparations and Precautions for the Exercise ECG Test, Methodology of the Exercise ECG Test: Technical Aspects, Problems Related to the Exercise ECG Test: Technical Aspects, Problems Related to the Exercise ECG Test, Effects of Drugs and Metabolic Abnormalities on the Exercise ECG Test, Indications of the Exercise ECG Test, Contraindications of the Exercise ECG Test, Protocols for the Exercise ECG Test, Exercise ECG Test in Children, Physiologic versus Abnormal Responses to Exercise, Interpretation of the Exercise ECG Test, Exercise-induced Cardiac Arrhythmias, Myocardial Perfusion Imaging with Thallium 201: Correlation with Exercise Electrocardiography and Coronary Angiography, Value of the Exercise ECG Test for Screening Asymptomatic Subjects for Latent Coronary Artery Disease, Circulatory Adjustments to Exercise, and Complications of the Exercise ECG Test and Some Aspects of Medico-Legal Problems.

The intention of this book is to describe every pertinent aspect of exercise electrocardiography, which is directly or indirectly related to the patient's care. The contents are intended to be clinical, concise and practical, so that this book will provide all physicians with up-to-date materials related to the exercise ECG test.

This book will be particularly valuable to all primary physicians, including family physicians, internists, cardiologists, cardiology fellows and medical residents. In addition, medical students, coronary care unit nurses and physicians in the field of rehabilitation medicine will obtain a great benefit by reading this book.

I am sincerely grateful to all authors for their valuable contributions to this book, EXERCISE ELECTROCARDIOGRAPHY: PRACTICAL APPROACH. I also wish to thank my personal secretary, Miss Theresa McAnally for her devoted and cheerful secretarial assistance. She has been most valuable in handling correspondence to all contributors in addition to

typing many of my chapters for this book. It has been my pleasure to share
the work to complete this valuable book with the Staff of the Williams and
Wilkins Company.

Lake Naomi,   EDWARD K. CHUNG, M.D.
Mt. Pocono, Pa.

Contributors

Elias Botvinick, M.D.
Assistant Professor of Medicine and Radiology
University of California, San Francisco
School of Medicine
San Francisco, California   94143

Edward K. Chung, M.D., F.A.C.P., F.A.C.C.
Professor of Medicine
Jefferson Medical College of
Thomas Jefferson University
Director of the Heart Station
Thomas Jefferson University Hospital
Philadelphia, PA.   19107

Lisa S. Chung, M.D.
Chief Medical Officer and Medical Director
U.S. Public Health Service
Philadelphia, PA. 19107

Jan Praetorius Clausen, M.D.
Department of Clinical Physiology
Frederiksberg Hospital, Ndr. Fasanvej 57
DK-2000 Copenhagen F. Denmark

Arthur W. Colbourn, M.D.
Fellow in Cardiology
Jefferson Medical College of
Thomas Jefferson University
Philadelphia, PA.   19107

James Conklin, M.D.
Staff Physician
Wilford Hall Air Force Medical Center
Lackland AFB, Texas

B. Don Franks, Ph.D., F.A.C.S.M.
Chairperson, Division of Physical Education
University of Tennessee
School of Health, Physical Education and Rehabilitation
1914 Andy Holt Avenue
Knoxville, Tennessee   37916

Victor F. Froelicher, M.D., F.A.C.C.
Assistant Professor of Medicine
University of California at San Diego
Director, Cardiac Rehabilitation and Exercise Testing
University of California at San Diego
School of Medicine
San Diego, Calif.   92103

Lewis W. Gray, M.D.
Fellow in Cardiology
Jefferson Medical College of
Thomas Jefferson University
Philadelphia, PA.   19107

Frederick W. James, M.D., F.A.C.C.
Associate Professor of Pediatrics
Head, Exercise Laboratory
Children's Hospital
Elland and Bethesda Avenue
Cincinnati, Ohio   45229

John P. Naughton, M.D., F.A.C.P., F.A.C.C.
Dean, School of Medicine
Professor of Medicine
State University of New York at Buffalo
101 Farber Hall
Buffalo, New York   14214

William W. Parmley, M.D., F.A.C.P., F.A.C.C.
Professor of Medicine
Chief, Cardiovascular Division
University of California, San Francisco
School of Medicine
San Francisco, Calif.   94143

David Shames, M.D.
Associate Professor of Radiology
University of California, San Francisco
School of Medicine
San Francisco, California   94143

Edward A. Solow, M.D.
Fellow in Cardiology
George Washington University
School of Medicine
Washington, D.C.

Contents

1

Introductory Remarks on Exercise Electrocardiography

Edward K. Chung, M.D., F.A.C.P., F.A.C.C.

General Considerations[1-9]

The exercise electrocardiography (stress ECG test or exercise ECG test) is one of the most important and valuable non-invasive diagnostic tests in the clinical evaluation and management of patients with suspected or known cardiovascular disease, particularly coronary artery disease. The exercise ECG test is also a very useful tool as a screening procedure for healthy individuals who are considered to be at possible risk of coronary heart disease.

Initially, the Master's two-step test was very popular, but it has been gradually replaced by the treadmill exercise ECG test in the past decade, primarily because only insufficient exercise can be performed by the former. Namely, there will be a lack of sufficient sensitivity by the Master's test leading to an extremely high incidence of false negative tests. In the United States of America, the exercise electrocardiography is performed by a motor-driven treadmill in most medical institutions and many private offices of physicians. In European countries, however, the treadmill exercise ECG test is much less popular, and instead, a bicycle ergometer is commonly used. The reason for this is probably that European life is more familiar with bicycle riding. In addition, other forms of exercise ECG tests have been evaluated, such as induced-hypoxia, isometric exercise and atrial pacing. These exercise tests have not gained wide popularity owing to difficulties in performance and standardization as well as a lack of sensitivity and specificity (sensitivity and specificity will be discussed later in this Chapter). At present, various multistage exercise protocols have been developed by different investigators for the exercise ECG test using either a motor-driven treadmill or an electrically-braked bicycle ergometer (see Chapter 9).

The exercise ECG test is primarily used for the assessment of the etiology of chest pain and for early detection of coronary heart disease. In addition, the exercise ECG test can provide valuable information in evaluating the functional capacity of the patients with coronary artery disease, and in evaluating the efficacy of medical as well as surgical therapy.

Historical Considerations

As far as a history of the exercise electrocardiography is concerned, Dr. Arthur M. Master's original contribution is truly legendary, and he unquestionably deserves invaluable credit and recognition.[10, 11] Before the introduction of Master's two-step test in 1929,[10] the earliest recognition in the field of the exercise ECG test should be credited to Bousfield.[12] The S-T segment depression was recorded in the 3 standard leads during a spontaneous angina in 1918 by Bousfield for the first time.[12] Later, in 1928, Feil and Siegel[13] demonstrated that angina was accompanied by a prolonged period of the S-T segment depression. They used the term "positive response" when the S-T, T wave changes were produced by the exercise along with the duplication of the anginal pain. They claimed that the ECG abnormalities in angina patients are due to a reduction of blood flow to the heart. Their published ECG tracings clearly revealed that the ECG findings returned to normal when the chest pain subsided and also when the nitroglycerin was administered in patients with angina pectoris. They performed their exercise tests by having the patients do sit-ups. Prior to these investigators' accomplishments, Einthoven[14] published an ECG tracing demonstrating the S-T segment depression after exercise, although he did not comment on this finding. He probably deserves credit in the field of exercise electrocardiography.

Master[10] published his first paper regarding the exercise test in 1929. He measured only pulse and blood pressure in evaluating the cardiac capacity, and he failed to recognize the value of the electrocardiographic findings to diagnose ischemia. It is interesting to note that Master and Jaffe[11] proposed the importance of taking an electrocardiogram before and after the exercise test to detect coronary insufficiency for the first time in 1941, 12 years after Master's original contribution[10] in 1929.

Wood and Wolferth[15] also described the S-T segment change in patients with coronary heart disease by exercise in 1931, and they pointed out the usefulness of the S-T segment changes in the diagnosis. They proposed that lead V_4 was more useful to detect ischemic changes than the standard limb leads.

In 1932, Goldhammer and Scherf[16] reported the S-T segment depression in 75% of 40 patients with angina, and they proposed the value of exercise to confirm the diagnosis of ischemia due to coronary heart disease.

In 1935, Katz and Landt[17] proposed that lead V_5 was the best lead to bring out the ischemic changes. They tried to standardize their exercise tests by having the patients lift dumbbells while lying on a table.

Missal[18] studied initially normal subjects by having them run up from

3–6 flights of stairs, but later, in 1938, he used Master's 9-inch steps to exercise his patients. He had his patients exercise to the point of anginal pain and stressed the importance of taking the ECG recording as quickly as possible thereafter.

In 1940, Riseman et al.[19] described the use of continuous monitoring for the first time, and they pointed out that S-T segment depression usually appeared before the onset of anginal pain and usually persisted for a time after the chest pain subsided. They also described the protective effects of O_2 breathing, and indicated the presence of mild S-T segment depression in healthy individuals up to 1 mm. as compared with marked (2–7 mm.) S-T segment depression in patients with coronary artery disease. Their conclusion, however, was that the exercise test was of little practical value because of its poor differentiation between the healthy individuals and the coronary patients.

Important recognition of the false positive exercise ECG test due to digitalis effect was described, for the first time, by Liebow and Feil[20] in 1941, and they emphasized that this finding would confuse the diagnosis of true ischemic changes in the exercise ECG.

In 1942, Johnson, et al.[21] developed the "Harvard step test" which was very similar to the original Master's test while they were working at the Harvard Fatigue Laboratory. The Harvard step test was used widely in athletic circles to assess the physical fitness, and a form of it (the Pack test) was utilized for military purposes. Pulse counts were used during recovery periods for an index of physical fitness.

In 1949, Hecht[22] reported that his experience with the anoxemia test showing 90% sensitivity in the diagnosis of coronary artery disease. He emphasized that the chest pain was an unreliable end point and accompanies ischemia in only 50% of the cases. Hecht also stressed that the S-T segment changes associated with anoxemia may not occur in patients with previous myocardial infarction.

In 1950, Wood et al.[23] described their experience with an effort test at the National Heart Hospital in London. They had patients run up 84 steps adjacent to their laboratory, and emphasized that it was necessary to push the patients to the maximal level of their capacity. They concluded that the sensitivity of their test was 88% reliable compared with a 39% reliability of the Master's test. They further emphasized that the amount of exercise should not be fixed but adjusted to the patient's capacity in order to bring out a higher percentage of positive tests in patients with coronary artery disease by giving the maximal exercise.

In 1952, Yu and Soffer[24] proposed the following ECG changes indicating myocardial ischemia by using the Master's test with continuous monitoring:

(1) S-T segment depression of 1.0 mm. or greater
(2) Alteration of the T wave direction from upright to inverted or vice versa

(3) Increased amplitude of the T wave of 50% or greater than the resting ECG finding

(4) Prolongation of the Q-T/T-Q ratio during exercise to more than two.

They again stressed the importance of continuous monitoring. In addition, Yu et al.[25] reported the exercise ECG test using a motor-driven treadmill elevated to a 10–20% grade with continuous monitoring. They proposed a bipolar lead from the right scapula to the lead V_5 position to be used for a treadmill exercise ECG test.

In 1953, Feil and Brofman[26] studied the effect of exercise on the electrocardiogram of bundle branch block. They indicated that transient bundle branch block developing with exercise was first described by Bousfield[12] in 1918. They also reported false positive exercise ECG tests in his patients with Wolff-Parkinson-White syndrome.

Until 1955, the Master's test had been the exercise ECG test of choice, and it is still widely used in many parts of the world where sophisticated and modern exercise laboratory facilities are not available. In 1956, modern exercise ECG tests using a motor-driven treadmill began to receive wide acceptance for research purposes as well as for clinical medicine. Recently, numerous investigators reported the data regarding the correlation between the result of the exercise ECG tests and the coronary arteriographic findings (will be discussed later).

Among many investigators, the following should be recognized as valuable contributors[1-9] in the field of modern exercise electrocardiography (in alphabetical order): Åstrand, Balke, Blackburn, Bruce, Clausen, Ellestad, Epstein, Fox, Froelicher, Kattus, McHenry, Naughton, Sheffield and many others.

Pathophysiologic Considerations

The exercise ECG test has two major roles. One role is to determine whether the coronary circulation is capable of increasing oxygen supply to the myocardium in response to increased demands. During physical exercise, myocardial oxygen demands are increased by the increment of systolic pressure, contractile state and the heart rate.[27] Another role of the exercise ECG test is to assess the exercise capacity. The major determining factor of the exercise capacity is considered to be the capability of the heart to increase the cardiac output, providing there is no evidence of anemia, pulmonary disease, nervous system or peripheral circulatory disorders.

The heart extracts approximately 70% of the oxygen from each unit of blood perfusing the myocardium at rest,[28] so that oxygen delivery cannot be significantly increased by increased extraction. For practical purposes, myocardial metabolism is entirely aerobic. Thus, coronary blood flow must increase in order to increase the myocardial oxygen supply.[29] It has been shown that coronary blood flow increases directly in proportion to increased demands by the myocardium for oxygen in healthy individuals.[30] On the other hand, coronary blood flow fails to increase adequately to meet the demands of the myocardium for oxygen in the patients with coronary artery disease leading to myocardial ischemia. Myocardial ischemia may be manifested by anginal pain, S-T, T wave changes, ventricular dysfunction, various cardiac arrhythmias and any combinations of the above.

It has been well demonstrated that the myocardial oxygen supply may not be reduced significantly at rest to cause myocardial ischemia, even in some patients with severe coronary artery disease. It is not yet settled regarding the degree of coronary artery stenosis to designate a "significant" obstruction. It has been shown in the experimental animal study that reduction of the resting coronary blood flow is produced by an 85% stenosis.[31] During exercise, however, a coronary blood flow is considered significantly reduced when there is at least 50% narrowing.[31, 32] Physical exercise leads to an increment of myocardial oxygen consumption via the increased heart rate, intramyocardial tension and the velocity of myocardial contraction.[33, 34] Acceleration of the heart rate is associated with a reasonably linear increment of myocardial oxygen consumption,[35, 36] and the heart rate during exercise provides a useful parameter of myocardial oxygen requirements. By measuring blood pressure during exercise, the simple product of the heart rate and systolic blood pressure can be calculated, and this result is considered to be a practical index of myocardial oxygen requirements.[34-37]

Detailed descriptions regarding physiologic versus abnormal responses to exercise are found in Chapter 11.

Preparations and Precautions[1-9]

Needless to say, all exercise ECG tests must be ordered by the physicians. When the order is accepted by the exercise laboratory, the exercise test is scheduled as an elective procedure on either an outpatient or inpatient basis. The patients are instructed to report for their exercise ECG tests either after an overnight fast or 2 hours after a light meal. All patients should be dressed comfortably and the exercise laboratory should be in a comfortable temperature, between 68 and 74°F., with 40–60% humidity. It is preferable to have the patient rest comfortably in the supine position for at least 10 minutes before the actual exercise is performed.

Prior to the exercise ECG test, a complete history should be taken and a thorough physical examination should be performed in order to determine whether the patient is suitable for the test. Indications versus contraindications of the exercise ECG test should be carefully considered (see Chapters 7 and 8). Careful consideration should also be given to whether the patient is taking any drug (e.g., digitalis, propranolol, etc.) which may influence the result of the exercise ECG test (see Chapter 6).

It is mandatory to obtain a 12-lead electrocardiogram in order to determine the presence or absence of any acute cardiac events (e.g., acute myocardial infarction) or any possible contraindications. This author routinely obtains two complete 12-lead ECGs, one before the test and one after the completion of the test for comparison. Chest X-ray is not essential immediately before the test; it is preferable to have a chest X-ray taken a few weeks prior to the exercise ECG test, especially when a possibility of heart failure is suspected.

It is an excellent idea to obtain an informed consent form (see Chapter 9) prior to the test, signed by the patient and witnessed by the physician, from the medico-legal point of view, although some institutions do not request a formal consent form.

The patient should be fully instructed regarding the entire procedure of the exercise ECG test, and the test should be supervised by a physician who is fully familiar with all aspects of the test, including the procedure and the interpretations.

The exercise ECG test should be terminated at the patient's request at any time. In addition, we have to stop the test when the patient develops significant symptoms (e.g., chest pain, dizziness, dyspnea, etc.), hypotension, cyanosis, bradycardia or other serious cardiac arrhythmias and/or marked S-T segment changes. The patient should be treated immediately as needed for significant symptoms, cardiac arrhythmias and any other untoward complications. It is essential to have all necessary cardiopulmonary resuscitative equipment, including a defibrillator and commonly used cardiac emergency drugs in the exercise laboratory. All physicians and assistants working in the exercise laboratory should be capable of handling any cardiopulmonary emergencies.

Methodology

Exercise Methods

As described previously, the most commonly used exercise ECG test, at present, is a motor-driven treadmill test, particularly in the United States of America. In Europe, however, the bicycle ergometer is more popular than the treadmill exercise test.

A less commonly used method is the arm-crank ergometer which is particularly valuable in patients who are unable to exercise on the treadmill or bicycle.[38, 39] This exercise test has been shown to be a reliable substitute for the more conventional methods.[38, 39]

Another method is right atrial pacing, which increases myocardial oxygen demand by increasing heart rate, and cardiac stress can be assessed without voluntary muscle exercise. A pacing catheter is introduced into the right atrium. It has been shown that the hemodynamics of exercise and atrial pacing are different significantly. At equivalent cardiac rates, afterload is much lower with atrial pacing than with exercise. Atrial pacing has been proven to be a less sensitive test to detect myocardial ischemia than the treadmill exercise test.[40] Thus, false positive and false negative tests have been reported to be high to compare with treadmill exercise ECG test in the same group of patients.[41] Nevertheless, the right atrial pacing may be useful for patients who are unable to perform treadmill or bicycle exercise tests, although its main value is in a research setting.

Protocols for the Exercise (Treadmill) ECG Tests

Although numerous multistage exercise protocols have been designed by different investigators,[1, 42–45] none of these protocols are ideal for every individual.

As far as the ideal exercise ECG test is concerned, the initial workload should be well within an individual's anticipated physical working capacity; the workloads should be increased gradually and not abruptly, and the workloads should be maintained for a sufficient length of time to attain a near physiologic steady state. It is essential to monitor symptoms (e.g., chest pain, dizziness, dyspnea, extreme fatigue, etc.), signs, blood pressure, heart rate and electrocardiographic changes, during the entire procedure, and throughout at least 6–8 minutes of post-exercise periods. The exercise should be terminated when significantly abnormal symptoms, signs, marked S-T segment changes or serious arrhythmias are detected, or when a pre-determined heart rate is reached.

In some exercise protocols, the workload is increased by changing speed alone with fixed grade (incline or elevation),[44] whereas in some other protocols, grade is increased with fixed speed.[1] In Bruce's protocol, however, the workload is increased by changing both speed and grade.[45] The four commonly used protocols by Balke,[42] Bruce,[45] Ellestad[44] and modified Åstrand[43] have been compared in 51 healthy men, and there was no significant difference between these tests at maximum oxygen intake (VO_2), heart rate and blood pressure.[9]

For the progressive increment of the workload, at least 3-minute intervals are preferable so that steady state blood pressure and heart rate responses can be achieved. When dealing with any exercise protocol requiring speed greater than 4.0 m.p.h., patients of shorter stature have to run or jog in order to keep up, and the end result is often an undesirable deterioration of the electrocardiogram in addition to giving an uncomfortable and awkward feeling to the patients.

When the maximum exercise test is compared with the submaximum (85–90% of the maximum test) exercise test, there appears to be no significant difference in the clinical and practical sense. This author prefers the submaximum exercise test because many patients with coronary heart disease are unable to perform the maximum exercise test (see Chapter 9).

Metabolic equivalents (METs) which are multiples of the basal metabolic rates, are commonly used to express the workload in various stages of the exercise protocols.[1, 9] In most patients with coronary heart disease, the workloads with 8 METs are sufficient for the evaluation of angina. Healthy, sedentary individuals seldom exercise beyond 10–11 METs workload. Physically active individuals such as athletes may be able to achieve the workloads beyond 16 METs.

When we evaluate the cardiovascular functional capacity to correlate with METs, functional Class III patients usually become symptom-limited at 3–4 METs; those with functional Class II at 5 or 6 METs; and those with Class I should be able to perform the exercise beyond 7 or 8 METs.

Various multistage exercise protocols, including this author's own, will be discussed in detail elsewhere in this book (see Chapter 9).

Lead System and Electrode Placement

It is extremely important to obtain high quality electrocardiographic recordings for proper interpretation of the exercise ECG tests. In order to obtain a high quality ECG recording, it is essential to use proper skin preparation at the site of electrode placement, and to use specially designed electrodes. The most reliable and optimal one is a light-weight silver-silver chloride electrode which provides a good skin contact by means of a liquid conductor. Disposable and reusable electrodes of this type are commercially available for clinical use. For proper skin preparation, the sites of electrode application should be cleaned with ethyl alcohol, and the superficial keratinized layer of epidermis can be removed by gentle abrasion with an emery board, fine-grain sandpaper or dental burr, or by vigorous rubbing with gauze. When the superficial epidermal layer is removed, it should be washed away by using light cleansing with acetone.

In female patients, particularly in obese individuals with large breasts, the exercise should be performed with the patient wearing an undergarment to support the breasts. Otherwise, motion artifacts as a result of the chest electrode movement by the breasts during exercise lead to extremely poor quality ECG recordings which commonly obscure the diagnostic S-T segment changes and potentially dangerous exercise-induced cardiac arrhythmias. It should be noted that approximately 10% of patients with exercise-induced S-T segment changes occur only during exercise.[41, 46]

The most widely utilized lead system is a modified bipolar lead V_5 when single-channel ECG recording equipment is available. The positive electrode is placed in the 5th intercostal space at the left anterior axillary line, and the negative electrode is placed in various locations including the forehead (CH_5), right infraclavicular region (CS_5), right scapular region (CB_5), manubrium (CM_5), left 5th intercostal space (CC_5) or the back (CA_5).[1–3, 8, 47] Among these combinations, CM_5 seems to be the most popular lead system, and this lead is reported to detect 89% of the ECG abnormalities to compare with 12-lead ECG recordings.[47] When 2-channel recordings are available an additional inferior lead (lead II, III or aVF) with a modified lead V_5 can increase the diagnostic possibility of the exercise ECG tests. When a multichannel recorder is available, 6 leads consisting of leads II, aVF and V_{3-6} are said to be ideal to detect more ECG abnormalities.[1] When limb leads are utilized in order to prevent motion artifacts, arm electrodes should be placed in both infraclavicular fossae, and the left leg electrode is placed just above the left anterior superior iliac spine. Orthogonal vector leads—X,Y,Z leads—have been used by some investigators[48, 49] for the exercise ECG tests, but this lead system has not been widely accepted.

Many investigators still use a single lead system—a modified bipolar lead V_5 with reasonably satisfactory clinical results. Although multiple lead recordings have not been widely employed as yet, this author utilizes a 2-channel recording—a combination of lead II and a modified V_5 (CM_5) with satisfying results. We are in the process of obtaining 3-channel ECG equipment in the near future at our exercise laboratory. The 3-lead system will consist of lead II, and modified V_3 and V_5. When a large R wave is not registered in the CM_5 lead in some cases, the modified V_5 position should be moved one intercostal space higher or lower until the largest R wave is recorded according to the ECG finding shown in the 12 lead ECG (control ECG tracing).

In most institutions, a complete 12-lead ECG is recorded before the exercise and another one taken 6–8 minutes after the termination of the exercise test. Some investigators, however, recommend another 12-lead ECG immediately after the end of exercise.

Most investigators are satisfied with visual observation and conventional interpretation of the exercise ECG tests. However, several exercise laboratories utilize a computerized interpretation of the exercise ECG test with impressive results, particularly for the S-T segment abnormalities.[3, 49, 50]

End Points To Terminate Exercise ECG Test

In order to obtain the greatest diagnostic information as well as proper assessment of the patient's cardiovascular function, the patient should perform the exercise to a near-maximum level. The exercise can be terminated when the patient reaches the predicted submaximum heart rate (see Chapter 9) providing that the patient remains asymptomatic throughout the entire procedure.[1-9]

The exercise must be terminated prematurely, however, at the patient's request when significant symptoms, particularly severe chest pain, marked dyspnea, dizziness and severe fatigue, are produced. The physician should not insist that the patient continue the exercise in order to reach the predicted heart rate and/or significant S-T segment abnormalities develop if he experiences symptoms of an intensity which would prompt him to stop his daily activities. When a lack of motivation by the patient is apparent and all parameters show normal findings, the physician may encourage him to continue the exercise in some cases. It is an excellent idea to observe the patient's facial expression during exercise to assess whether he is in any unusual distress because some patients try to overcome serious symptoms and do not report them to the physician.

The exercise should be terminated promptly when the patient develops marked horizontal S-T segment depression or elevation and/or significant cardiac arrhythmias (e.g., multifocal ventricular premature contractions, ventricular group beats, ventricular tachycardia, various bradyarrhythmias) regardless of symptoms. In addition, the exercise should be stopped prematurely when the patient develops elevation of blood pressure (systolic, 220 mm. Hg. or more) or hypotension.

When the patient develops paroxysmal cough during exercise, the finding may be an early sign of impending pulmonary edema. The exercise may have to be terminated under this circumstance. A physician who supervises the test should make a correct and instant decision carefully on every individual whether the exercise should be terminated or continued.

Detailed descriptions regarding the endpoints for the exercise ECG test are found in Chapter 9.

Indications Versus Contraindications

The major indications of the exercise ECG test include:[1-9]

(1) Confirmation or exclusion of coronary heart disease—assessment of etiology of chest pain
(2) Assessment of functional capacity—exercise tolerance, and
(3) Evaluation of the efficacy of medical and/or surgical treatment for coronary heart disease.

The minor indications of the exercise ECG test are as follows:[1-9]

(1) Assessment of the nature of certain cardiac arrhythmias
(2) Assessment of a possible etiology of various symptoms (e.g., dizziness, fainting episode, etc.)
(3) Screening purposes for general population or life insurance companies
(4) Rehabilitation of cardiac patients and
(5) Research purposes in conjunction with other laboratory tests.

As far as the contraindications of the exercise ECG test are concerned, they may be divided into absolute versus relative contraindications, or they may be divided into cardiac versus non-cardiac contraindications.[1-9] For example, absolute cardiac contraindications should include acute myocardial infarction, acute congestive heart failure, cardiogenic shock, unstable angina pectoris, etc. On the other hand, absolute non-cardiac contraindications may include amputee, high fever, mentally disturbed patients, and any acute or serious non-cardiac disorders (e.g., acute hepatitis, renal failure, pneumonia, etc.).

Detailed descriptions of indications and contraindications of the exercise ECG test are found elsewhere in this book (see Chapters 7 and 8).

Interpretations of the Exercise ECG Test

Although there is a significant controversy regarding the interpretations of the exercise ECG test, the most important and reliable criterion for a positive test is horizontal (square wave) or down-slope S-T segment depression of 1 mm. or greater. Less common finding of a positive exercise ECG test is the S-T segment elevation which is often termed "Prinzmetal or atypical angina." It has been shown that exercise-induced S-T segment elevation is frequently observed due to areas of abnormal myocardial wall motion in patients with previous myocardial infarction.[51, 52]

Functional S-T segment depression (J-point depression) up to 2 mm. is considered to be insignificant. If the depression is more than 2 mm. with duration beyond 0.08 second, however, the term, "slow rising" S-T segment depression is often used,[2] and this finding is considered to be "probable positive." Another probable positive criterion is inverted U waves induced by exercise.[3, 5]

Some ECG findings such as isolated T wave change, development of bundle branch block or peaked P waves during or after exercise are insignificant clinically.

The incidence of a false positive or false negative exercise ECG test varies markedly depending upon the diagnostic criteria used, the prevalence of coronary heart disease, and many other factors. For example, a false positive exercise ECG test is much more common in women than men. Numerous factors may cause a false positive test—e.g., digitalis, mitral valve prolapse syndrome, Wolff-Parkinson-White syndrome, hyperventilation syndrome, etc. It is also interesting to note that a "borderline" or "equivocal" exercise ECG test is extremely common in middle-aged women to compare with men.

Detailed descriptions regarding the interpretations of the exercise ECG test are found in Chapter 12.

Factors Influencing the Result of the Exercise ECG Test

As indicated previously, there are numerous factors which may influence the result of the exercise ECG test. A typical example is digitalis preparation which commonly causes a false positive test. Another example is propranolol (Inderal) which frequently produces a false negative exercise ECG test.

Detailed descriptions regarding the effects of drugs and metabolic abnormalities on the exercise ECG test are found in Chapter 6. In addition, various problems related to the exercise ECG test are discussed in Chapter 5.

Clinical Values of the Exercise ECG Test

Every physician should be familiar with commonly used terms, such as "sensitivity" and "specificity" for the better understanding of the clinical value of the exercise ECG test.

* *Sensitivity* of a test is the percentage of patients with disease who are detected correctly, i.e.,

$$\text{Sensitivity} = \frac{\text{true positives}}{\text{true positives + false negatives}}$$

* *Specificity* of a test refers to the ability of a negative test to correctly identify normal subjects, or the percentage of normal subjects with negative tests, i.e.,

$$\text{Specificity} = \frac{\text{true negatives}}{\text{false positives + true negatives}}$$

* *Predictive value* of an abnormal test is the percentage of patients with abnormal tests which is indicative of disease, i.e.,

$$\text{Predictive value} = \frac{\text{true positives}}{\text{true positives + false positives}}$$

Without doubt, the multistage treadmill exercise ECG test provides useful information in the evaluation and management of the patients with known or suspected coronary artery disease in terms of the diagnosis as well as the assessment of functional capacity. However, the value of the exercise ECG test is limited when dealing with asymptomatic and healthy individuals because of the extremely high incidence of false positive tests. Nevertheless, there is not much doubt that an abnormal ECG response to exercise in asymptomatic subjects is predictive of an increased incidence of future coronary events. Namely, the risk of developing clinical manifestation of coronary heart disease in subsequent years has been shown to be 10–15 times greater in asymptomatic subjects with abnormal exercise ECG tests than a group with negative tests.[54-57]

The sensitivity and specificity of the exercise ECG test result will vary markedly according to numerous factors, including the patient population studied, the exercise protocol used, the end points to terminate the test, the diagnostic criteria for the exercise ECG test, the monitoring lead system and criteria for "significant" coronary artery lesion. The prevalence of the abnormal S-T segment response to exercise in symptomatic patients with documented coronary artery disease is reported to be between 54 and 85%.[51] It should be noted that abnormal S-T segment changes by exercise represent myocardial ischemia and *not* the anatomy of coronary vessels. Thus, advanced coronary artery disease is not always associated with exercise-induced myocardial ischemia.

Numerous studies have documented that there is a definite correlation between the number and location of coronary artery lesions and the S-T segment changes induced by exercise.[46, 58] In one study using 112 patients, the incidence of positive exercise ECG test was directly proportional to the number of coronary arteries involved with more than 75% stenosis.[51] There was only a 44% incidence of positive exercise ECG test in patients with either right or left circumflex coronary artery lesion (single vessel disease), whereas the incidence of positive test was 77% in patients with isolated lesion of the left anterior descending artery. The incidence of positive test increased to 91% when any two vessels are involved. It was interesting to note that the incidence of positive test was 100% in 23 patients (out of 112 subjects) with severe, 3-vessel lesions.[51]

The correlation between the coronary arteriography and exercise ECG test is discussed in detail in Chapter 14. Clinical value of the exercise ECG test is fully discussed in Chapter 12.

Cardiac Arrhythmias and the Exercise ECG Test

Various cardiac arrhythmias may be induced or abolished by exercise. Ventricular arrhythmias are extremely common with exercise in both healthy subjects and patients with organic heart disease.[59, 60] In general, the prevalence rate of all forms of ventricular arrhythmias increases proportionately with the exercise heart rate obtained. Ventricular premature contractions, particularly multifocal or grouped, are uncommon in individuals without organic heart disease at the exercise heart rate below 70% of the predicted maximum rate.[8] Myocardial ischemia may be strongly suspected when serious ventricular arrhythmias develop in conjunction with the onset of exercise-induced angina even in the absence of the S-T segment changes. An isolated finding of exercise-induced ventricular arrhythmias alone is not diagnostic of coronary heart disease. Exercise-induced ventricular arrhythmias are common in patients with mitral valve prolapse syndrome or cardiomyopathy.

Supraventricular arrhythmias are uncommon during exercise, and their occurrence is not diagnostic of organic heart disease. Atrial premature contractions are the most common supraventricular arrhythmia associated with exercise. Detailed descriptions regarding the cardiac arrhythmias and the exercise ECG test are found in Chapter 13.

Hemodynamic Responses to Exercise

A continuous oscilloscopic display of the exercise ECG with periodic (usually 1-minute interval) ECG write-outs is mandatory during the entire procedure and for at least 6 minutes during the post-exercise period for detection of the S-T segment changes and cardiac arrhythmias. In addition, it is essential to measure blood pressure at minute intervals by applying a blood pressure cuff on the upper extremity during exercise and at least 6 minutes post-exercise. Furthermore, it is extremely important to record these parameters whenever any symptoms, physical signs or arrhythmias develop.

It has been reported that there is an increased risk of overt coronary events in patients who demonstrate less than expected acceleration of the heart rate during multistage exercise.[61] Some cases with advanced coronary heart disease may develop actual slowing of the heart rate during progressive exercise. This finding is usually associated with angina, but not necessarily with S-T segment abnormality. It should be noted, however, that less than expected increment of the sinus rate during exercise may actually be due to sick sinus syndrome, especially in older individuals.

When a reproducible and sustained reduction of systolic blood pressure of over 10 mm. Hg. occurs during exercise in association with angina and/or S-T segment changes, multiple-vessel coronary lesions should be suspected.[51, 62] This type of blood pressure response is encountered in approximately 5% of the patients with coronary artery disease at the exercise laboratory. The majority of these patients have advanced triple-vessel lesions with well preserved ventricular function. In some cases, however, the abnormal blood pressure response may also be seen in patients with marked ventricular dysfunction.

It is extremely important to distinguish the above-mentioned pathological responses of the heart rate and blood pressure during exercise from similar findings which occur during the first stage of exercise in normal individuals who are quite anxious prior to the exercise ECG test.

Complications and Potential Risks

It is well documented that there is extremely low risk of morbidity and mortality associated with multistage treadmill exercise ECG test (either maximum or submaximum). Morbidity-mortality data collected by Rochmis and Blackburn[63] in 1971 using the 73 multicenter questionnaire analysis, which included 170,000 exercise ECG tests (treadmill, bicycle ergometer and Master's tests), demonstrated only 16 deaths (mortality approximately 0.01%—1 per 10,000 tests), and 40 patients requiring hospitalization for non-fatal complications (morbidity approximately 0.02%—2.4/10,000 tests). Among the 16 deaths reported, all occurred within 1 week following the exercise ECG test, and 8 were immediate deaths. Mortality was not related to the type and/or severity of the exercise test. Among the 170,000 tests, 73% were of the multistage variety. In another study involving 15,000 maximum exercise ECG tests over a 10 year period, there were no fatalities.[64] In this report, two patients developed post-exercise cardiac arrest without subsequent myocardial infarction. In the same study, another two patients developed myocardial infarction following a hot shower. One of these patients was an apparently normal subject, whereas the other individual had a history of angina pectoris. Both patients survived.

Likewise, no fatality was encountered among 5,500 submaximum exercise ECG tests performed at our exercise laboratory in the past 5 years. No patient developed acute myocardial infarction during or immediately after exercise ECG tests. No episode of ventricular fibrillation was observed at our exercise laboratory, although 15 patients developed paroxysmal ventricular tachycardia (6 or more consecutive ventricular premature contractions). No patient suffered from serious outcome and only a small number of patients required active treatment (e.g., intravenous lidocaine injection) for ventricular tachycardia because in the majority of cases, the arrhythmia subsided spontaneously upon resting.

From available data, the reported mortality and morbidity of the exercise ECG test are very low. Nevertheless, potential risks of developing serious cardiac arrhythmias, particularly ventricular tachyarrhythmias, acute myocardial infarction and even death, are always possible in every individual during or after exercise. Therefore, every available precaution should be taken, and possible contraindications should be carefully considered in order to prevent any major complication. It is mandatory to have all necessary cardiopulmonary resuscitative equipment including defibrillator and commonly used cardiac drugs in the exercise ECG laboratory. All personnel working in the exercise ECG laboratory should be capable of providing cardiopulmonary resuscitative measures.

Complications of the exercise ECG test are described in detail in Chapter 17.

Summary

Exercise electrocardiography (exercise ECG test or stress ECG test) is one of the most important non-invasive diagnostic methods in the field of cardiology. The exercise ECG test is summarized as follows:

1. The exercise ECG test should be performed under direct supervision by a physician who is fully familiar with the entire procedure of the test.

2. The entire procedure should be explained to the patient before the test and a consent form must be obtained.

3. Availability of cardiopulmonary resuscitative equipment and drugs is essential in the exercise ECG laboratory.

4. False negative exercise ECG tests may be observed during anti-anginal drug therapy, in individuals under a regular physical training program and even in proven coronary patients.

5. False positive exercise ECG tests may be observed during digitalis therapy, during hyperventilation, in individuals with mitral valve prolapse syndrome, the WPW syndrome and hypokalemia, and even in perfectly healthy persons, particularly women.

6. On rare occasions, exercise may produce serious arrhythmias or acute myocardial infarction and even death. The mortality is reported to be only 0.01%.

7. The exercise ECG test is indicated for every individual with chest pain due to unknown cause.

8. The primary value of the exercise ECG test is for an early detection of coronary heart disease, and for the assessment of functional capacity (exercise tolerance).

9. It should be noted that a positive exercise ECG test does not necessarily indicate the presence of coronary heart disease, whereas a negative exercise ECG test does not necessarily exclude the possibility of coronary heart disease.

10. The exercise ECG test is contraindicated in many clinical circumstances, particularly acute myocardial infarction, unstable angina, severe aortic stenosis, digitalis toxicity and acute or serious non-cardiac disorders (e.g., pulmonary embolism, physical handicaps, mental disorders, etc.).

11. Exercise ECG test must be stopped at the patient's request or when significant S-T segment alterations, serious cardiac arrhythmias and/or significant symptoms (e.g., chest pain, severe dyspnea, dizziness or fatigue, etc.) occur.

12. There are several exercise ECG test protocols proposed by different investigators, but 7-stage-graded protocol (Chung's protocol) is utilized in our laboratory.

13. The most common and important diagnostic criterion for a positive exercise ECG test is a horizontal or downslope S-T segment depression of 1 mm. or more during and/or after exercise.

14. The S-T segment elevation induced by exercise is rare but its clinical significance is much more serious than the S-T segment depression. Previous myocardial infarction with or without ventricular aneurysm is frequently responsible for the S-T segment elevation during exercise.

15. Ventricular arrhythmias induced by exercise are considered to be abnormal response during minimum exercise (less than 70% of the predicted maximum), but the finding is *not* necessarily indicative of coronary heart disease.

16. Development of atrial or A-V junctional premature beats, or transient atrial tachyarrhythmias induced by exercise is considered to be insignificant clinically.

17. Peaking P waves, or alteration of the T wave configuration or direction alone during and/or after exercise is insignificant clinically.

18. The best leads utilized for the exercise ECG test include lead II (or aVF), modified V_3 and V_5 if a 3-channel recorder is available.

19. The best two leads will be lead II (or aVF) and modified V_5 when a 2-channel recorder is used.

20. When a single-channel recorder is used, modified lead V_5 is the best lead to choose.

REFERENCES

1. Naughton, J.: Stress electrocardiography in clinical electrocardiographic correlations, *in* Cardiovascular Clinics, Vol. 8, pp. 127–139, Philadelphia, F. A. Davis, 1977.
2. Fortuin, N. J. and Weiss, J. L.: Exercise stress testing. Circulation, *56:*699, 1977.
3. Faris, J. V., McHenry, P. L. and Morris, S. N.: Concepts and applications of treadmill exercise testing and the exercise electrocardiogram. Am. Heart J., *95:*102, 1978.
4. Kattus, A. A.: Exercise electrocardiography: Recognition of the ischemic response, false-positive and false-negative patterns, *in* Exercise In Cardiovascular Health and Disease, edited by E. A. Amsterdam, J. H. Wilmore and A. N. DeMaria, New York, Yorke Medical Books, 1977.
5. Redwood, D. R., Borer, J. S. and Epstein, S. E.: Whither the ST segment during exercise? Circulation, *54:*703, 1976.
6. Sheffield, L. T., Reeves, T. J., Blackburn, H. et al.: The exercise test in perspective. Circulation, *55:*681, 1977.
7. Ellestad, M. H.: Stress Testing. Principles and Practice. Philadelphia, F. A. Davis, 1976.
8. McHenry, P. L. and Fisch, C.: Clinical applications of the treadmill exercise test. Mod. Concepts Cardiovasc. Dis., *46:*21, 1977.
9. Pollock, M. L., Bohannon, R. L., Cooper, K. H. et al.: A comparative analysis of four protocols for maximal treadmill stress testing. Am. Heart J., *92:*39, 1976.
10. Master, A. M. and Oppenheimer, E. J.: A simple exercise tolerance test for circulatory efficiency with standard tables for normal individuals. Am. J. Med. Sci., *177:*223, 1929.
11. Master, A. M. and Jaffe, H. L.: The electrocardiographic changes after exercise in angina pectoris. J. Mt. Sinai Hosp., *7:*629, 1941.
12. Bousfield, G.: Angina pectoris. Changes in electrocardiogram during paroxysm. Lancet, *2:*457, 1918.
13. Feil, H. and Siegel, M.: Electrocardiographic changes during attacks of angina pectoris. Am. J. Med. Sci., *175:*255, 1928.
14. Einthoven, W.: Weiteres über das elektrokardiogram. Arch. Ges. Physiol., *172:*517, 1908.
15. Wood, F. C. and Wolferth, C. C.: Angina pectoris: The clinical and electrocardiographic phenomena of the attack and their comparison with the effects of experimental temporary coronary occlusion. Arch. Intern Med., *47:*339, 1931.
16. Goldhammer, S. and Scherf, D.: Elektrokardiographische untersuch ungen bei kranken mit angina pectoris. Z. Klin. Med., *122:*134, 1932.
17. Katz, L. and Landt, H.: Effect of standardized exercise on the four-lead electrocardiogram: Its value in the study of coronary disease. Am. J. Med. Sci., *189:*346, 1935.
18. Missal, M. E.: Exercise tests and the electrocardiograph in the study of angina pectoris. Ann. Intern Med., *11:*2018, 1938.
19. Riseman, J. E. F., Waller, J. and Brown, M.: The electrocardiogram during attacks of angina pectoris: Its characteristics and diagnostic significance. Am. Heart J., *19:*683, 1940.
20. Liebow, I. M. and Feil, H.: Digitalis and the normal work electrocardiogram. Am. Heart J., *22:*683, 1941.
21. Johnson, R. E., Brouha, L. and Darling, R. C.: A practical test of physical fitness for strenuous exertion. Rev. Can. Biol., *1:*491, 1942.
22. Hecht, H. H.: Concepts of myocardial ischemia. Arch. Intern. Med., *84:*711, 1949.
23. Wood, P., McGregor, M., Magidson, O. and Whittaker, W.: The effort test in angina pectoris. Br. Heart J., *12:*363, 1950.

24. Yu, P. N. G. and Soffer, A.: Studies of electrocardiographic changes during exercise (Modified double two-step test). Circulation, 6:183, 1952.
25. Yu, P. N. G., Bruce, R. A. Lovejoy, F. W., Jr. and McDowell, M. E.: Variations in electrocardiographic responses during exercise (studies of normal subjects under unusual stresses and of patients with cardiopulmonary diseases). Circulation, 3:368, 1951.
26. Feil, H. and Brofman, B. L.: The effect of exercise on the electrocardiogram of bundle branch block. Am. Heart J., 45:665, 1953.
27. Sonnenblick, E. H., Ross, J. and Braunwald, E.: Oxygen consumption of the heart: Newer concepts of its multifactorial determination. Am. J. Cardiol., 22:328, 1968.
28. Brachfield, N., Bozer, J. and Gorlin, R.: Action of nitroglycerin on the coronary circulation in male cardiac subjects. Circulation, 19:697, 1959.
29. Khouri, E. M., Gregg, D. E. and Rayford, C. R.: Effect of exercise on cardiac output, left coronary flow and myocardial metabolism in the unanesthetized dog. Circ. Res., 17:427, 1965.
30. Kitamura, K., Jorgensen, C. R., Gobel, F. L. et al.: Hemodynamic correlates of myocardial oxygen consumption during upright exercise. J. Appl. Physiol., 32:516, 1972.
31. Gould, K. L., Lipscomb, K. and Hamilton, G. W.: Physiologic basis for assessing critical coronary stenosis: instantaneous flow response and regional distribution during coronary hyperemia as measures of coronary flow reserve. Am. J. Cardiol., 33:87, 1974.
32. Roitman, D., Jones, W. B. and Sheffield, L. T.: Comparison of submaximal exercise ECG test with coronary cineangiocardiogram. Ann. Intern. Med., 72:641, 1970.
33. Sarnoff, S. J., Braunwald, E., Welch, G. H., Jr. et al.: Hemodynamic determinants of oxygen consumption of the heart with special reference to the tension-time index. Am. J. Physiol., 192:148, 1958.
34. O'Brien, K. P., Higgs, L. M., Glancy, D. L. and Epstein, S. E.: Hemodynamic accompaniments of angina: A comparison during angina induced by exercise and by atrial pacing. Circulation, 39:735, 1969.
35. Blomquist, C. G.: Use of exercise testing for diagnostic and functional evaluation of patients with arteriosclerotic heart disease. Circulation, 44:1120, 1971.
36. Sheffield, L. T. and Roitman, D.: Systolic blood pressure, heart rate, and treadmill work at anginal threshold. Chest, 63:327, 1973.
37. Robinson, B. F.: Relation of heart rate and systolic blood pressure to the onset of pain in angina pectoris. Circulation, 35:1073, 1967.
38. Hermansen, L., Ekblom, B. and Saltin, B.: Cardiac output during submaximal and maximal treadmill and bicycle exercise. J. Appl. Physiol., 29:82, 1970.
39. Shaw, D. J., Crawford, M. H., Karliner, J. S. et al.: Arm-crank ergometry: A new method for the evaluation of coronary artery disease. Am. J. Cardiol., 33:801, 1974.
40. Rios, J. C. and Hurwitz, L. E.: Electrocardiographic responses to atrial pacing and multistage treadmill exercise testing. Am. J. Cardiol., 34:661, 1974.
41. Kelemen, M. H., Gillilan, R. E., Bouchard, R. J. et al.: Diagnosis of obstructive coronary disease by maximal exercise and atrial pacing. Circulation, 48:1227, 1973.
42. Balke, B. and Ware, R.: An experimental study of physical fitness of air force personnel. U.S. Armed Forces Med. J., 10:675, 1959.
43. Åstrand, P. O. and Rodahl, K.: Textbook of Work Physiology. New York, McGraw-Hill, 1970.
44. Ellestad, M. H., Allen, W., Wan, M. C. K. and Kemp, G.: Maximal treadmill stress testing for cardiovascular evaluation. Circulation, 39:517, 1969.
45. McDonough, J. R. and Bruce, R. A.: Maximal exercise testing in assessing cardiovascular function. J. S. C. Med. Assoc., 65:26, 1969.
46. McHenry, P. L., Phillips, J. F. and Knoebel, S. B.: Correlation of computer-quantitated treadmill exercise electrocardiogram with arteriographic location of coronary artery disease. Am. J. Cardiol., 30:747, 1972.
47. Blackburn, H.: The exercise electrocardiogram, in Measurement in Exercise Electrocardiography, The Ernst Simonson Conference, edited by H. Blackburn, p. 220, Springfield, Ill., Charles C Thomas, 1969.
48. Simoons, M. L. and Hugenholtz, P. G.: Gradual changes of ECG wave form during and after exercise in normal subjects. Circulation, 52:570, 1975.
49. Blomqvist, G. C.: The Frank lead exercise electrocardiogram: Quantitative study based on

averaging technical and digital computer analysis. Acta Med. Scand., *178* (suppl 440), 1965.

50. Sheffield, L. T., Holt, J. H., Lester, F. M. et al.: On-line analysis of the exercise electrocardiogram. Circulation, *40:*935, 1969.
51. McHenry, P. L. and Morris, S. N.: Exercise electrocardiography: Current state of the art, *in* Advances in Electrocardiography, edited by R. C. Schlant and J. W. Hurst, Vol. 2, Ch. 14, New York, Grune & Stratton, 1976.
52. Chahine, R. A., Raizner, A. E. and Ishimori, T.: The clinical significance of exercise-induced ST-segment elevation. Circulation, *54:*209, 1976.
53. Chung, E. K.: Clinical Electrocardiography, Part 9, Exercise Electrocardiography, New York, Medcom, 1978.
54. Bruce, R. A. and McDonough, J. R.: Stress testing in screening for cardiovascular disease. Bull. N.Y. Acad. Med., *45:*1288, 1969.
55. Aronow, W. S.: Five year follow-up of Double Master's test, maximal treadmill stress test, and resting and post-exercise in asymptomatic persons. Circulation, *52:*616, 1975.
56. Froelicher, V. F., Thomas, M., Pillow, C. and Lancaster, M. C.: An epidemiological study of asymptomatic men screened with exercise testing for coronary heart disease. Am. J. Cardiol., *34:*770, 1974.
57. Cummings, G. R., Samm, J., Borysyk, L. and Kich, L.: Electrocardiographic changes during exercise in asymptomatic men: 3 year follow-up. Can. Med. Assoc. J., *112:*578, 1975.
58. Goldschlager, N., Selzer, A. and Cohn, K.: Treadmill stress tests as indicators of presence and severity of coronary artery disease. Ann. Intern. Med., *85:*277, 1976.
59. McHenry, P. L., Morris, S. N., Kavalier, M. and Jordan, J. W.: Comparative study of exercise-induced ventricular arrhythmias in normal subjects and patients with documented coronary artery disease. Am. J. Cardiol., *37:*609, 1976.
60. Kennedy, H. L. and Underhill, S. J.: Frequent or complex ventricular ectopy in apparently healthy subjects. Am. J. Cardiol., *38:*141, 1976.
61. Ellestad, M. H. and Wan, M. K. C.: Predictive implications of stress testing: Follow-up of 2,700 subjects after maximum treadmill stress testing. Circulation, *51:*363, 1975.
62. Thompson, P. D. and Kelemen, M. H.: Hypotension accompanying the onset of exertional angina: A sign of severe compromise of left ventricular blood supply. Circulation, *52:*28, 1975.
63. Rochmis, P. and Blackburn, H.: Exercise tests: A survey of procedures, safety, and litigation experience in approximately 170,000 tests. J.A.M.A., *217:*1061, 1971.
64. Bruce, R. A.: Progress in exercise cardiology, *in* Progress in Cardiology, edited by P. N. Yu and J. F. Goodwin, pp. 113–172, Philadelphia, Lea & Febiger, 1975.

2

Master's Two-Step Test

Edward A. Solow, M.D. and
Edward K. Chung, M.D., F.A.C.P., F.A.C.C.

General Considerations

Since Master and Jaffe published their report on the electrocardiographic response to exercise,[1] the Master's two-step test, and later the double Master's two-step test, have become the most widely used exercise ECG test,[2,3] and a vast body of long-term follow-up data has been accumulated on patients undergoing these tests.

Even though the shortcomings of the Master's two-step exercise test have been well demonstrated,[3-6] its inherent simplicity, lack of expensive equipment and safety continue to make it an attractive alternative to the newer (e.g., treadmill) exercise ECG tests. In order to derive the maximum usefulness from the test it is necessary that:

(1) a strict protocol be adhered to,
(2) technical factors be standardized, and
(3) the physician who interprets the test should be fully familiar with the meaning of a positive or negative result for each patient tested.[7]

In this chapter we will examine some of the clinical data accumulated in the more than 30 years dealing with the Master's test, and review some of the studies regarding the correlation between the Master's test and coronary angiographic data. The technique of the Master's two-step test will be reviewed, and those points which require strict standardization will be identified. Finally, the significance of a positive and a negative Master's test will be discussed.

Unless otherwise specified, whenever the term Master's test or Master's two-step test is used in this chapter, we are referring to the double Master's test; that is, twice the originally prescribed number of trips over the stairs in 3 minutes, which is twice the original time limit.

Method of the Master's Two-Step Test

The potential for erroneous results from a Master's two-step ECG test is great.[4] Consequently, careful attention to the technical details of the test is essential in order to provide the maximum usefulness. Full details of the test and its evolution are available,[3, 7-11] and a brief review will be presented.

The test should be administered by a physician or other medical personnel who are well trained in the test itself and in the treatment of the potential complications, under direct supervision of a physician. Before the test begins the physician must review each patient's medical history, perform a physical examination with special reference to the cardiovascular system, and review the pre-exercise ECG to determine if the patient is a suitable candidate for the exercise ECG test. A detailed discussion of the contraindications to the exercise ECG test can be found in Chapter 8; but, in brief, any sign of acute cardiovascular disease should alert the physician to cancel the test. Also, before the test begins, the physician must be certain that the necessary equipment and drugs for cardiopulmonary resuscitation are available in the room where the test is to be done because, even though the Master's test has been found extremely safe,[12] many of the patients examined will have significant coronary artery disease, and the potential for a serious emergency is always present. Finally, the test is fully explained to the patient and he (or she) should sign an informed consent form (see Chapter 3), witnessed by the physician.

After the control (pre-exercise resting) 12-lead ECG is taken, adhesive electrodes are affixed to the torso as first described by Abarquez and colleagues[13] so that a lateral precordial ECG (lead V_4 or V_5) lead can be monitored during the test. The patient is then asked to walk to the top of the standardized two-step staircase and down the other side.[7-9] This counts as one trip. The patient then turns toward the examiner who stands next to the stairs with the ECG equipment and walks back over the stairs. By always turning toward the examiner, the patient will alternate his direction of turning and prevent dizziness or entanglement in the ECG cable. The method of the Master's test is shown in Figure 2-1. The patient now traverses the stairs the proper number of times for his (or her) age and sex (see Table 2-1) in 3 minutes. Since the ECG response to myocardial ischemia may be very short lived in some patients,[13, 14] lead V_5 (or V_4) should be sampled for 5-10 seconds every minute during exercise. As soon as the subject completes the test, or at the first appearance of chest pain or visible signs of any distress (pallor, ataxic gait, undue tachypnea, etc.), the test should be terminated and the subject quickly lies down, and a modified ECG is taken in the following order: leads V_6, V_5, V_4, V_3, II and aVF. This will assure the physician of the highest possible chance of detecting ischemic ECG changes,[15, 16] but should be made quickly so as not to miss any transient

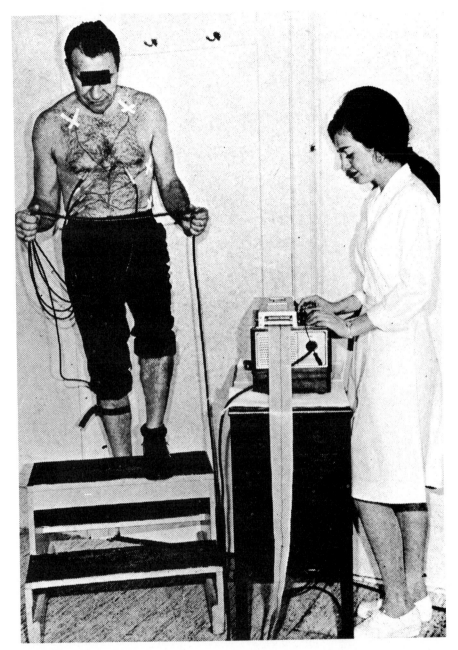

Fig. 2-1 Method of the Master's test (Reproduced with permission from Master, A.M. and Rosenfeld, I.: The "two-step" exercise test brought up to date. Dis. Chest, *51:*347, 1967).

Table 2-1. Trips Performed in Master Double Two-Step Exercise Test*†

Weight (lb.)	Age (yr.)												
	15–19	20–24	25–29	30–34	35–39	40–44	45–49	50–54	55–59	60–64	65–69	70–74	75–79
50–59	64(64)												
60–69	62(60)												
70–79	60(58)												
80–89	58(56)	58(56)	58(56)	56(54)	54(52)	54(48)	52(46)	50(44)	50(42)	48(42)	46(40)	46(38)	44(36)
90–99	56(52)	56(54)	56(52)	54(50)	54(48)	52(46)	50(44)	50(44)	48(42)	46(40)	44(38)	44(38)	42(36)
100–109	54(50)	56(52)	56(52)	54(50)	52(48)	50(46)	50(44)	48(42)	46(40)	44(38)	44(36)	42(36)	40(34)
110–119	52(46)	54(50)	54(50)	52(48)	50(46)	50(44)	48(42)	46(40)	46(38)	44(36)	42(36)	42(34)	4:'
120–129	50(44)	52(48)	54(48)	52(46)	50(44)	48(42)	46(40)	46(38)	44(38)	42(36)	40(34)	40(32)	38(30)
130–139	48(40)	50(46)	52(46)	50(44)	48(42)	46(40)	46(38)	44(38)	42(36)	40(34)	40(32)	38(30)	36(30)
140–149	46(38)	48(44)	50(44)	48(42)	48(40)	46(38)	44(38)	42(36)	40(34)	40(32)	38(32)	36(30)	36(28)
150–159	44(34)	48(42)	50(40)	48(40)	46(38)	44(38)	42(36)	40(34)	40(32)	38(32)	36(30)	36(28)	34(26)
160–169	42(32)	46(40)	48(38)	46(38)	44(36)	44(36)	42(34)	40(32)	38(32)	36(30)	36(28)	34(26)	34(24)
170–179	40(28)	44(38)	46(36)	46(36)	44(34)	42(34)	40(32)	38(32)	36(30)	36(28)	34(26)	34(26)	32(24)
180–189	38(26)	42(36)	46(34)	44(34)	42(34)	40(32)	38(32)	38(30)	36(28)	34(28)	32(26)	32(24)	30(22)
190–199	36(24)	40(34)	44(32)	42(32)	42(32)	40(30)	38(30)	36(28)	34(26)	32(26)	30(24)	30(24)	28(22)
200–209		38(32)	42(30)	42(30)	40(30)	38(28)	36(28)	34(26)	32(26)	32(24)	30(22)	28(22)	28(20)
210–219		36(30)	42(28)	40(28)	38(28)	36(26)	34(26)	34(26)	32(24)	30(22)	28(22)	28(22)	26(20)
220–229		34(28)	40(26)	40(26)	38(26)	36(26)	34(24)	32(24)	30(22)	28(22)	26(20)	26(20)	24(18)

* Master, A. M. and Rosenfeld, I.: The "two-step" exercise test brought up to date, New York J. Med., *61:*1850 (June 1), 1961; Dis. Chest, *51:*347, 1967.

† Figures for male patients are followed by those for female patients in parentheses.

ischemic changes. This modified ECG is repeated at 2 and 6 minutes during post-exercise period (while the patient rests), or until the tracing has returned to its control state, at which time a full 12-lead ECG is obtained.

This protocol is intended for those physicians who use single channel ECG equipment. If multi-channel equipment is available, then the leads checked during exercise should include one over the lateral precordium (lead V_4, V_5 or V_6) and one over the inferior wall of the heart (lead II or aVF most commonly).

Interpretation of the Master's Two-Step Test

As can be expected, a "positive" or "negative" result in a Master's test obviously largely depends on the criteria of an ischemic electrocardiographic response to exercise. During the formative years of exercise ECG tests, a number of such definitions were advanced, ranging from an S-T segment depression of as little as 0.1 mm.[10] to S-T segment depression of over 1.0

mm.[17] When the minimum S-T segment depression is used for a positive diagnostic criterion, of course, there will be a very high incidence of a false positive result and vice versa. The most popular criterion acceptable by most physicians for a positive Master's test is a horizontal or downsloping S-T segment depression of 0.5 mm.[5, 18] (Figure 2-2). An S-T segment elevation of a similar degree also signifies a positive Master's test, but the S-T segment elevation is very rare (Figure 2-3).

The appearance of frequent, grouped or multifocal ventricular premature contractions, although certainly abnormal response to exercise, is not clearly indicative of an ischemic response to exercise if the S-T segment criterion is not met. The clinical significance of atrial arrhythmias induced by exercise

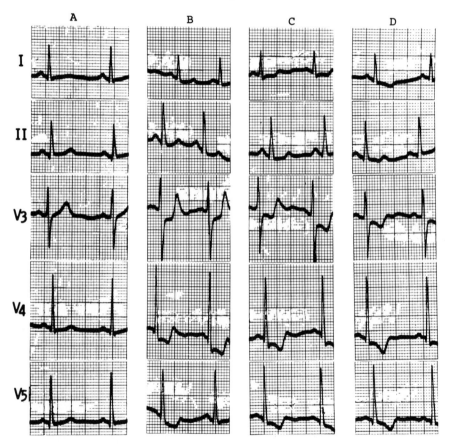

Fig. 2-2 Positive Master's test. Note marked S-T segment depression with biphasic T waves in tracings B, C and D. The tracing A represents a resting (control) ECG. The tracings B, C and D were obtained after exercise with 2-minute interval.

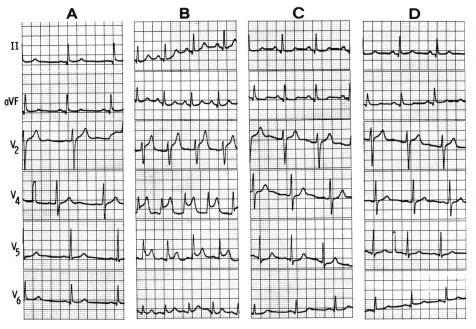

Fig. 2-3 Positive Master's test. Note marked S-T segment elevation in tracing B. The tracing A represents a control (resting) ECG. The tracing B, C and D were recorded after exercise with 2-minute interval.

is even less clear,[19, 20] and the finding is generally considered to be insignificant clinically.

In the early 1960's, certain measurements of the post-exercise ECG interpretation were suggested in an effort to increase the sensitivity and specificity of the Master's test.[11] There were 3 of these:

(1) the ratio of the duration of the S-T segment depression measured from the Q wave until the S-T segment returns to the baseline (Q-X interval) to the duration of electrical systole (Q-T interval) in the same beat (the Q-X/Q-T ratio),

(2) the ratio of the Q-T intervals before and after exercise, and

(3) the measurement of the J-point depression.

Although used briefly, these measurements failed to provide any useful information, and have generally been abandoned.[10, 21] The only exception is a J-point (i.e., "functional") depression of 2.0 mm. or more in the post-exercise ECG. This is probably indicative of a positive response, but not at the same level of confidence as the horizontal S-T segment depression.[7, 18] One final criterion of a probably positive Master's test is an inverted U wave during or after exercise (Figure 2-4).

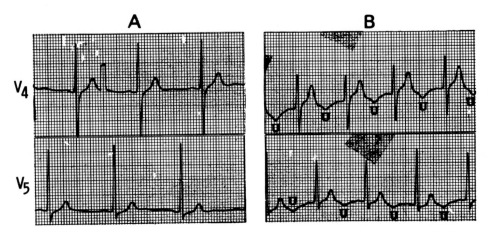

Fig. 2-4 Probable positive Master's test. Note inverted U waves in tracing B. The tracing A represents a control ECG whereas the tracing B is a post-exercise ECG.

It is important to view the significance of a positive Master's test in the perspective of the total patient. We emphasize that the exercise ECG test does not stand alone in the evaluation of chest pain or in the diagnosis of coronary artery disease. In other words, the test result must be interpreted in conjunction with the history, the physical findings and other laboratory values in the total evaluation of a given patient.

In the middle-aged man with chest pain, a positive Master's test is generally indicative of significant coronary artery disease.[17, 22-25] An S-T segment depression of 2.0 mm. or more in the post-exercise ECG, furthermore, has been shown to very frequently coincide with significant obstruction of all three coronary arteries.[23, 25]

On the other hand, similar, if not identical, exercise ECG finding—positive response in asymptomatic young individuals, especially females, may not indicate the presence of definite coronary heart disease. Nevertheless, it has been pointed out that the risk of future coronary events is significantly high in the asymptomatic young man with a positive Master's test.[10, 18, 26, 27] The significance of a positive Master's test in a young woman is unknown.

The question of "false positive" Master's tests is confusing. Although it has been demonstrated in some series that up to 30% of patients without coronary artery disease demonstrable by coronary angiography had positive Master's tests,[4, 17] the incidence of future coronary events in asymptomatic males with positive Master's tests is as high as 50%.[26] We feel quite strongly that, in view of the relatively low workload of the double Master's two-step exercise ECG test compared with the treadmill exercise ECG test (see Chapter 9), any unequivocal positive response in a young or middle-aged man, or even middle-aged woman implies the presence of coronary artery disease in the majority of cases.

An important point to remember is that the S-T segment changes indistinguishable from what we have been calling an "ischemic" change (i.e., horizontal or downsloping depression of 0.5 mm. or more) can be seen in patients with rheumatic heart disease, hypertensive heart disease, cardiomyopathies, mitral valve prolapse syndrome, in patients taking digitalis glycosides, in patients with thyrotoxicosis, in patients during hyperventilation and in patients with electrolyte abnormalities, particularly of serum potassium.[5] All of these factors must be taken into account when interpreting a positive Master's test (see also Chapters 6 and 12).

Contrary to widely held belief, a negative Master's test does not exclude the presence of coronary artery disease.[4, 17, 25-27] Even though Robb and Marks[10] showed one-tenth the coronary death rate in patients with negative Master's tests when compared to those with positive Master's tests, a negative Master's test cannot rule out coronary artery disease.[21] The explanation is that, although the workload on the subject of a Master's test is standardized for age, sex and weight, the heart rate response varies widely,[2] and it is the product of the heart rate and blood pressure which chiefly determines myocardial oxygen consumption.[3, 5] Therefore, the likelihood of a positive response to an exercise ECG test is directly proportional to the heart rate. Since the workload of the Master's test may be insufficient to raise the heart rate to the point where myocardial oxygen demand outstrips supply, a negative result in even a well-performed Master's test cannot rule out coronary artery disease. Such a false negative result has been estimated to occur in about one-third of patients with angiographically proven coronary artery disease[4, 25] or with typical anginal pain diagnostic of angina pectoris.[21] It is our opinion that if an individual with chest pain or with a history that makes him particularly coronary prone should have a negative Master's test, then he should still undergo a more aggressive exercise ECG test (e.g., treadmill) utilizing a protocol which produces maximal or submaximal exercise (see Chapter 9). Such a test is more likely to uncover an ischemic ECG response to exercise than is a Master's test.[3, 5, 20]

Zohman and Kattus[28] have recently pointed out that if typical angina pain is produced during an exercise test, it is very suggestive of a positive response even in the absence of S-T segment changes. Once again, we would like to emphasize that the patient must be evaluated in the perspective of his entire clinical situation, and not in the light of just one test.

The diagnostic criteria for a positive and a probably positive Master's test are found in Table 2-2.

Clinical Investigations

Many investigators have looked at the prognostic significance of the Master's test.[10, 18, 19, 26, 29] Direct comparison between these studies is difficult

Table 2-2. Criteria of Master's Test

A. Criteria of Positive Master's Test

1. S-T segment depression (horizontal or downsloping) of 0.5 mm. during or after exercise
2. S-T segment elevation (horizontal or upsloping) of 0.5 mm. during or after exercise

B. Criteria of Probably Positive Master's Test

1. Junctional (J-point) depression of 2.0 mm. or more during or after exercise
2. Inversion of the U wave during or after exercise
3. Typical angina pain during or immediately after exercise with or without S-T segment changes.

since there is no uniformity of patient population and diagnostic criteria for a positive or negative Master's test. Nevertheless, a review of the results of selected investigations will be helpful in gaining an appreciation of the significance of the Master's test.

Investigation by Brody

Brody[19] presented a 3–10 year follow-up of 756 unselected middle-aged businessmen who had had two-step tests at the Greenbrier Clinic from 1948 to 1955. Twenty-three (3%) of these 756 men had positive results, defined as at least 0.5 mm. of horizontal or downsloping S-T segment depression on the post-exercise ECG. Seventy percent of these 23 men suffered new coronary events during the follow-up period (10 cases of new angina and 6 acute myocardial infarctions), while only 4% of the 733 subjects with negative two-step tests had new coronary events.

Investigation by Mattingly

In reviewing the histories of 300 healthy army officers who had had Master's tests from 1942 to 1951, Mattingly[26] found that of the 6 who had an abnormal post-exercise ECG (more than 0.5 mm. horizontal S-T segment depression), 3 (50%) suffered a new coronary event within the 10 year follow-up period. Only 3 events occurred in the remaining 294 officers who had had negative Master's tests. He went on to review the histories of 1,000 subjects with suspected coronary artery disease who had Master's tests, and he found that those with a positive test had an incidence of subsequent coronary events 8 times that of subjects with negative tests. The difference is even more striking when only men over age 30 at the time of inclusion into the study were reviewed.

Investigation by Robb and Marks

Robb and Marks[10] presented the Metropolitan Life Insurance Company's experience with 1,659 insurance applicants who had Master's tests between 1949 and 1961 and followed through 1962. The majority underwent the Master's test because they had atypical chest pain or abnormal ECG. The criterion of an abnormal test was a horizontal S-T segment depression of 0.1 mm. or greater. Of the 16% of subjects who had ischemic post-exercise ECG the mortality rate was 23/1,000 person-years of follow-up, whereas the rate was 4/1,000 person-years in those with a negative response. The coronary artery disease death rates were 21/1,000 for an abnormal result and only 2–3/1,000 for normal post-exercise ECG. In analyzing their data further, they showed that the incidence of coronary events roughly paralleled the degree of S-T segment depression. That is, the chance of sustaining a fatal myocardial infarction was greater as the degree of S-T segment depression increased.

Investigation by Robb and Seltzer

The initial large series of Robb and Marks was enlarged by Robb and Seltzer[18] to 3,325 subjects followed through 1971. They found an even closer correlation between the degree of S-T segment depression and the risk of future death from myocardial infarction. Their results are as follows: with depression between 0.1 mm. and 0.9 mm., the death rate per 1,000 person-years of follow-up was 10.1; with a depression of 1.0–1.9 mm., 28.6; and with a depression of greater than 2.0 mm., the chance of death from coronary artery disease was 83.4/1,000 person-years of follow-up, or even twenty times the coronary death rate for individuals with a negative test.

Investigation by Bellet et al.

Bellet and co-workers[29] used radiotelemetry of the ECG during and after Master's two-step tests in 795 Bell Telephone Company employees who had normal resting ECGs. In the 3 year follow-up period, they found that 14% of those with positive tests (more than 1.0 mm. horizontal S-T segment depression during or after exercise) suffered new manifestations of coronary artery disease. Only 1.4% of the individuals with negative tests did.

Conclusion from Various Investigative Studies

Even though these studies are not entirely comparable, certain conclusions can be drawn:

(1) In middle-aged individuals without other signs of coronary artery disease, an ischemic response to a Master's two-step test means a greatly increased (about 10 times) chance of a new coronary event in the subsequent 3–10 years.[19, 26, 29]

(2) In patients evaluated because of suspected coronary artery disease, the incidence of new coronary events is again up to 10 times greater for individuals with positive Master's tests.[10, 18, 26]

(3) The incidence of a new coronary event roughly parallels the degree of S-T segment depression in the post-exercise ECG.[10, 18]

(4) A negative response to exercise by the Master's test means a low chance of coronary events (about 1–2%) in the follow-up period of 3–10 years, but does not exclude the possibility of coronary artery disease in any individual patient.

Correlation with Coronary Angiography

As the technique of coronary angiography became widely employed in the 1960's, the results were naturally compared to the Master's two-step test, and it was demonstrated that in patients found to have "significant" coronary artery disease by angiography, between 45 and 80% had positive Master's two-step tests.[4, 17, 22-25] Comparisons between these series are even more difficult than they are between the clinical studies since not only does the definition of a positive Master's test vary from study to study, but there is no agreement as to what constitutes "significant" coronary artery obstruction. At the time these studies were done it was not known that the hemodynamic consequences of coronary artery disease were nil until the coronary lumen was narrowed by at least 70%.[30] It should therefore be borne in mind that many of the conclusions coming out of these studies may not be accurate in light of present knowledge, since these investigations used 50% obstruction as a definition of "significant" coronary artery disease. We have arbitrarily divided the larger angiographic studies into two groups: those that appeared between 1960 and 1966, and those between 1966 and 1971.

Earlier Studies (1960–1966)

Early in the 1960's, Kattus and his group[22] showed that 14 patients with angina pectoris diagnosed clinically all had coronary artery lesions demonstrated by arteriography and ischemic ECG response to exercise. The first large series was presented in 1966 by Cohen et al.[23] Of 34 patients with angiographically proven coronary artery disease, 27 had abnormal Master's tests; an 80% detection rate. They also found that an ischemic S-T segment depression of 2.0 mm. or more was usually indicative of triple vessel coronary artery disease. Subsequently, Hultgren et al., however, could find no correlation between the degree of S-T segment depression and the angiographic findings in 55 patients with coronary artery disease.[24] They found the Master's test to be positive in 69% of patients with coronary artery disease, and found no positive tests in patients with negative coronary arteriograms.

Recent Studies (1967–1971)

The "excellent" specificity of the earlier studies could not be confirmed by Demanny and co-workers.[17] Again using 50% narrowing as indicative of significant obstruction, they found a rate of positive Master's test in patients with abnormal angiograms of only 43%, and also found positive Master's tests in 24% of patients in whom no significant coronary lesions could be found.

Late in the 1960's, Most et al.[25] looked at the sensitivity of the Master's test as it relates to: (1) the criterion of a positive Master's test and (2) the type of coronary artery disease to which it is compared. Only 58% of 65 patients with significant coronary lesions (again 50% obstruction) had positive Master's tests if an S-T segment depression of 1.0 mm. or greater was used as positive result. However, this number rose to 66% if 0.5 mm. depression was considered a positive test. Looking at the type of coronary lesion, it was found that the Master's test was positive in only about one-third of cases of single vessel disease, but was positive in over 70% of triple vessel cases.

Finally, Fitzgibbon et al.[4] showed a positive rate of 67% in patients with proven coronary artery disease, and a false positive rate of 15%.

Summary

The Master's two-step exercise ECG test was the first standardized test of cardiac reserve and continues as the double Master's test to be the most widely used exercise ECG test in the country. It is simple, inexpensive and safe; but there is a large potential for both false positive and false negative results unless a strict protocol is followed and unless the physician interpreting the test clearly understands the significance of the results obtained.

Long-term follow-up of patients undergoing the Master's test has shown that a positive result is a reliable indicator of an increased risk of subsequent coronary artery disease in asymptomatic subjects. Overall, there is a false positive rate of between 10 and 20% in large groups of asymptomatic subjects, this number being much lower when populations of symptomatic patients are considered.

Although numerous investigations comparing the Master's test to coronary angiographic findings have been presented in the literature, most, if not all, suffer from an imprecise definition of "significance" of coronary artery obstruction, making the conclusions reached difficult to apply clinically, and of uncertain value.

The most important and unavoidable limitation of the Master's test is obviously that the amount of exercise given is usually insufficient to compare with modern exercise ECG methods such as treadmill exercise. Consequently, significant numbers of false negative tests can not be avoided. Nevertheless, the Master's test is still a useful non-invasive diagnostic tool for the detection of coronary artery disease when modern sophisticated equipment is not available. It can be said that the diagnosis of significant coronary artery disease is certain when the Master's test is unequivocally positive.

REFERENCES

1. Master, A. M. and Jaffe, H. L.: The electrocardiographic changes after exercise in angina pectoris. J. Mt. Sinai Hosp., 7:629, 1941.
2. Rougraff, M. E. and Baker, J. C.: Heart rate response to exercise by double Master test. Tex. Med., 66:54, 1970.
3. Sheffield, L. T. and Roitman, D.: Stress testing methodology. Progr. Cardiovasc. Dis., 19:33, 1976.
4. Fitzgibbon, G. M., Burggraf, G. W., Groves, T. D. and Parker, J. O.: The double Master's two-step test: clinical, angiographic and hemodynamic correlations. Ann. Intern. Med., 74:509, 1971.
5. Bruce, R. A. and Hornsten, T. R.: Exercise stress testing in evaluation of patients with ischemic heart disease. Progr. Cardiovasc. Dis., 11:371, 1969.
6. Rowell, L. B., Taylor, H. L., Simonson, E. and Carlson, W. S.: The physiologic fallacy of adjusting for body weight in performance of the Master two-step test. Am. Heart J., 70:461, 1965.
7. Master, A. M.: The Master two-step test. Am. Heart J., 75:809, 1968.
8. Master, A. M. and Rosenfeld, I.: Two-step exercise test: Current status after twenty five years. Mod. Concepts Cardiovasc. Dis., 36:19, 1967.
9. Master, A. M. and Rosenfeld, I.: The "two-step" exercise test brought up to date. Dis. Chest, 51:347, 1967.
10. Robb, G. P. and Marks, H. H.: Latent coronary artery disease, determination of its presence and severity by the exercise electrocardiogram. Am. J. Cardiol., 13:603, 1964.
11. Master, A. M. and Rosenfeld, I.: Criteria for the clinical application of the two-step exercise test. J.A.M.A., 178:129, 1961.
12. Rochmis, P. and Blackburn, H.: Exercise tests: A survey of procedures, safety, and litigation experience in approximately 170,000 tests. J.A.M.A., 217:1061, 1971.
13. Abarquez, R. F., Freiman, A. H., Reichel, F. and LaDue, J. S.: The precordial electrocardiogram during exercise. Circulation, 22:1060, 1960.
14. Bellet, S., Deliyiannis, S. and Eliakim, M.: The electrocardiogram during exercise as recorded by radioelectrocardiography. Am. J. Cardiol., 8:385, 1961.
15. Blackburn, H. and Katigbak, R.: What electrocardiographic leads to take after exercise? Am. Heart J., 67:184, 1964.
16. Mason, R. E., Likar, I., Biern, R. O. and Ross, R. S.: Multiple lead exercise electrocardiography. Experience in 107 normal subjects and 67 patients with angina pectoris, and comparison with coronary cinearteriography in 84 patients. Circulation, 36:517, 1967.
17. Demanny, M. A., Tambe, A. and Zimmerman, H. A.: Correlation between coronary arteriography and the post-exercise electrocardiogram. Am. J. Cardiol., 19:526, 1967.
18. Robb, G. P. and Seltzer, F.: Appraisal of the double two-step exercise test, a long term follow-up study of 3,325 men. J.A.M.A., 234:722, 1975.
19. Brody, A. J.: Master two-step exercise test in clinically unselected patients. J.A.M.A., 171:1195, 1959.
20. Bellet, S. and Roman, L.: Stress electrocardiography in the diagnosis of arrhythmias. Geriatrics, 25:102, 1970.
21. Friedberg, C. K., Jaffe, H. L., Pordy, L. and Chesky, K.: The two-step exercise electrocardiogram. A double blind evaluation of its use in the diagnosis of angina pectoris. Circulation, 26:1254, 1962.
22. Kattus, A. A., MacAlpin, R., Longmire, W. P. et al.: Coronary angiograms and the exercise electrocardiogram in the study of angina pectoris. Am. J. Med., 34:19, 1963.

23. Cohen, L. S., Elliott, W. C., Klein, M. D. and Gorlin, R.: Coronary heart disease: clinical, cinearteriographic, and metabolic correlations. Am. J. Cardiol., 17:153, 1966.
24. Hultgren, H., Calciano, A., Platt, F. and Abrams, H.: A clinical evaluation of coronary arteriography. Am. J. Med., 42:228, 1967.
25. Most, A. S., Kemp, H. G. and Gorlin, R.: Post-exercise electrocardiography in patients with arteriographically documented coronary artery disease. Ann. Intern. Med., 71:1043, 1969.
26. Mattingly, T. W.: The post-exercise electrocardiogram. Its value in the diagnosis and prognosis of coronary arterial disease. Am. J. Cardiol., 9:395, 1962.
27. Froelicher, V. F.: The application of electrocardiographic screening and exercise testing to preventive cardiology. Prev. Med., 2:592, 1973.
28. Zohman, L. R. and Kattus, A. A.: Exercise testing in the diagnosis of coronary heart disease: A perspective. Am. J. Cardiol., 40:243, 1977.
29. Bellet, S., Roman, L. R., Nichols, G. J. and Muller, O. F.: Detection of coronary-prone subjects in a normal population by radioelectrocardiographic exercise test. Am. J. Cardiol., 19:783, 1967.
30. Gould, K. L. and Lipscomb, K.: Effects of coronary stenosis on coronary flow reserve and resistance. Am. J. Cardiol., 34:48, 1974.

3

Preparations and Precautions for the Exercise ECG Test

Edward K. Chung, M.D., F.A.C.P., F.A.C.C. and
Lisa S. Chung, M.D.

General Considerations

It is extremely important to provide proper preparation and follow careful precautions (see Table 3-1). This is essential not only for the production of the best quality exercise electrocardiogram which can provide all necessary information for the interpretation of the test, but also for the prevention of untoward complications, including sudden death. For example, the exercise electrocardiogram with the best quality can *not* be expected when proper skin preparation with the use of proper electrodes is not done. Similarly, the most suitable lead system which can detect the S-T segment change in the maximal degree must be utilized. Needless to say, careful considerations of indications versus contraindications of the exercise ECG test are essential. The purpose of the exercise ECG test in a given patient should be clearly known. When a high chance of false positive exercise ECG test in a given patient (e.g., in the presence of digitalis effect, left bundle branch block, WPW syndrome, etc.) is expected, the test should be cancelled unless the test is intended for the assessment of a functional capacity.

It is mandatory that a physician who supervises the exercise ECG test be fully familiar with the entire procedure as well as the interpretation of the test. Ready availability of cardiopulmonary resuscitative facilities, including a defibrillator and commonly used cardiac emergency drugs, is essential. In addition, medical as well as paramedical personnel working in the exercise laboratory must be capable of providing cardiopulmonary resuscitative measures. It is generally agreed that an informed consent form should be obtained before the exercise ECG test in order to protect the individual physician as well as the medical institution involved, especially in the United States of America.

Preparations and Precautions[1-11]

Preparations and precautions for the exercise ECG test are summarized in Table 3-1.

1. Patient Preparations

Patients should be instructed to come to the exercise laboratory for their exercise ECG test either after an overnight fast or at least 2 hours after a light meal. All patients should be free of any recognizable illness or discomfort other than known or suspected coronary artery disease before the test. They should be dressed comfortably with light-weight shoes (e.g., tennis shoes), and the exercise laboratory should be kept at a comfortable temperature ranging from 68–74° F., with 40–60% humidity. The exercise room should have ample space so that a physician can take a good history and perform an adequate physical examination. Ideally, the patient should rest comfortably in the supine position for at least 10 minutes before the actual exercise test. In most cases, however, taking the control (resting) 12-lead electrocardiogram before the exercise test is often sufficient for a resting period.

2. Complete History and Physical Examination

Although the attending physician (private physician) and house staff take a complete history and perform a complete physical examination in most situations, the physician who is going to supervise the exercise test must do the same just prior to the test. By taking a careful history, one may be able to assess the nature of chest pain (typical versus atypical). As emphasized repeatedly, the reproducibility of typical angina by exercise is one of the most reliable clues to diagnose coronary artery disease. On the other hand, many anxious individuals may have atypical chest discomfort, and in this circumstance, exercise-induced S-T segment change may represent a normal variant (e.g., neurocirculatory asthenia) or false positive result. False positive exercise ECG test is common in apparently healthy young to middle-aged women.

Not uncommonly, unrecognized myocardial infarction may be diagnosed by a careful history. When congestive heart failure is diagnosed, by history or physical examination, needless to say, the exercise ECG test must be cancelled. For example, various findings such as gallop rhythm, pulmonary rales, cardiomegaly and exertional dyspnea are certainly strongly suggestive of significant congestive heart failure.

Many other factors which may be contraindications for the exercise ECG test (see Chapter 8) can be recognized. By inspection or superficial physical examination, physical handicap (e.g., severe arthritis, deformity of lower extremities, etc.) is readily appreciated. Abnormal vital signs (e.g., fever,

Table 3-1. Exercise ECG Test: Preparations and Precautions

1. Patient preparations
2. Complete history and physical examination
3. Careful consideration of indications and contraindications
4. Careful consideration of various factors which may cause false positive or false negative exercise ECG test
5. Careful consideration of various drug effects (e.g., digitalis, propranolol) and electrolyte imbalance (e.g., hypokalemia)
6. Control (resting) 12-lead ECG before the test and another 12-lead ECG at the end of the test
7. Chest X-ray(?)
8. Informed consent form signed by the patient and witnessed by a physician
9. Instruct the procedure to the patient fully
10. Proper skin preparations and electrodes placement
11. Proper lead systems
12. Periodic blood pressure measurement and recording
13. Direct supervision of the test by a physician who is fully familiar with the procedure and interpretation of the exercise ECG test
14. Stop the test when acute symptoms, serious arrhythmias, significant S-T segment changes and/or hypotension occur
15. Treat the patient for any serious symptoms or arrhythmia as needed
16. Ready availability of cardiopulmonary resuscitative equipments (e.g., defibrillator) and drugs with well-trained medical and paramedical staff

unusually rapid or slow resting heart rate, hypotension or severe hypertension beyond 220 mm. Hg., and rapid respiratory rate) are usually considered to be contraindications to the exercise testing.

On auscultation a loud systolic murmur at the base suggestive of severe aortic stenosis should be considered to be a contraindication. When midsystolic click with or without mitral systolic murmur is heard, mitral valve prolapse syndrome is strongly suspected. In this case, a high chance of false positive exercise ECG test should be expected. In general, there is higher incidence of false positive exercise ECG test in any patient with significant valvular heart disease. In case of mitral stenosis (diastolic rumble with or without opening snap), exercise-induced atrial fibrillation may be anticipated.

Various non-cardiac disorders interfere with exercise testing. By and large, the exercise ECG test is contraindicated (see Chapter 8) in any individual with significant non-cardiac disorders (e.g., pulmonary emphysema, renal failure, severe anemia, malignancy, etc.). These problems can be recognized easily by physical examination and history.

By taking a careful history, detailed information regarding drug therapy can be obtained. As repeatedly emphasized, many drugs interfere with the result of the exercise ECG test. The best examples are that digitalis commonly causes false positive exercise ECG test, whereas propranolol (Inderal) frequently causes a false negative exercise ECG test (see Chapter 6). Thus, the exercise ECG test has no diagnostic value when the patient is taking digitalis prior to the test, and, therefore, the test should be cancelled. The above-mentioned important history and physical findings may not be fully appreciated by the attending physician.

Careful physical examination is also important during the post-exercise period, because certain findings (e.g., clearly audible S_3 or S_4 gallop) are diagnostic for coronary artery disease in most cases (see Chapter 12).

3. Careful Consideration of Indications and Contraindications

It is essential to consider indications and contraindications of the exercise ECG test carefully before the test. The physician who will supervise the exercise ECG test must evaluate the purpose of the test. Indications and contraindications of the exercise ECG test are discussed in Chapters 7 and 8, respectively.

4. Careful Consideration of Various Factors Which May Cause False Positive or False Negative Exercise ECG Test

Various factors which may produce false positive or false negative exercise ECG test should be carefully evaluated (see Chapters 5, 6 and 12). In particular, when any factor which frequently causes false positive exercise ECG test (e.g., digitalis, left ventricular hypertrophy, left bundle branch block, WPW syndrome, etc.) is present, the test may be cancelled unless the functional capacity is to be assessed. Table 3-2 briefly summarizes various problems associated with the exercise ECG test.

5. Careful Consideration of Various Drug Effects and Electrolyte Imbalance

As described elsewhere (see Chapter 6), various drugs and electrolyte imbalance may cause false positive or false negative exercise ECG test (see Table 3-2). The best example is digitalis which most commonly causes false positive exercise ECG test. Various psychotropic drugs influence similar effects on the exercise ECG test. Hypokalemia is the most common electrolyte imbalance causing false positive exercise ECG test. Propranolol (Inderal) and other anti-anginal drugs often cause false negative exercise ECG test.

6. 12-Lead Electrocardiogram

It is mandatory to obtain a control (resting) 12-lead electrocardiogram before the exercise testing. Two or three unexpected cases showing recent myocardial infarction have been documented annually in our exercise laboratory by a resting 12-lead ECG in conjunction with a careful history

Table 3-2. Exercise ECG Test—Problems

1. *False negative test*: Drugs (anti-anginal drugs—Nitroglycerin, propranolol etc.), physical training (e.g., athletes), proven coronary patients, left axis deviation of the QRS complex
2. *False positive test*: Digitalis, hypokalemia, hyperventilation, Wolff-Parkinson-White syndrome, mitral valve prolapse syndrome, healthy persons (i.e., women)
3. Influence of drugs and electrolyte imbalance
4. *Influence of pre-existing ECG abnormalities*: Right bundle branch block, left bundle branch block, left ventricular hypertrophy, right ventricular hypertrophy, Wolff-Parkinson-White syndrome, artificial pacemaker-induced ventricular rhythm, nonspecific abnormality of ST-T waves
5. Exercise-induced myocardial infarction, hypotension, serious cardiac arrhythmias and even death.

taking. Exercise ECG test is considered to be contraindicated when recent myocardial infarction is diagnosed. The result of the exercise ECG test is difficult or impossible to interpret, as far as the diagnostic aspect is concerned, when there are various ECG abnormalities including left bundle branch block (LBBB), left ventricular hypertrophy (LVH), digitalis effect and WPW syndrome (see Table 3-2). In addition, exercise ECG test is considered to be contraindicated when resting ECG shows significant cardiac arrhythmias such as ventricular tachycardia or acquired complete A-V block (see Chapter 8). Furthermore, it is essential to compare the pre-exercise ECG and post-exercise ECG.

In our exercise laboratory, a complete 12-lead ECG is taken before the test and another one after the termination of the exercise ECG test. When a new 3-channel recorder is available, a complete 12-lead ECG may be obtained any time during or after exercise as needed.

7. Chest X-Ray

It is *not* essential to take a chest X-ray immediately before exercise ECG test, but it is preferable to evaluate recent chest film. By doing so, the presence or absence of various findings (e.g., cardiomegaly, pulmonary congestion, pulmonary emphysema, calcifications, etc.) can be assessed, and some findings may be valuable to determine the contraindication of exercise testing.

8. Informed Consent Form

The absolute necessity of obtaining an informed consent form for the exercise ECG test is *not* universally recognized. However, many exercise laboratories, particularly in the United States of America, emphasize the value of the consent form in order to protect an individual physician as well as the medical institution involved. It is preferable to explain the possible risks involved with the exercise testing by the physician before the patient signs the consent form. The consent form should be witnessed by the physician who will supervise the test. Nevertheless, the exact value of the consent form for the exercise ECG test is not certain from the medico-legal viewpoint (see Chapter 17).

An example of the informed consent form for the exercise ECG test which is currently used in our exercise laboratory is shown in Table 3-3.

9. Instruct the Procedure to the Patient

The entire procedure of the exercise ECG test should be explained to the patient in detail by a technician under the supervision of a physician or

Table 3-3. Thomas Jefferson University Hospital Exercise ECG Laboratory Consent Form

I, _____, authorize Edward K. Chung, M.D., Director of the Heart Station, and such assistants (physicians) as he may designate, to administer and conduct the exercise (stress) electrocardiography (ECG) test which was requested by my physician.

This test is designed to evaluate the presence or absence of significant heart disease; and/or to evaluate the efficacy of my current therapy, and/or to measure my physical fitness for work and/or sport.

I understand that I will walk on a motor-driven treadmill. During the performance of the exercise ECG test, my electrocardiogram will be monitored and my blood pressure will be measured and recorded at periodic intervals. The exercise will be progressively increased according to the standard schedule until I attain a predetermined end point corresponding to moderate exercise stress, or become distressed in any way or develop any abnormal response, whichever of the above occurs first. I may request that the test be discontinued at any time.

Every effort will be made to conduct the test in such a way as to minimize discomfort and risk. However, I understand that just as with other diagnostic tests there are possible potential risks associated with the exercise ECG test. These include weakness, transient lightheadedness, fainting, chest discomfort, leg cramps and palpitations. On rare occasions (approximately 2 to 3 per 10,000) heart attack (myocardial infarction) or sudden death (approximately 1 per 10,000) may occur. In addition, my physician may request that Thallium-201 (a radioactive element in solution for purposes of heart scanning) be administered intravenously as part of the exercise ECG test. This adds no additional risks to the exercise ECG test and there are no known side effects from its administration. I further understand that the laboratory is properly equipped for such situations and that its professional personnel are trained to administer any emergency care necessary.

Signature _____

Date   _____

Witness _____

directly by a physician. For anxious individuals, the physician should explain the procedure directly. When the patient is not familiar with the exercise testing, a brief demonstration of actual walking on the treadmill by a technician may be of great value. The patient should be instructed to report immediately when he experiences unusual or significant symptoms (e.g., chest pain, dizziness or feeling of impending syncope, etc.) during exercise. In addition, the patient should be assured that he may request the termination of exercise prematurely whenever necessary.

When any individual is extremely anxious and reluctant to perform the exercise test, it may be necessary to postpone or even cancel the test. By and large, various untoward problems tend to occur when dealing with uncooperative individuals who are reluctant to perform the test. In addition, the exercise ECG test should be given with extreme caution or even avoided when unusually excessive questions are raised before signing the consent form. This type of individual often creates the medico-legal problem in the future.

10. Skin Preparation and Electrodes Placement

It is extremely important to apply proper skin preparation and to use specially designed electrodes in order to produce high quality electrocardiographic recordings during and after exercise. Otherwise, it will be difficult to interpret the exercise ECG result because of excessive artifacts. For proper skin preparation, the superficial keratinized layer of epidermis should be removed by gentle skin abrasion by using an emory board, dental burr, fine-grain sandpaper or vigorous rubbing with gauze. To eliminate excessive lipid content, it should be washed away by light cleansing with acetone or other organic solvent. Excessively vigorous debridement should be avoided in order to prevent edema formation and an increase in electrical resistance at the electrode-skin interface.

The most reliable electrodes for the exercise ECG testing are light-weight silver-silver chloride electrodes in which the skin contact occurs by means of a liquid conductor. This will minimize the loss of contact which often occurs with motion, particularly during peak exercise period. The optimal electrode should be 1 cm. in diameter or less, and encased in a light-weight plastic well which is 2–3 mm. in depth. Disposable electrodes manufactured by different companies are available in the market for clinical use. Electrode cables designed to reduce motion artifact are also available, obviating the need for telemetered monitoring of the ECG recordings. The electrocardiographic machine must meet the minimal specifications proposed by the American Heart Association in order to avoid an excessive distortion of the S-T segment.

In women, particularly obese individuals with large breasts, the exercise ECG test should be performed with the patient wearing an undergarment to support the breasts. By doing so, excessive motion artifacts due to movement of the chest electrode by the breasts during exercise can be minimized or even be avoided.

11. Proper Lead Systems

In addition to the proper skin preparations with the use of specially designed electrodes, proper selection of a lead system is equally important. When a proper lead system is not utilized, an excessive incidence of false positive or false negative tests can not be avoided.

When a single-channel ECG recorder is available, various modified bipolar lead V_5 positions are the best selection. Namely, the positive electrode is placed in the 5th left intercostal space at the anterior axillary line, whereas the negative electrode is placed in a variety of positions including the forehead (CH_3), right infraclavicular areas (CS_5), manubrium (CM_5), left 5th intercostal space (CC_5), or on the back (CA_5). Among these modified bipolar lead V_5 positions, the most popular and the best lead system with the highest sensitivity is lead CM_5. It has been shown that lead CM_5 will identify 89% of abnormal ECG responses when compared to full 12-lead electrocardiogram.[12] In patients with dextrocardia, the exactly opposite site of the lead CM_5 should be the ideal electrode placement location. When lead CM_5 does not record the highest R wave amplitude, the electrode placement in some subjects (e.g., chest deformity, abnormal electrical axis, etc.) may be modified further in order to register the tallest R wave amplitude.

Various lead systems for exercise ECG test are summarized in Table 3-4. When a 2-channel ECG recorder is available, lead CM_5 plus lead II (or aVF) will be the best combination. In addition, a combination of leads CM_5, modified V_3 and II (or aVF) will be even superior when 3-channel ECG recorder is available. It has been also suggested a combination of 6-lead system including leads II, aVF and modified V_{3-6} may detect 100% of abnormal ECG responses.[5] It is not certain whether a full 12-lead ECG is superior to the above-mentioned 6-lead system as far as the diagnostic sensitivity is concerned. Other multilead systems such as X,Y,Z lead, modified leads I, aVF and V_5, modified leads V_{4-6}, modified leads V_{3-6} and modified leads V_{3-6} plus II, have been utilized by different authors, but these lead systems are not widely accepted.

12. Periodic Blood Pressure Measurement and Recordings

It is essential to measure and record blood pressure during and after exercise with a regular interval. It has been known that the so-called double product or systolic blood pressure multiplied by the heart rate is an excellent index of myocardial O_2 consumption. Recent experience indicated that the development of hypotension during exercise is an important sign strongly sugges-

Table 3-4. Lead Systems for Exercise ECG Test

Single-channel recorder: Modified V_5 (e.g., CM_5)
2-Channel recorder: Modified V_5 and II (or aVF)
3-Channel recorder: Modified V_5, V_3 and II (or aVF)
6-Channel recorder: Leads II, aVF and V_{3-6}
Other multi-lead systems: X,Y,Z,-lead,
                              Modified I, aVF and V_5
                              Modified leads V_{4-6}
                              Modified leads V_{3-6}
                              Modified leads V_{3-6} plus II
                              Modified 12-lead

tive of coronary artery disease (see Chapter 12). Nevertheless, an accurate measurement of blood pressure is often difficult, especially during a peak exercise period. For this reason, specially designed blood pressure apparatus manufactured by different companies is available for the exercise ECG test.

In most exercise laboratories, blood pressure is measured at 1-minute intervals during exercise and at least 8 minutes during the post-exercise period or until the ECG finding returns to the resting ECG value. When any patient develops hypotension or significant hypertension (systolic pressure above 220 mm. Hg.), the exercise ECG test should be terminated prematurely.

13. Direct Supervision by a Physician

From the medico-legal viewpoint, it is highly recommended that the exercise ECG testing be supervised directly by a physician. The physician should be fully familiar with the entire procedure as well as the interpretations of the exercise ECG test. This is especially so when dealing with high prevalence of coronary artery disease in the cardiology referral centers such as our exercise laboratory. When the high risk patient is involved, the physician should be extremely alert so that he can determine the optimal time to terminate the test prematurely as needed. Physical presence of the physician during and after exercise, however, is not uniformly practiced at every exercise laboratory, especially when dealing with a large population with healthy individuals for various exercise programs.

14. Terminate the Test Prematurely as Needed

The physician who supervises the test must terminate the exercise testing prematurely when the patient develops significant symptoms (e.g., severe chest pain, feeling of impending syncope, etc.), abnormal physical findings (e.g., cyanosis, pallor, etc.), serious cardiac arrhythmias (e.g., ventricular tachycardia), marked horizontal or downsloping S-T segment depression of 2 mm. or more and/or hypotension (see Chapter 9). This is the most important role of the physician who supervises the exercise testing.

15. Administration of Treatment as Needed

The supervising physician has to determine whether immediate treatment is necessary for significant symptoms, particularly chest pain and serious cardiac arrhythmias. Not uncommonly, sublingual nitroglycerine is needed for exercise-induced angina, and at times, nasal O_2 is required. For serious ventricular arrhythmias, intravenous injection of lidocaine (Xylocaine) should be considered. On rare occasions, the patient may require hospitalization because of severe chest pain and/or serious cardiac arrhythmias.

16. Ready Availability of Cardiopulmonary Resuscitative Facilities with Commonly Used Cardiac Drugs and Well Trained Medical and Para-Medical Personnel

It is mandatory that all exercise laboratories be equipped with cardiopulmonary resuscitative facilities, including a defibrillator and commonly used cardiac drugs (e.g., lidocaine, atropine, isoproterenol, epinephrine, digoxin, etc.). In addition, every individual working in the exercise laboratory should be capable of delivering cardiopulmonary resuscitative measures. Recently, in our exercise laboratory, a patient with previous myocardial infarction developed cardiac arrest due to ventricular fibrillation during exercise. Fortunately, he was successfully resuscitated and he recovered uneventfully. Among other things, he required intracardiac injection of epinephrine, 4 applications of defibrillator, intravenous lidocaine, etc. in addition to closed cardiac massage and mouth-to-mouth resuscitation. This patient would not have been saved if a defibrillator had not been immediately available in the exercise laboratory.

Summary

Proper preparations and precautions must be followed for the exercise ECG testing. They may be summarized as follows:

1. Complete history and physical examination are essential before the exercise ECG test. Various factors which may be considered as contraindications should be detected. In addition, factors which may cause false positive or false negative test may be identified.

2. Indications and contraindications of the exercise ECG test should be carefully considered. It is essential to determine the purpose of the test.

3. Digitalis most commonly causes false positive exercise ECG test, whereas propranolol often produces false negative test.

4. The exercise ECG test has no diagnostic value in the presence of LBBB, or WPW syndrome.

5. It is essential to take 2 sets of complete 12-lead electrocardiograms—pre-exercise ECG and post-exercise ECG.

6. Chest X-ray is not essential immediately before the exercise test, but recent chest film provides various useful information.

7. An informed consent form should be obtained before the exercise ECG test for medico-legal protection, particularly in the United States of America.

8. The patient should be fully instructed regarding the entire procedure of the exercise testing.

9. Direct supervision by a physician who is fully familiar with the entire procedure as well as the interpretation of the exercise ECG test is essential.

10. Proper skin preparations and the use of specially designed electrodes are extremely important for the best quality exercise ECG recordings.

11. The best single lead system is a bipolar modified lead V_5 (CM_5). A combination of CM_5 and lead II (or aVF) seems to be the best when a 2-channel recorder is available. When a 3-channel recorder is used, leads II (or aVF), modified V_3 and V_5 seem to be the best combination.

12. Blood pressure should be measured and recorded at 1-minute intervals during exercise and at least 8 minutes during the post-exercise period.

13. ECG should be monitored without interruption during the after exercise until completion of the test (usually 8–10 minutes during recovery period).

14. The exercise testing should be terminated prematurely when the patient develops significant symptoms, serious cardiac arrhythmias and/or hypotension. Appropriate treatment should be given as needed.

15. It is essential to have all necessary cardiopulmonary resuscitative facilities in the exercise laboratory, including a defibrillator. Every individual working in the exercise laboratory must be capable of delivering cardiopulmonary resuscitative measures.

REFERENCES

1. Naughton, J.: Stress electrocardiography, *in* Clinical Electrocardiographic Correlations, edited by J. C. Rios, Cardiovasc. Clin., *8*:127–139, 1977.
2. Fortuin, N. J. and Weiss, J. L.: Exercise stress testing. Circulation, *56*:699, 1977.
3. Faris, J. V., McHenry, P. L. and Morris, S. N.: Concepts and applications of treadmill exercise testing and the exercise electrocardiogram. Am. Heart J., *95*:102, 1978.
4. McHenry, P. L. and Morris, S. N.: Exercise electrocardiography. Current state of the art, *in* Advances in Electrocardiography, edited by R. C. Schlant and J. W. Hurst, pp. 265–304, New York, Grune & Stratton, 1976.
5. Ellestad, M. H.: Stress Testing. Principles and Practice. Philadelphia (pp. 25—46), F. A. Davis, 1976.
6. Markiewicz, W., Houston, N. and DeBusk, R. F.: Exercise testing soon after myocardial infarction. Circulation, *56*:26, 1977.
7. Sivarajan, E., Snydsman, A., Smith, B. et al.: Low-level treadmill testing of 41 patients with acute myocardial infarction prior to discharge from the hospital. Heart and Lung, *6*: 975, 1977.
8. Simoons, M. L., Van Den Brand, M. and Hugenholtz, P. G.: Quantitative analysis of exercise electrocardiograms and left ventricular angiocardiograms in patients with abnormal QRS complexes at rest. Circulation, *55*:55, 1977.
9. Linhart, J. W.: Stress testing in angina. Resident & Staff Physician, pp. 79–89, Feb., 1978.

10. Chung, E. K.: Clinical Electrocardiography (Part 9), Exercise Electrocardiography. New York, Medcom, 1978.

11. Chung, E. K.: Sick sinus syndrome and brady-tachyarrhythmia syndrome, *in* Artificial Cardiac Pacing: Practical Approach, edited by E. K. Chung, Baltimore, Williams & Wilkins, 1978.

12. Blackburn, H. and Katybok, R.: What electrocardiographic leads to take after exercise. Am. Heart J., *67:*184, 1964.

4

Methodology of the Exercise ECG Test: Technical Aspects

B. Don Franks, Ph.D., F.A.C.S.M.

General Considerations

The technical aspects of exercise tolerance testing depend on the purpose(s) of the test, the type of patient and the work task available.

Testing purposes include determination of cardiorespiratory function, the presence or absence of coronary heart disease, work performance ability and/or the basis for a program of physical activity. These purposes are accomplished by determining the patient's cardiorespiratory response to different intensities of work. The test protocol depends upon the medical and activity history of the patient. Younger, more active patients start at higher intensities and progress at greater increments.

The ECG is monitored continuously. Selected leads of the ECG, blood pressure and other variables of interest are recorded at each level of work. Skin preparation and placement of electrodes are important prerequisites for good ECG records during work.

There is no one correct way to conduct an exercise tolerance test. This chapter will present the issues related to testing methods in relation to the purposes of the test.

Reasons for Testing

The primary reasons for testing an individual's responses to exercise are to:

- Evaluate cardiorespiratory function
- Screen for coronary heart disease (CHD)
- Provide a basis for exercise prescription
- Determine ability to perform a specific work task(s).

Cardiorespiratory Function

Figure 4-1 lists the components of cardiorespiratory function. Historically, medical tests have evaluated cardiorespiratory efficiency at rest, while testing of athletes has concentrated on maximal ability and endurance. Physical fitness testing has included all components of cardiorespiratory function. Although there are moderate relationships among the different components of cardiorespiratory function, it is clear from the research literature that one should measure directly the component(s) of cardiorespiratory function which are considered important for a particular patient. If there is interest in maximal ability, it should be measured directly, not estimated from resting or submaximal efficiency. If one is interested in efficiency during submaximal work, then it should be measured directly, not estimated from resting or maximal measures.

If absolute levels of cardiorespiratory function are important, as in comparisons among subpopulations, then careful standardization of the testing protocol, pre-test activities, familiarization of the patient with the task, adequate rest between work levels, all become essential characteristics of the test. If the evaluation of specific exercise or other intervention programs is the objective, then a similar control group is necessary for comparison.

Table 4-1 describes the variables that can be used in testing cardiorespiratory efficiency, endurance and maximal ability. It should be noted that heart rate is a good measure of cardiorespiratory function at rest and in response to a standard level of work; whereas, oxygen uptake, work done or time are good measures of cardiorespiratory response to maximal work, or work up to a specific percent of maximum or set heart rate (as in the physical working capacity tests). Oxygen uptake at rest or in response to the same work level and heart rate response to maximal work are not recommended because they do not differentiate among different levels of cardiorespiratory function.

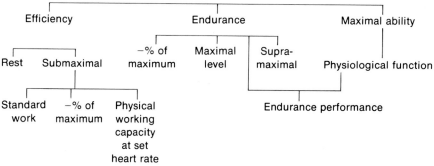

Fig. 4-1.   Components of cardiorespiratory function

Table 4-1. Tests of Cardiorespiratory Function

Components	Condition	Laboratory Tests*	Field Tests**
Efficiency, rest	Inactive	Measures of heart, lungs, blood vessels, and biochemical aspects of muscle	Heart rate
Submaximal	Standard external work load	Same as rest	Heart rate
	% of maximum	Work level	Time or work done
	Progressive work load to set heart rate	Work done, or time	Time
Endurance			
	% of maximum	Work done, or time	Time or distance
	Maximum	Work done, or time	Time or distance
	Supramaximum	Work done, or time	Time or distance
Maximal ability	Work to limit	Measures of heart, lungs, blood vessels, and biochemical aspects of muscle	
Endurance —maximum ability			Time for endurance run

   * Laboratory work tasks = treadmill, bicycle ergometer, bench step.
  ** Field work tasks = bench step, endurance run.

Screening for Coronary Heart Disease (CHD)

A second reason for administering an exercise ECG test is to screen for signs of coronary heart disease. This may be done in persons as a regular part of a medical or fitness examination, or the high risk patients referred for the test by their physician. If this is the sole purpose for the test, then the use of standardized protocol, pre-test activities, etc. is less important because the purpose of the test is to put increasing stress on the person to determine if there are abnormal ECG responses.

There are intuitively attractive arguments for including maximal stress in this situation. One would be more confident of negative results of a stress test if the test had gone to maximal effort. However, although there is convincing evidence that persons who show abnormalities at low levels of work have poorer prognosis than persons with a negative test, the evidence is unclear concerning the relative prognosis between those with a negative test and those with abnormalities at near maximal levels of work.

In testing to determine whether or not ECG abnormalities are present in response to stress, some of the testing methods used to minimize the stressfulness of the test, such as warm-up and taper-down, may be purposely omitted in order to observe the person's response to the more stressful situation.

Exercise Prescription (see Chapter 9)

A third reason for determining physiological response to exercise is to establish a program of regular physical activity. This is often done as a follow-up of the cardiorespiratory evaluation or the CHD screening. If it is essential to precisely quantify the physical activity program, as in a research study, then a maximal test is used and the activity program set at a certain percent of maximum. If, however, the prescription is primarily in a clinical or service program, the percent of estimated maximum can be utilized. The exercise test should obviously exceed the proposed exercising level to ensure that the patient can exercise at that level without abnormal responses.

Work Performance

Another reason for exercise tests is to determine one's ability to perform, and/or continue to perform, a specific task or series of tasks. The most common examples would be in industry or athletics. In those large muscle activities which continue beyond several minutes, the cardiorespiratory function is an important ingredient. However, the main interest is in the performance rather than the underlying cardiorespiratory function. The test should therefore measure the endurance performance directly, or in a test that is similar to the performance.

Summary

Exercise tolerance tests are given to determine cardiorespiratory function, work performance, to screen for CHD and/or as a basis for recommending an exercise program. Although these reasons have been separated to illustrate the different elements of the testing protocol for specific purposes, in practice, there is usually more than one reason for administering a test to a patient. It is often desirable to include determination of cardiorespiratory function, screen for CHD and provide a basis for exercise prescription all at the same time.

Personnel

The most important part of any testing situation is the personnel. There are four types of people necessary to conduct an exercise tolerance test:

- Patient
- Testing technician
- Program director
- Physician

Each of these roles has certain competencies related to it, although one person may perform more than one of the roles.

Patient

The patient is ready for the test only after it has been indicated from background information, interview and resting tests that he/she should have the test and there are no contraindications to an exercise test (see Chapter 8). The patients must have given informed consent (see Chapter 3) to take the test, have had previous experience with the type of work to be performed, have followed the pre-test instructions concerning food, drink, smoking, medication and activity, and be in suitable clothing.

Testing Technician

The person who administers the test must be able to set up the testing situation, administer the test to the patient obtaining accurate data, care for and calibrate the equipment, be familiar with testing and emergency procedures, including cardiopulmonary resuscitation (CPR), and be able to relate to the patient. Of course, the entire procedure must be conducted under the direct supervision of the physician-in-charge. In other words, the technician should be fully familiar with the entire procedure of the exercise ECG test, even in the absence of a physician.

Program Director

The program director confirms that the patient is cleared to take the test, that the testing technician has the competencies to safely administer the test and the information necessary to determine the appropriate protocol. It is the director's responsibility to ensure that emergency equipment and procedures are operative. The program director may supervise the exercise ECG test directly or he (or she) can assign a physician to conduct the test.

Physician

The physician is trained in the interpretation of exercise ECG and advanced CPR, including the use of the defibrillator and various drugs. He/she helps the program director establish indications, contraindications for testing and the criteria for stopping the exercise test. A physician may conduct the entire exercise ECG test when he (or she) is designated by the program director.

Work Tasks

There are numerous large muscle group activities which can be used to elicit an elevated cardiorespiratory response. These include stepping up and down on a bench or stair; pedaling a bicycle ergometer with legs and/or arms; walking or running on a treadmill; carrying loads on a hike; skipping rope; doing a series of jumps or hops; running in place; running a set distance for time or a set time for distance.

If the sole purpose is to determine if there are abnormal ECG responses to increased levels of cardiorespiratory function, then any of the tasks could be used. Some tasks provide easier division into levels of work and facilitate obtaining good records. If performance or prescription for a particular activity is the purpose of the test, then a similar activity should be used for the test. If one wants to prescribe a general level of activities, then work tasks easily quantified are needed. Tasks which can be quantified and replicated are needed for evaluating cardiorespiratory function or determining the longitudinal progress of individuals.

Table 4-2 ranks the most common work tasks (bench, bike, treadmill and endurance run) in terms of their reproducibility and feasibility. A treadmill test is the most reproducible but also the most expensive. The bicycle ergometer can be quantified easily, allows recording of variables with little movement of the upper body and is less expensive than the treadmill, but

Table 4-2. Advantages of Different Work Tasks

Work Task	Reproducible	Quantifiable	Economical	Group Test	Natural Activity
Treadmill	++++	+++	+		++
Bicycle ergometer	+++	++++	++		+
Bench stepping	++	++	+++	+++	+
Endurance runs	+	+	++++	++++	+++

local muscular fatigue in the legs may cause the patient to stop before maximal stress to the cardiorespiratory systems is reached in non-cycling populations. It is most difficult to replicate and record variables during the bench step; however, it is the least expensive. The endurance run is not recommended except to test the endurance of those patients who have already been active and whose cardiorespiratory efficiency has been tested.

Pre-Test

The testing personnel establish the procedures to be used prior to, during and following the exercise tolerance test. As indicated in Table 4-3, the first step is to determine whether or not an exercise test should be administered and for what purpose(s) (see Chapters 7 and 8). If a test is indicated, then the patient's informed consent is obtained. At that time the patient is given an exact description of the test, risks and the pre-test instructions (see Chapter 3).

Informed Consent

An example of an informed consent form is found in Chapter 3. The primary ingredients include a clear description of the test, its potential risks and benefits; the patient's right to stop at any time without penalty; and the assurance of confidentiality of the data.

Pre-test Instructions

At the time the patient is scheduled for the test, instructions are given concerning what should and should not be done prior to the test. These instructions usually include such things as prohibition of eating, drinking (except water), smoking and vigorous physical activity for several hours prior to the test if it is desirable to get accurate data. Continuing or discontinuing medication depends on the test purpose and is decided in consultation with the patient's physician, if he (or she) is not the test

Table 4-3. Pre-test Steps

1. Test indicated for this patient
2. Specific purposes of the test
3. Informed consent
4. Pre-test instruction
5. Set work task and test protocol
6. Calibrate equipment
7. Practice by patient
8. Instruction in task; include stopping procedure
9. Emergency care ready

administrator. If the purpose is exercise prescription which will be carried out while the patient is on medication, then the medication need not be halted. If the purpose of the test is to determine the cardiorespiratory level, or screen for abnormal response as an indication of CHD, then the medication should be stopped except when contraindicated.

Work Task and Protocol

The work task is determined based on the test purpose and available equipment. If one wants to compare data with other studies, the protocols found in Figure 4-2 have been widely used. Table 4-4 recommends the starting level and increments for different stages for different populations (modified from American College of Sports Medicine Guidelines). The three protocols found in Table 4-5 apply these recommendations for different populations to estimated energy levels needed for bench, bike or treadmill tasks. In most situations, 2-minute intervals for each stage and a continuous test are recommended because one gets the essential information for cardiorespiratory function, screening for CHD and exercise prescription in a relatively short time. However, if the primary purpose is to determine the "true" maximal ability, or the physiological response to a particular level of work, then each work bout should be continued 5 minutes with intermittent intervals of light activity (e.g., slow walking).

1. Progressive Test

There is no reason to use a single level test. The progressive, graded test includes warm-up, information about the patient's response to a variety of intensities of exercises and can be done efficiently in terms of time. It can include both submaximal and maximal variables.

2. Warm-up

There is evidence that warm-up improves performance and decreases the stressfulness of a set level of exercise. Therefore, unless one is interested in the effects of sudden high levels of stress (as one might be in the case of emergency workers), then one would normally include a low level of activity as the first stage.

3. Taper-down

A warm-down period is routinely included in conditioning sessions. However, many testing protocols have failed to include an active recovery after the most stressful part of the test. Abrupt stopping is more stressful than hard exercise and should be avoided except in the case where one wants to examine the ability to withstand this type of stress.

FUNCTIONAL CLASS	CLINICAL STATUS	O_2 REQUIREMENTS ml O_2/kg/min	STEP TEST	TREADMILL TESTS				BICYCLE ERGOMETER**
			NAGLE, BALKE, NAUGHTON*	BRUCE†	KATTUS‡	BALKE**	BALKE**	
			2 min stages 30 steps/min	3-min stages	3-min stages	% grade at 3.4 mph	% grade at 3 mph	For 70 kg body weight
NORMAL AND I	PHYSICALLY ACTIVE SUBJECTS	56.0	(Step height increased 4 cm q 2 min)			26		
NORMAL AND I	PHYSICALLY ACTIVE SUBJECTS	52.5			mph %gr	24		kgm/min
NORMAL AND I	PHYSICALLY ACTIVE SUBJECTS	49.0		mph %gr	4 22	22		
NORMAL AND I	PHYSICALLY ACTIVE SUBJECTS	45.5	Height (cm)	4.2 16		20		1500
NORMAL AND I	PHYSICALLY ACTIVE SUBJECTS	42.0	40		4 18	18	22.5	1350
NORMAL AND I	PHYSICALLY ACTIVE SUBJECTS	38.5	36			16	20.0	1200
NORMAL AND I	PHYSICALLY ACTIVE SUBJECTS; SEDENTARY HEALTHY	35.0	32		4 14	14	17.5	1050
NORMAL AND I	PHYSICALLY ACTIVE SUBJECTS; SEDENTARY HEALTHY	31.5	28	3.4 14		12	15.0	900
NORMAL AND I	PHYSICALLY ACTIVE SUBJECTS; SEDENTARY HEALTHY	28.0	24		4 10	10	12.5	
NORMAL AND I	PHYSICALLY ACTIVE SUBJECTS; SEDENTARY HEALTHY; DISEASED, RECOVERED; SYMPTOMATIC PATIENTS	24.5	20	2.5 12	3 10	8	10.0	750
II	PHYSICALLY ACTIVE SUBJECTS; SEDENTARY HEALTHY; DISEASED, RECOVERED; SYMPTOMATIC PATIENTS	21.0	16			6	7.5	600
II	PHYSICALLY ACTIVE SUBJECTS; SEDENTARY HEALTHY; DISEASED, RECOVERED; SYMPTOMATIC PATIENTS	17.5	12	1.7 10	2 10	4	5.0	450
III	PHYSICALLY ACTIVE SUBJECTS; SEDENTARY HEALTHY; DISEASED, RECOVERED; SYMPTOMATIC PATIENTS	14.0	8			2	2.5	300
III	DISEASED, RECOVERED; SYMPTOMATIC PATIENTS	10.5	4				0.0	
III	DISEASED, RECOVERED; SYMPTOMATIC PATIENTS	7.0						150
IV	SYMPTOMATIC PATIENTS	3.5						

*Nagle FS, Balke B, Naughton JP: Gradational step tests for assessing work capacity. *J Appl Physiol* **20**:745-748, 1965.

†Bruce RA: Multi-stage treadmill test of submaximal and maximal exercise. Appendix B, this publication.

‡Kattus AA, Jorgensen CR, Worden RE, Alvaro AB: S-T-segment depression with near-maximal exercise in detection of preclinical coronary heart disease. *Circulation* **41**:585-595, 1971.

Fox SM, Naughton JP, Haskell WL: Physical activity and the prevention of coronary heart disease. *Ann Clin Res* **3:404, 1971.

Fig. 4-2. Work tasks and protocols. (Reprinted with permission from *Exercise Testing and Training of Apparently Healthy Individuals: A Handbook for Physicians,* the American Heart Association, 1972.)

4. Stopping

The test may be terminated by the physician who supervises the exercise ECG test. The test may be terminated prematurely at the patient's request because of intolerable symptoms, such as severe chest pain, dyspnea, dizzi-

Table 4-4. Suggested Starting Levels and Increments for Exercise Tolerance Testing

	Starting MET* Level	Increments for Each Stage
Active, young, healthy	6–7	3
Inactive or older "normal," healthy	4–5	2
Questionable health or CHD Patient	2–3	1

* The MET level is the multiple of the resting metabolism (VO_2), estimated to be 3.5 ml/kg. of body weight/minute. Thus, the CHD patient would begin an exercise test at 2 or 3 times his/her resting level, or an activity costing 7–10.5 ml. of oxygen/kg. of body weight/minute.

ness, fatigue, etc. In addition, the physician may stop the test when there are significant S-T segment alterations, cardiac arrhythmias and/or hypotension during exercise. At any rate, the physician-in-charge determines whether the test should be continued or stopped in a given moment.

5. Calibration

All equipment must be carefully maintained and checked with known standards preceding testing sessions. The speed and percent grade of the treadmill, resistance of the bicycle ergometer, accuracy of timing devices, gas analysis equipment are all continuously checked. It must be emphasized that no dial setting or meter can be assumed to be accurate. Only in those rare cases where the level of work, the ability to compare the response to work, or to later replicate the work are unimportant can one disregard calibration.

6. Practice on test

Individuals show "improvement" on new work tasks by repeating the task. Therefore, if the purpose of a test is to provide accurate baseline data to compare with tests following some type of intervention, or simply as a function of time, it is important to provide pre-test practice on the task. The attachments, mouthpiece, etc. should be included as part of the practice. When the accuracy of a particular testing period is important, the average of more than one trial increases the reliability.

7. Instructions (see also Chapter 3)

In addition to the general description of the task, the patient is given specific information just prior to the test administration. This includes a

Table 4-5. Recommended Protocol for Different Types of Patients

Stages in the Test (2 min. each)*			MET Level	Bench Step Ht. Rate		Bicycle Ergometer Work‡	Treadmill	
Young, active healthy	"Normal" inactive healthy	Questionable health or CHD		(cm)†	(step/min.)	(KPM/min.)	Speed (km/hr.§)	Grade (%)
		1	2	0	24	0 (50 rpm)	3.2	0
		2	3	16	12	150	4.8	0
	1	3	4	16	18	300	4.8	2.5
		4	5	16	24	450	4.8	5.0
	2	5	6	16	30	600	4.8	7.5
		6	7	36	18	750	4.8	10
1	3	7	8	36	24	900	5.5	10
		8	9	36	27	1050	5.5	12
	4		10	36	30	1200	9.7	0
2			11	36	33	1350	9.7	1.75
	5		12	36	36	1500	9.7	3.5
			13	50	27	1650	11.3	3.0
3			14	50	30	1800	11.3	5.0

* After the patient is stopped, the final stage is to return to stage one for a taper-down. In the case of the young, active patients, the taper-down may be at an even lower level.

† 16 cm. = 6.3 inches
  36 cm. = 14.2 inches
  50 cm. = 20 inches

‡ Kilopound meters/min.

§ 3.2 km/hr. = 2 m.p.h.
  4.8 km./hr/ = 3 m.p.h.
  5.5 km./hr. = 3.4 m.p.h.
  9.7 km./hr. = 6 m.p.h.
  11.3 km./hr. = 7 m.p.h.

review of what to expect, when to start, what kind of things to report to the tester, what to do when the end of the highest level of work is obtained and what to do after the taper-down period.

8. Emergencies

The emergency equipment and supplies are checked, and procedures for all staff are reviewed and practiced.

Exercise ECG

Good exercise ECG tracings depend primarily on two things: skin preparation and placement of electrodes. The skin should be cleaned with alcohol, or similar solution, then roughed up by light sandpaper or similar substance, until the skin in the area of the electrode is red. A popular placement is to place the arm electrodes in the relatively flat space just below the midpoint of the clavicle; the leg electrodes between the iliac crest and the umbilicus; and the chest electrode in the V_5 position.

The multiple lead recording has the same advantage during exercise as during rest; namely, the ability to find abnormalities that might normally be missed with a single lead.

During Test

Setting and changing the work task, recording the selected variables at specified times, monitoring the ECG and observing the patient are the important elements of the exercise tolerance test.

Patient

Continual communication with the patient helps reduce anxiety related to the test, reminds the patient of the next step in the test and alerts the tester to any unusual reactions to the test. If the patient has a mouthpiece (e.g., for VO_2 determination), then hand signals are established prior to the test.

Recordings

Variables such as heart rate, blood pressure and the ECG are normally recorded at least once during each stage of the test. In order to compare the test results with later tests, it is important to determine exactly when each variable will be recorded and adhere to that schedule. Table 4-6 is a rating of perceived exertion, established by Borg, which is a good addition to the normal variables. It is especially useful in knowing when the end point is being approached in maximal tests.

Monitoring

The ECG should be continually monitored on the scope with periodic and frequent determinations of blood pressure by the physician. The tester monitors the patient in terms of any symptoms throughout the test.

Stopping

In maximal tests, the patient continues until he/she decides they have reached their maximal work, until one of the pre-determined end points is reached or until there are symptoms or ECG abnormalities which cause the physician to stop the test. Some standards which have been used for

Table 4-6. Rating of Perceived Exertion*

6	
7	Very, very light
8	
9	Very light
10	
11	Fairly light
12	
13	Somewhat hard
14	
15	Hard
16	
17	Very hard
18	
19	Very, very hard
20	

* Reproduced with permission from G. Borg: Perceived exertion as an indicator of somatic stress. Scand. J. Rehabil. Med., 2:92, 1970.

stopping tests are systolic blood pressure (SBP) of 250 mm. Hg., or when SBP goes down with an increase in work; diastolic blood pressure (DBP) of 120 mm. Hg.; excessive breathing or sweating, unsteadiness, loss of mental alertness or pains in the chest, arm or jaw.

In submaximal tests, one procedure widely used is to predict the patient's maximum heart rate (see Chapter 9), then to exercise the person until either 85% of the predicted maximum heart rate is attained or one of the other reasons for stopping occurs.

Following Test

Patient

Following the taper-down there is normally a short recovery period where additional data may be collected. When the patient feels comfortable and the ECG abnormality returns to the resting value, the physician-in-charge can determine whether to dismiss the patient. In general, a personal physician who ordered the test should be notified immediately by the physician who conducted the exercise ECG test when the patient suffers from severe symptoms (e.g., chest pain, dyspnea, etc.) or when marked S-T, T wave alterations and/or cardiac arrhythmias are produced by the exercise. A formal interpretation of the exercise ECG test will be reported by the physician who is in charge of the exercise ECG laboratory. When the exercise ECG test is given for non-diagnostic purposes, the proper exercise program will be prescribed by the personal physician (the exercise program director is often consulted) based on the test data.

Table 4-7. Sequence of Testing

1. Medical clearance
2. Informed consent
3. Non-stressful tests
    (a) Background information
    (b) Body composition
    (c) Resting cardiorespiratory efficiency
    (d) Psychological tests
4. Submaximal cardiorespiratory efficiency
5. Begin light activity program
6. Maximal cardiorespiratory function and endurance
7. Revise activity program
8. Include games and sports
9. Periodic retest and activity revision

Reports

The data are recorded on the permanent record sheet, along with any comments by the tester and/or attending physician. Reports are prepared for the patient, the patient's physician(s), the program director (for exercise prescription) and the permanent files.

Follow-up

Periodic follow-ups are made to retest the patient and to revise the exercise prescription as needed.

Sequence of Testing and Activity

Table 4-7 illustrates the sequence of testing and activity recommended for those patients who are available to the testing center on a continual basis. The non-stressful tests are administered first, followed by submaximal efficiency tests. If there are no contraindications, then an activity program is begun at low levels in activities easily quantified and controlled, such as walking or cycling. Following adaptation to that program, the maximal test is given, and the activity program is revised. It is at this point that a variety of sports and games can safely be recommended for the patient, followed by periodic retests and exercise program revisions.

Summary

Exercise tolerance tests are administered to evaluate cardiorespiratory efficiency, endurance and/or maximal ability; as screening for coronary heart disease; to determine performance ability; and/or provide a basis for exercise prescription. The program director, in consultation with the attending physician, determines the test protocol to be administered to a given patient.

Treadmill walking or running is the most natural and reproducible work task for most patients. However, riding the bicycle ergometer or bench stepping are more economical and can be utilized for exercise tolerance testing.

Prior to the test the patient voluntarily agrees to the test procedures which have been clearly described and the testing technician checks the test and emergency equipment and procedures. For most situations, a continuous, progressive, multistage test is recommended. The starting level is 3, 5 or 7 METS for de-conditioned, normal/sedentary and young/active patients, respectively. Increments for each stage are 1, 2 or 3 METS for the same three groups, respectively. An active recovery follows the highest work level determined by the patient, the test technician or the physician. The recommended sequence of testing begins with non-stressful tests, submaximal testing and a light activity program of quantifiable activities. After the person adjusts to the light activity program, then maximal tests can be administered and, if there is no contraindication, games and sports can then be included in the program.

The skin is roughed up and the electrodes are placed where multileads can be recorded with a minimum of movement artifact. Arm leads placed just below the midpoint of the clavicle, leg electrodes placed between the iliac crest and the umbilicus, and the chest leads at V_4 or V_5 provide locations with minimal artifact, allowing selected leads to be recorded during exercise.

It is essential that the exercise ECG test be performed under the supervision of a physician who is fully familiar with the entire procedure of the test and the interpretation of the exercise ECG test.

REFERENCES

1. American College of Sports Medicine: Guidelines for Graded Exercise Testing and Exercise Prescription. Philadelphia, Lea & Febiger, 1975.
2. American Heart Association, Committee on Exercise: Exercise Testing and Training of Apparently Healthy Individuals: A Handbook for Physicians. New York, American Heart Assoc., 1972.
3. American Heart Association, Committee on Exercise: Exercise Testing and Training of Individuals with Heart Disease or at High Risk for its Development: A Handbook for Physicians. New York, American Heart Assoc., 1975.
4. Astrand, P. O. and Rodahl, K.: Textbook of Work Physiology. New York, McGraw-Hill, 1970.
5. Barnard, R. J., Gardner, G. W. and Diaco, N. V.: Cardiovascular responses to sudden strenuous exercise. J. Appl. Physiol., 34:833, 1973.
6. Borg, G.: Perceived exertion as an indicator of somatic stress. Scand. J. Rehabil. Med., 2:92, 1970.
7. Cooper, K.: The New Aerobics. New York, Bantam Books, 1970.
8. Cureton, T. K., Jr.: Physical Fitness and Dynamic Health. New York, Dial Press, 1965.
9. DeVries, H.: Physiology of Exercise, Second Edition. Dubuque, W. C. Brown, 1974.

10. Fox, S. M., Naughton, J. P. and Gorman, P. A.: Physical activity and cardiovascular health. Mod. Concepts Cardiovasc. Dis., *41*:17, 1972.
11. Franks, B. D.: Athletics and cardiovascular health. J. Sports Med., *3*:172, 1975.
12. Franks, B. D.: Physical warm-up, *in* Ergogenic Aids and Muscular Performance, edited by W. P. Morgan, New York, Academic Press, 1972.
13. Franks, B. D. and Deutsh, H.: Evaluating Performance in Physical Education. New York, Academic Press, 1973.
14. Gualtiere, W. S., Delman, A. J., Becker, R. J. and Neupert, G. K.: Submaximal or maximal exercise testing of asymptomatic individuals? Sports Med. Bull., *11*:6, 1976.
15. Naughton, J. P. and Hellerstein, H. K.: Exercise Testing and Exercise Training in Coronary Heart Disease. New York, Academic Press, 1973.
16. Pollock, M. K.: The quantification of endurance training programs, *in* Exercise and Sport Sciences Reviews, Vol. 1, edited by J. H. Wilmore, New York, Academic Press, 1973.
17. Proceedings of the International Symposium on Physical Activity and Cardiovascular Health. Can. Med. Assoc. J., Vol. 96, March 25, 1967.
18. Proceedings of the National Workshop on Exercise in the Prevention, in the Evaluation, and in the Treatment of Heart Disease. J. S. C. Med. Assoc. (Suppl), *65*:1, 1969.
19. Wiley, J., Franks, B. D. and Molnar, S.: Time components of the left ventricle during work. N. Zealand J. Health Phys. Educ. Recreation, *2*:67, 1969.
20. Wilmore, J. H.: Maximal vs. submaximal exercise testing. Sports Med. Bull., *10*:10, 1975.
21. Wilson, P. K.: Adult Fitness and Cardiac Rehabilitation. Baltimore, University Park Press, 1975.

5

Problems Related to the Exercise ECG Test

Arthur W. Colbourn, M.D. and
Edward K. Chung, M.D., F.A.C.P., F.A.C.C.

General Considerations

The exercise ECG test is perhaps the most useful non-invasive cardiac study in the evaluation of patients with chest pain. It is of particular value in those patients with atypical chest pain, and is of lesser usefulness in patients with established coronary heart disease. Its role as a screening test for coronary artery disease in the asymptomatic population is open to question.

Important decisions regarding the management of patients with suspected or proven coronary artery disease are often based on the results of the exercise ECG test. Significant controversy exists, however, concerning many areas both in methodology and interpretation. The limitations of the exercise ECG test are well recognized, and the physician must be aware of this fact when management of the patient is based in part on conclusions from the exercise ECG test.

This Chapter will review commonly encountered problems in the exercise ECG test which may be limiting factors in usefulness for the diagnosis as well as the treatment of cardiac patients.

Problems Related to Sensitivity and Specificity

The sensitivity and specificity of the exercise ECG test when used in the diagnosis and management of coronary artery disease remains an area of controversy. The exercise ECG test is by no means perfect, and false positive as well as false negative tests can not be avoided in certain circumstances. The generally accepted criteria for a positive ischemic response is 1 mm. of horizontal or downsloping S-T segment depression persisting for 0.08 second beyond the J point (see Chapter 12). Using these criteria, and comparing the results to coronary arteriography, the overall sensitivity and specificity of the exercise ECG test is in the range from 75–90% (see Chapter 14).

One factor affecting the sensitivity and specificity of the exercise ECG test is the electrocardiographic criteria used for a positive result. Specificity can obviously be increased by requiring more S-T segment depression for a positive result, but this must naturally occur at the expense of sensitivity and the risk of missing significant numbers of patients with critical coronary artery disease. Another factor affecting sensitivity and specificity is population variation. In the asymptomatic population where the incidence of coronary artery disease is expected to be low, the chance of a positive result being false positive is obviously higher than in a population with typical anginal discomfort due to coronary artery disease. In this asymptomatic population, Froelicher et al.[1] found only 44%, and Borer et al.[2] 37% of positive tests to be true positive tests. Conversely, Goldschlager et al.[3] found the treadmill exercise ECG test to have a sensitivity of 64% (36% false negative), and a specificity of 93% (7% false positive) in a population heavily weighted with patients with proven coronary artery disease. From coronary angiography studies, it is apparent that the exercise ECG test correlates directly with the number of vessels critically obstructed. Goldschlager et al.[3] found only 9% false negative results with the exercise ECG test in patients with triple vessel disease, but 63% false negative results in patients with single vessel disease. A consensus from the literature indicates that approximately 75% of patients with three vessel critical coronary disease will have a positive exercise ECG test, 60% with two vessel disease and 50% with single vessel disease.

In addition to these more general problems related to testing methodology and patient population selection, there are many other factors known to cause false positive and false negative responses to the exercise ECG test which are more easily identified.

1. False Positive Exercise ECG Responses

Using coronary arteriography as the standard for the determination of critical coronary obstruction, an estimated 10–20% positive responses during exercise ECG test are false positive.

(a) Drug Effects and Metabolic Abnormalities

Digitalis administration is a common cause of false positive exercise ECG tests. Phenothiazines and lithium may also have effects which complicate the exercise ECG test interpretation. Hypokalemia, commonly encountered secondary to diuretic administration or to the alkalosis in chronic hyperventilation, is another common cause of false positive exercise tests. In addition, estrogen administration is reported to cause false positive exercise ECG tests.[4] These particular problems are discussed in more detail in Chapter 6.

(b) Women

Several reports have suggested that women have a higher incidence of false positive responses to exercise than men. Sketch et al.[5] studied 251 patients, 195 men and 56 women. Using coronary angiography as the standard, with 75% obstruction indicating significant coronary artery disease and less than 50% obstruction indicating no significant coronary artery disease, Sketch et al. found that women had 67% false positive results as compared to only 8% in men. They found 37% false negatives in men and 12% false negative results in women. These investigators concluded that a positive exercise ECG result in a female was of little predictive value for the presence of coronary artery disease.[5] Other studies, however, have had differing results. Linhart et al.[6] studied 98 consecutive women by exercise ECG test and coronary angiography. They found no significant difference between male and female exercise ECG responses when resting ECG abnormalities and concomitant cardiovascular drug therapy were eliminated. Ellestad[7] has found the rate of equivocal tests (marginal changes in the S-T segment response to exercise) to be higher in women than in men, but found that the incidence of coronary pathology in patients with definite positive responses was similar for both sexes. Ellestad concluded that the marginal exercise ECG response must be viewed critically when occurring in females, but that definite positive results have the same validity as in males.

(c) Mitral Valve Prolapse Syndrome

Patients with mitral valve prolapse syndrome have been noted to have a high incidence of false positive exercise ECG tests. The precise reason for this phenomenon is uncertain, but one study has suggested that true myocardial ischemia does exist in these patients. Natarajan et al.[8] studied 23 patients with mitral valve prolapse syndrome with normal coronary arteries confirmed by angiography. Seven of these 23 patients (30%) showed myocardial lactate abnormalities with atrial pacing (abnormalities at rest were present in 2 of these patients). This result would suggest that myocardial ischemia may exist in these patients in the absence of coronary artery disease, and that the ischemic exercise ECG response in patients with mitral valve prolapse is valid. The etiology of the ischemia is uncertain under this circumstance, but theories relating to "small vessel disease" or a cellular metabolic abnormality secondary to cardiomyopathy have been suggested.

(d) Vasoregulatory Abnormalities

Friesinger et al.[9] have identified a group of patients who are felt to have abnormal autonomic responses to ordinary cardiovascular stress. These patients may or may not exhibit additional symptoms typical of the neurocirculatory asthenia syndrome: chest pain, sighing respirations, easy fatigability, poor exercise tolerance and frequently a positive family history of similar complaints. They reported a group of 40 patients who had positive exercise ECG test results, but who did not fulfill the usual criteria for coronary heart disease. The group was characterized by a relatively young age, lack of risk factors for coronary artery disease and lack of typical ischemic chest discomfort symptoms. During exercise, there was an unusual rapid increase in heart rate on standing, S-T segment and T wave abnormalities immediately on standing and S-T segment changes compatible with ischemic change unaccompanied by chest discomfort occurring early during exercise, with disappearance of these changes as exercise progressed. Followup studies indicate that the clinical course in these patients is benign, and that the usual prognostic implications accorded to a positive exercise test are not applicable.

(e) Pre-existing ECG Abnormalities

A false positive exercise ECG test is common when dealing with various pre-existing ECG abnormalities, particularly left bundle branch block, left ventricular hypertrophy and Wolff-Parkinson-White syndrome. These problems will be discussed later in this Chapter.

2. False Negative Exercise ECG Responses

Various clinical circumstances, when false negative exercise ECG tests are expected to occur frequently, will be discussed as follows.

(a) Protocol for the Exercise ECG Test

Factors in the exercise ECG protocols favoring a false negative result would be regimens allowing for insufficient exercise, and protocols utilizing single ECG lead monitoring. When ECG monitoring is limited to a single chest lead, ischemia limited to the diaphragmatic (inferior) wall will be missed, reducing the sensitivity of the exercise ECG. Insufficient exercise obviously causes a false negative exercise ECG test in proven coronary patients. The best example to typify this statement is that a false negative Master's test is much more common than the result of the treadmill exercise ECG test because the exercise given by Master's test is frequently insufficient to produce ischemic change even in many proven coronary patients (see Chapter 2).

(b) Drug Effects

Nitrates and propranolol improve both exercise performance and the exercise ECG response in patients with coronary artery disease. Because of this dampening of the ischemic response, these drugs are potential causes for false negative exercise ECG results. These effects are discussed more completely in Chapters 6 and 16.

(c) Physical Training

Redwood et al.[10] studied 7 patients with documented coronary artery disease with exercise ECG tests before and after a 6 week exercise training program. Following training, exercise capacity increased, the length of time before onset of angina increased by an average of 7 minutes and the intensity of exercise before onset of angina (as measured by total body O_2 consumption) increased by 56%. Using the triple product (heart rate/systolic blood pressure/ejection time) as a measure of myocardial oxygen consumption (MVO_2), they found this to be less at any given level of exercise following training. Detry and Bruce[11] found that submaximal exercise ECG tests following physical training resulted in less increase in heart rate, systolic blood pressure, heart rate-systolic blood pressure product and less S-T segment depression. The relationship between the magnitude of S-T segment depression and heart rate-blood pressure product, however, was unchanged. These studies imply that improvement in the S-T segment response to submaximal and maximal exercise following physical training results from changes in the hemodynamic response to exercise, rather than from alterations in myocardial oxygen supply. It is apparent that physical training can improve exercise capacity, and result in fewer ischemic S-T changes at any given exercise load. Physical training is a potential cause for false negative exercise ECG test results, especially when the exercise effort is submaximal.

Influence of Pre-existing ECG Abnormalities

1. Non-specific Abnormalities of S-T Segment and T Waves

The diagnostic criteria for exercise ECG test interpretation assume the baseline ECG to be normal with respect to the S-T segment and T wave. Problems in interpretation arise when ECG abnormalities exist in this respect. Linhart and Turnoff[12] studied 121 patients with abnormal control ECG and 57 control patients with normal baseline ECG by exercise ECG tests to correlate with coronary angiography. Using angiography as the standard, they found that an additional 1.0 mm. of exercise-induced S-T segment depression requirement over baseline resulted in a sensitivity and specificity comparable to patients with a normal control ECG. Harris et al.[13] reported a similar study with 44 patients, but found that an additional 2.0 mm. of S-T segment depression over baseline was necessary for comparable validity. Both of these studies indicate that valid conclusions can be made with exercise ECG tests in patients with an abnormal baseline ECG, providing these abnormalities are not secondary to cardiovascular drug therapy, particularly digitalis. Nevertheless, the incidence of false positive exercise ECG tests is expected to be high when the resting ECG shows significant S-T segment depression.

2. Left Ventricular Hypertrophy (LVH)

Patients with systemic hypertension, but without evidence of LVH by ECG, have been found to have normal exercise capacity and normal S-T segment response to exercise.[14] Wong et al.[14] have noted, however, that if typical ECG changes of LVH are present in the hypertensive patients, there is a 42% incidence of significant S-T segment depression with exercise. If a history typical of angina is present, in addition, they found an incidence of 63% with significant S-T segment depression. The implication that LVH can be a frequent cause of false positive exercise ECG tests has been confirmed by several studies. Harris et al.[15] reported 21 patients with LVH by ECG criteria, and normal coronary arteries by angiography. Twenty of these 21 patients have some degree of resting horizontal S-T segment depression. Six of 16 patients who were able to obtain 90% of maximal predicted heart rate had a positive exercise ECG test. They concluded that typical ischemic S-T segment depression during exercise in patients with LVH does not necessarily imply underlying coronary artery disease.

Marked ventricular hypertrophy may increase myocardial oxygen demands beyond the capacity of an even normal coronary supply. Ellestad[7] feels that the abnormal S-T segment response to exercise in patients with LVH does represent ventricular dysfunction, and may represent true myocardial ischemia, even in the absence of coronary artery disease. Ellestad agrees, however, that the S-T segment response compatible with ischemic change to exercise in patients with LVH cannot be used to implicate coronary artery disease.

In our experience, the exercise ECG test is not reliable in diagnosing coronary artery disease when the resting ECG demonstrates a typical systolic overloading LVH even when 2 mm. or more S-T segment depression is observed during and/or after exercise. This is because an extremely high incidence of false positive results is observed under this circumstance due to the fact that the secondary S-T, T wave changes are markedly exaggerated by the exercise. In fact, the positive result of the exercise ECG test in patients with LVH on the resting ECG is considered meaningless by many cardiologists. On the other hand, no significant alteration of the S-T segment, during and/or after exercise in patients with LVH, is strong evidence against the presence of coronary artery disease.

3. Left Bundle Branch Block (LBBB)

Patients with LBBB commonly have left ventricular dysfunction. Because of the repolarization abnormalities (secondary S-T, T wave changes) associated with LBBB, however, exercise-induced S-T segment changes cannot discriminate between patients with and without coronary artery disease. Ellestad[7] feels that neither exercise-induced S-T segment changes in the patient with LBBB, or exercise-induced LBBB, can be used to support the diagnosis of coronary artery disease. It should be emphasized that exercise-induced LBBB has nothing to do with the presence or absence of coronary artery disease. In fact, LBBB caused by exercise is usually rate-dependent.

The body of medical literature supports Ellestad's view concerning the limitations of exercise testing in patients with LBBB. Cooksey et al.[16], however, in a report of 10 patients with LBBB, found that an additional 1.5 mm. S-T segment depression over baseline was suggestive of significant underlying coronary disease. They noted that a negative test using these same modified criteria could not be used to exclude coronary artery disease.

Recently, it has been pointed out that the exercise ECG test is unreliable in asymptomatic patients with pre-existing LBBB because significant S-T segment depression occurs with exercise in the absence of coronary artery disease.[17] We would like to endorse our view on this report, emphasizing that the exercise ECG test is invalid in the diagnosis of coronary artery disease when dealing with individuals with pre-existing LBBB because of the extremely high incidence of false positive results. Even when the exercise ECG reveals 2 mm. or more S-T segment depression to compare with the resting ECG, in patients with LBBB, the finding cannot be interpreted as a true positive result. A false positive result is almost the rule rather than the exception in LBBB because the secondary S-T, T wave changes become markedly exaggerated by exercise. This finding is analogous to the exercise ECG result in patients with LVH.

4. Right Bundle Branch Block (RBBB)

As a rule, RBBB does not interfere with the interpretation of the exercise ECG test. In RBBB, the S wave encroaches on the S-T segment but does not mask ischemic changes. Johnson et al.[18] reported 62 patients with RBBB and exercise ECG test analysis, and concluded that RBBB did not alter the sensitivity or specificity of the S-T segment response to exercise. Ellestad[7] reported 58 cases of exercise-induced RBBB in 6,358 consecutive exercise

ECG tests. He noted that RBBB may occur in patients with normal coronary arteries, and indicates the presence of coronary artery disease only when there is the typical ischemic S-T segment response. Exercise-induced RBBB is again due to increased heart rate (rate-dependent) as seen in LBBB, and the finding has nothing to do with the presence or absence of coronary artery disease. Whinnery et al.[19] reported 40 asymptomatic men with acquired RBBB who were studied by exercise ECG test and coronary angiography. There was a low prevalence of coronary artery disease in this group, with only 8 of 40 having lesions greater than 50% obstruction. None of the patients had left ventricular dysfunction by ventriculography. They found the sensitivity of the exercise ECG test to be low in this group (but 6 of the 8 patients had single vessel disease), but the specificity to be high. There were no false positive results. These investigators also concluded that the S-T segment response to exercise in patients with RBBB should be interpreted by the usual criteria (see Chapter 12).

5. Hemiblocks

The presence of pure left anterior hemiblock (LAHB) does not interfere with the exercise ECG test interpretation, but false positive exercise ECG test can be expected when LVH is a coexisting abnormality on the resting ECG. There is an increased incidence of positive exercise ECG tests in patients with LAHB, which relates to the increased incidence of coronary artery disease in this group. Exercise-induced LAHB or LPHB is again a rate-dependent phenomenon. Nevertheless, exercise-induced LPHB has been reported,[20] and in all cases it occurred in patients with severe coronary artery disease. The pre-existing LPHB does not interfere with the exercise ECG test interpretation.

6. Wolff-Parkinson-White (WPW) Syndrome

When anomalous A-V conduction occurs during and/or after exercise in patients with the WPW syndrome, a false positive exercise ECG test is extremely common. Gazes[21] studied 23 patients with WPW syndrome who were asymptomatic, and without evidence of coronary artery disease. Using the Master's two-step test, he found that 20 of the 23 patients had a positive exercise ECG test when interpreted by the usual criteria.

Exercise has a variable effect on anomalous A-V conduction in the WPW syndrome. It may initiate it, cause it to disappear, or have no effect. Ellestad[7] has not noted exercise to precipitate an episode of reciprocating tachycardia in patients with the WPW syndrome. Likewise, in our own series of 16 individuals with WPW syndrome who underwent submaximal exercise ECG tests (see Chapter 9), there were no instances of any exercise-induced tachyarrhythmias.[22]

We would like to emphasize that the exercise ECG test is invalid for the diagnosis of coronary artery disease in individuals with the WPW syndrome when anomalous A-V conduction occurs during exercise. The reason for this is that the secondary S-T, T wave changes in the WPW syndrome become markedly exaggerated by the exercise, leading to a false positive result. This finding is analogous to the exercise ECG results seen in individuals with LVH or LBBB. In our study, all patients (12 out of 16 individuals) who demonstrated anomalous A-V conduction during exercise showed marked S-T segment depression diagnostic of positive exercise ECG tests in the absence of coronary artery disease (false positive exercise ECG test).[22] The exercise ECG test was clearly negative in all 4 subjects who had normal A-V conduction during exercise.[22]

Risks in the Exercise ECG Test

Rochmis et al.,[23] in a multicenter review of 170,000 exercise tests, found the mortality to be 0.01% and the combined morbidity-mortality to be 0.04%. There were 16 deaths in the 170,000 exercise ECG tests, and approximately 40 patients were hospitalized for short-term observation following exercise ECG test because of problems of chest pain and/or cardiac arrhythmias. Acute myocardial infarction was strongly suspected in 6 of the deaths. Ventricular fibrillation was documented in only 3 patients. Irving and Bruce,[24] in a separate review of 10,700 exercise ECG tests, documented 5 cases of post-exertional ventricular fibrillation. The feature common to all of these cases was "exertional hypotension," defined as a decrease or limited increase (10 mm. Hg. or less) in systolic blood pressure with exercise. Lingten[25] has reported a death following a negative exercise ECG test, apparently from hemorrhage into an intimal atherosclerotic coronary plaque.

Special precaution should be taken when exercising patients with suspected variant (atypical or "Prinzmetal") angina. Detry et al.[26] reported results of exercising 6 patients with angina and associated S-T segment elevation. Five of the 6 patients developed serious ventricular arrhythmias (ventricular tachycardia in 2, ventricular fibrillation in one during exercise, and ventricular tachycardia in one patient in the post-exercise period). These ventricular arrhythmias were all preceded by S-T segment elevation. Detry concluded that important information may be gained by exercising these patients, but that the associated risks must be appreciated.

The risks of exercise ECG tests are discussed in detail in Chapter 17.

Summary

Commonly encountered problems in exercise ECG tests have been reviewed. Differences both in testing methodology and patient population sampling are responsible for some of the interstudy variations of specificity and sensitivity in the exercise ECG test. Specific causes of false positive results include drug effects, particularly digitalis, metabolic abnormalities, especially hypokalemia, hyperventilation syndromes, vasoregulatory abnormalities, LBBB, LVH and the WPW syndrome. Women, and patients with mitral valve prolapse syndrome, have a disproportionately high percentage of positive results. False negative results may result from drug administration, particularly nitrates and propranolol, insufficient exercise and physical training.

Baseline ECG abnormalities as they relate to the exercise ECG test interpretation are discussed. It is extremely difficult to interpret the exercise ECG test when the resting ECG shows non-specific S-T, T wave abnormalities. RBBB, LAHB and LPHB do not interfere with the usual exercise ECG interpretation. On the other hand, the exercise ECG test in individuals with LBBB, LVH and WPW syndrome is invalid in most cases because of the extremely high incidence of false positive results. Exercise-induced LBBB, RBBB, LAHB or LPHB has nothing to do with the diagnosis of coronary artery disease, and these findings are usually rate-dependent.

The risk of the exercise ECG test is minimal when appropriate precautions in application are followed. In one large multicenter study involving approximately 170,000 exercise tests, the mortality was 0.01%. Special precaution is indicated in patients with suspected variant (atypical) angina.

The exercise ECG test is a useful tool in the evaluation of the patient with chest pain syndromes. Important limitations to the exercise ECG test exist, however, and awareness of these problems is essential so that proper precautions can be taken both in the administration and interpretation of the exercise ECG test.

REFERENCES

1. Froelicher, V., Yanowitz, F., Thompson, A. and Lancaster, M.: The correlation of coronary angiography and electrocardiographic response to maximal treadmill testing in 76 asymptomatic men. Circulation, 48:597, 1973.
2. Borer, J., Brensike, J., Redwood, D. et al.: Limitations of the electrocardiographic response to exercise in predicting coronary artery disease. New Engl. J. Med., 293:367, 1975.
3. Goldschlager, N., Selzer, A. and Cohn, K.: Treadmill stress tests as indicators of presence and severity of coronary artery disease. Ann. Intern. Med., 85:277, 1976.
4. Jaffe, M. D.: Effect of oestrogens on postexercise electrocardiogram. Br. Heart J., 38:1299, 1977.
5. Sketch, M., Mohiuddin, S., Lynch, J. et al.: Significant sex differences in the correlation of electrocardiographic exercise testing and coronary arteriograms. Am. J. Cardiol., 36:169, 1975.
6. Linhart, J., Laws, J. and Satinsky, J.: Maximal treadmill exercise electrocardiography in female patients. Circulation, 50:1173, 1974.
7. Ellestad, M.: Stress Testing: Principles and Practice. Philadelphia, F. A. Davis, 1975.
8. Natarajan, G., Nakhjavan, F., Kahn, D. et al.: Myocardial metabolic studies in prolapsing mitral leaflet syndrome. Circulation, 52:1105, 1975.
9. Friesinger, G., Biern, R., Likar, I. and Mason, R.: Exercise electrocardiography and vasoregulatory abnormalities. Am. J. Cardiol., 30:733, 1972.
10. Redwood, D., Rosing, D. and Epstein, S.: Circulatory and symptomatic effects of physical

training in patients with coronary artery disease and angina pectoris. New Engl. J. Med., *286:*959, 1972.

11. Detry, J. and Bruce, R.: Effects of physical training on exertional S-T segment depression in coronary heart disease. Circulation, *44:*390, 1971.

12. Linhart, J. and Turnoff, H.: Maximum treadmill exercise test in patients with abnormal control electrocardiograms. Circulation, *49:*667, 1974.

13. Harris, F., Mason, D., Lee, G. et al.: Value and limitations of exercise testing in detecting coronary disease in the presence of ST-T abnormalities on standard 12-lead electrocardiogram. Am. J. Cardiol., *37:*141, 1976.

14. Wong, H., Kasser, I. and Bruce, R.: Impaired maximal exercise performance with hypertensive cardiovascular disease. Circulation, *39:*633, 1969.

15. Harris, C., Aronow, W., Parker, D. and Kaplan, M.: Treadmill stress test in left ventricular hypertrophy. Chest, *63:*353, 1973.

16. Cooksey, J., Parker, B. and Bahl, O.: The diagnostic contribution of exercise testing in left bundle branch block. Am. Heart J., *88:*482, 1974.

17. Whinnery, J. E., Froelicher, V. F., Jr., Stewart, A. J. et al.: The electrocardiographic response to maximal treadmill exercise of asymptomatic men with left bundle branch block. Am. Heart J., *94:*316, 1977.

18. Johnson, S., O'Connell, J., Becker, P. et al.: The diagnostic accuracy of exercise ECG testing in the presence of complete RBBB. Circulation, *52:*II–48, 1975.

19. Whinnery, J. E., Froelicher, V., Longo, M. and Triebwasser, J.: The electrocardiographic response to maximal treadmill exercise of asymptomatic men with RBBB. Chest, *71:*335, 1977.

20. Bobba, P., Salerno, J. and Casari, A.: Transient left posterior hemiblock: Report of four cases induced by exercise test. Circulation, *46:*931, 1972.

21. Gazes, P.: False positive exercise test in the presence of Wolff-Parkinson-White syndrome. Am. Heart J., *78:*13, 1969.

22. Zuckerman, G. L. and Chung, E. K.: The exercise response in Wolff-Parkinson-White syndrome. (In press), 1978.

23. Rochmis, P. and Blackburn, H.: Exercise tests: A survey of procedures, safety, and litigation experience in approximately 170,000 tests. J.A.M.A., *217:*1061, 1971.

24. Irving, J. and Bruce, R.: Exertional hypotension and postexertional ventricular fibrillation in stress testing. Am. J. Cardiol., *39:*849, 1977.

25. Lingten, A.: Death from myocardial infarction after exercise test with normal result. J.A.M.A., *235:*837, 1976.

26. Detry, J., Mengeot, P., Rousseau, M. et al.: Maximal exercise testing in patients with spontaneous angina pectoris associated with transient ST segment elevation: Risks and electrocardiographic findings. Br. Heart J., *37:*897, 1975.

6

Effect of Drugs and Metabolic Abnormalities on the Exercise ECG Test

Arthur W. Colbourn, M.D. and
Edward K. Chung, M.D., F.A.C.P., F.A.C.C.

General Considerations

The exercise ECG test has gained wide popularity as a means of detecting asymptomatic ischemic heart disease. It is also of proven value in the management of established coronary heart disease, both by assessing impairment due to ischemia and by evaluating the efficacy of medical as well as surgical therapy. Increasing awareness is being given to the problem of specificity regarding the S-T segment response to exercise. This is a particular problem in the asymptomatic population undergoing the exercise ECG test, where as many as 60% of positive responses may be false positive.[1] It is in the asymptomatic patients that the greatest potential benefit exists in accurate early detection of coronary heart disease.

The myocardial response to ischemia is not an all or none phenomenon, and obviously the ECG response to ischemia cannot be expected to be any more specific. It is not possible to classify all exercise ECG tests as either clearly positive or negative. There are numerous extracardiac factors, however, which are known to cause false positive S-T segment responses to exercise. Awareness of these factors is essential not only for accurate interpretation, but also to maximize the inherent specificity of the exercise ECG test.

Drug Effects

Various drugs may affect the exercise ECG both by direct electrophysiologic and by hemodynamic alterations in the myocardial response to exercise.

A. Digitalis

Digitalis is a well recognized cause of false positive exercise ECG test. Digitalis will accentuate pre-existing ischemic S-T segment depression in patients with established coronary heart disease, and will cause S-T segment depression during and/or after exercise in patients with no evidence of coronary heart disease. Nordstrom-Ohrberg[2] found S-T segment depression in 89% of 64 volunteers following digitalis administration, and Goldbarg[3] found that digitalis produced abnormal S-T segments and T waves during exercise in 50–60% of young healthy males. Digitalis effect refers to shortening of the Q-T interval and either sagging or depression of the S-T segment. If the resting ECG shows this digitalis effect, as a rule, the abnormality will be more pronounced during and/or after exercise leading to frequent occurrence of false positive exercise ECG tests (Figures 6-1 and 2). However, it should be emphasized that a true positive exercise ECG test is, of course, expected to be observed frequently in digitalized patients because many of them suffer from coronary heart disease. In general, exercise ECG tests should be considered true positive, even during digitalis therapy, when marked (2 mm. or more) horizontal or downslope S-T segment depression

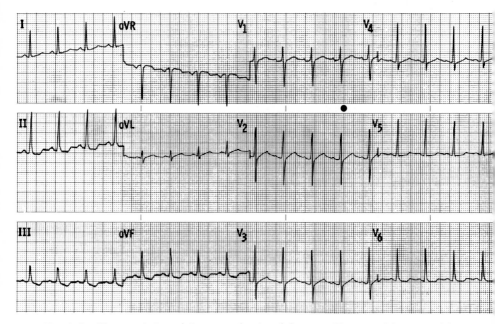

Fig. 6-1 Figures 6-1 and 2 were obtained from a 45-year-old man with no demonstrable coronary heart disease. His 12-lead ECG shown in Figure 6-1 reveals nonspecific S-T segment and T wave abnormalities due to digitalis effect.

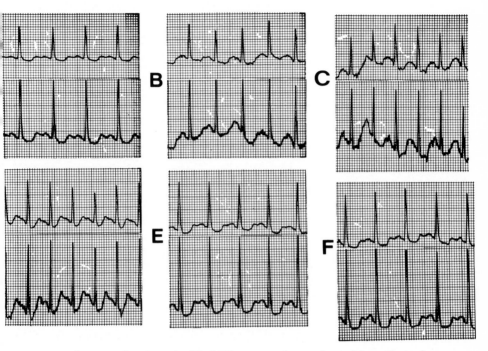

Fig. 6-2 The exercise (treadmill) ECG test performed on this patient demonstrates a false positive exercise ECG test. The rhythm strip A represents a control tracing, whereas the strips B and C are taken during exercise. The strips D to F represent post-exercise ECG. Each rhythm strip consists of leads V_5 (top) and II (bottom).

occurs during and/or after exercise (Figures 6-3 and 4). The diagnostic criteria for positive exercise ECG tests are described in detail in Chapter 12.

If the resting ECG in the digitalized patient is normal, the response of the S-T segment to exercise is unpredictable. Administration of 100% oxygen or potassium salts will lessen digitalis-induced S-T segment changes, hypoxia will exaggerate them and pre-administered nitroglycerin will not affect their appearance.[3] As the S-T segment is similarly affected both by digitalis and myocardial ischemia in the patient with coronary heart disease, a negative ECG response to exercise in the digitalized patient is strong evidence against the presence of myocardial ischemia.

In distinguishing the digitalis effect from true myocardial ischemia, Phillips[4] noted that Q-T interval analysis may be of some value. Both exercise and digitalis normally shorten the Q-T interval, whereas ischemia prolongs it. Accordingly, if rate-adjusted Q-T interval prolongation occurs during exercise in the patient taking digitalis, it can be assumed to represent an ischemic response.

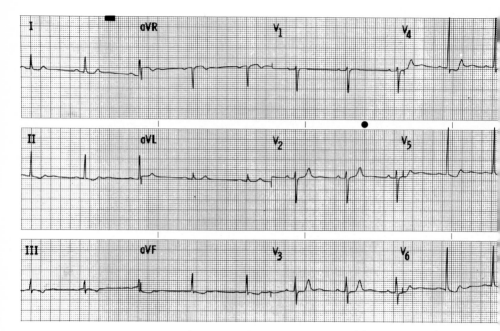

Fig. 6-3   Figures 6-3 and 4 were taken on a 57-year-old woman with angina and hypertension. She has been taking digoxin 0.25 mg. daily. Her 12-lead ECG shown in Figure 6-3 demonstrates a characteristic digitalis effect.

Digitalis-induced cardiac arrhythmias recorded at rest are characteristically exacerbated by exercise. For this reason suspected digitalis toxicity is a relative contraindication to the exercise ECG test (see Chapters 8 and 13).

The etiology of the digitalis-induced S-T segment alteration with exercise is uncertain. Ellestad[5] theorizes that digitalis may aggravate an intrinsic ventricular dysfunction, which, even though non-ischemic in nature, simulates ischemic change. It should be noted that the so called "digitalis effect" on the electrocardiogram is not necessarily present in every patient during digitalis therapy.

B. Nitrates

Nitroglycerin and the long-acting nitrates relieve the discomfort of myocardial ischemia, and allow the patient with coronary heart disease to exercise longer with less ischemic S-T segment change during exercise. Although nitroglycerin is a coronary vasodilator in normal coronaries, it is doubtful that diseased vessels with fixed obstructions are similarly affected. Nitrates appear to exert their beneficial effects in coronary patients by alterations in the peripheral circulation. Nitroglycerin lowers peripheral resistance decreasing afterload, and causes dilatation of the capacitance

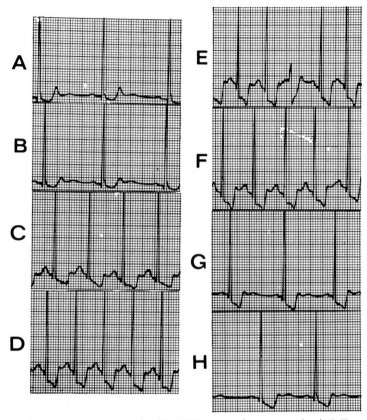

Fig. 6-4 Her exercise (treadmill) ECG test shows marked S-T segment depression with T wave inversion which most likely represents a true positive test. Lead V_5 was recorded during the entire exercise ECG test. The rhythm strips A and B were taken at rest in the supine and standing position, respectively. The strips C to E were recorded during exercise, whereas strips F to H were taken after exercise. Note a ventricular premature contraction in the strip E. The test was terminated prematurely because of severe chest pain.

vessels lowering pre-load. These changes reduce myocardial oxygen demand at any given workload. The primary peripheral action of nitrates was further emphasized by the studies of Ganz and Marcus[6] where direct injection of nitroglycerin into the coronary arteries failed to relieve artificial pacing-induced ischemic pain, in contrast to the systemic administration of nitroglycerin which proved effective.

Goldbarg[3] has noted that the response to nitroglycerin may be used to enhance the specificity of the exercise ECG test. Exercise performance and exercise ECG response both improve in the coronary patient after nitroglycerin. If this improvement does not occur, it is likely that either no coronary heart disease exists or that the disease is very extensive.

The effectiveness of nitroglycerin and isosorbide dinitrate by the sublingual route has been long recognized. More recently studies have shown isosorbide to be effective orally. Glancy[7] has demonstrated that 2 hours after taking isosorbide by mouth, patients were able to exercise longer and attain higher heart rates before the onset of angina as compared to control periods.

It is apparent that nitrates dampen the ischemic response to exercise both clinically and electrocardiographically. For these reasons, nitrates are a potential cause of false negative exercise ECG tests in patients with significant coronary artery disese. The relationship between nitrates and the exercise ECG test has also been discussed in Chapter 16.

C. Beta-adrenergic Blocking Drugs

Propranolol (Inderal), the prototype of the beta-blockers, causes a decrease both in heart rate and contractility. A lowering of blood pressure and cardiac output results, with a resultant decrease in myocardial oxygen consumption for any given workload. There is in addition a prolongation of ejection time and increase in ventricular volumes. Propranolol allows patients with coronary heart disease to exercise longer and to develop less ischemic S-T segment response to exercise. Frishman[8] studied propranolol effect on patients with stable but severe angina. He found that work performance increased at moderate doses (80–160 mg./day) with an associated decrease in the product of heart rate and blood pressure. At higher dosage levels, however, left ventricular function deteriorated and exercise capacity decreased. Fatigue became the endpoint to exercise in these patients rather than angina.

Propranolol, like the nitrates, may cause a false negative exercise ECG test in the patient with coronary heart disease because of its hemodynamic effects. Propranolol causes an additional problem in that its negative chronotropic effect may make the submaximal heart rate unobtainable, negating this conventional endpoint to exercise. The influence of beta-blocking agents on the exercise ECG test has also been discussed in Chapter 16.

D. Atropine

Despite a vagolytic action of atropine in increasing heart rate, it probably exerts no effect on the exercise ECG test. The patient's own circulating catecholamine level is the major determinant of heart rate and contractility during exercise, and overrides any effect of atropine.

E. Phenothiazines

In chronic usage, phenothiazines have been implicated in the development of a cardiomyopathic process characterized histologically by fibrous replacement of myocardial cells. Clinically, weakness and tachycardia commonly accompany phenothiazine usage, complicating the exercise ECG test in these patients. Ellestad[5] has reported T wave flattening, S-T segment depression and Q-T prolongation during the exercise ECG test in patients taking chlorpromazine (Thorazine). Giles[9] studied the effect of thioridazine (Mellaril) in high dosages, and noted not only S-T segment and Q-T interval changes, but also severe ventricular arrhythmias and sudden death. Ventricular irritability associated with phenothiazine usage is felt in part to be related to their ability to block the uptake of catecholamines with resultant high plasma levels. Because of these problems, Ellestad[5] feels that even maintenance dosage levels of chlorpromazine or thioridazine (approximately 400 mg./day) are a relative contraindication to the exercise ECG test.

F. Lithium

Lithium is a drug commonly used for the treatment of manic-depressive illness. All patients taking lithium show T wave flattening or inversion in the resting ECG simulating changes of hypokalemia.[10] Lithium has also been demonstrated to aggravate and even precipitate ventricular arrhythmias.[11] Lithium accumulates intracellularly, causing displacement of sodium and potassium, its electrophysiologic effects being secondary to the intracellular potassium depletion. Some authors report Q-T prolongation and S-T segment depression during exercise when lithium is used at high dosages.[5] Tilkian,[12] however, obtained different results. He performed the exercise ECG test in patients on long-term lithium therapy. He documented the T wave changes in the resting ECG previously noted, but found no S-T segment displacement either in the resting or exercise ECG. Exercise performance was unchanged, and no increase in cardiac arrhythmias was documented during exercise.

G. Alcohol

Alcohol has a detrimental effect on cardiac output, reducing it in normal hearts when large amounts are ingested. If underlying heart disease exists in the form of hypertensive or coronary heart disease, smaller amounts may have a similar effect. A decrease in cardiac output results in a decrease in exercise capacity. Alcohol has also been noted to cause ventricular repolarization abnormalities. Patients with established alcoholic cardiomyopathy may exhibit S-T segment depression or may develop bundle branch block with the progression of exercise. Ellestad[5] feels that the repolarization abnormalities are the rule with exercise in alcoholic cardiomyopathy. Similar abnormalities can be expected in patients with normal cardiac status following recent consumption of large amounts of alcohol.

H. Reserpine and Guanethidine

Reserpine inhibits the storage of norepinephrine within vesicles of adrenergic nerve endings leading to catecholamine depletion, and guanethidine blocks the release of norepinephrine from sympathetic nerve endings. Both of these agents cause a decrease in the availability of catecholamines during the stimulation of exercise, and decrease the maximal obtainable heart rate. This effect, however, is not as marked as that of propranolol, and is not usually of clinical significance in the exercise ECG test.

I. Quinidine and Procainamide (Pronestyl)

Neither quinidine nor procainamide has been documented to affect exercise capacity or ECG response to exercise.

Metabolic Abnormalities

A. Alkalosis

The problem of alkalosis occurs frequently in the clinical setting of chronic hyperventilation. This is seen commonly in ambulatory patients, particularly those who are emotionally labile with atypical chest pain. The state of chronic alkalosis leads to intracellular potassium depletion, increased urinary potassium loss and decrease in total body potassium stores. Fatigue, weakness and characteristic ECG changes result. The ECG shows "ischemic" S-T segment depression at rest, with exacerbation of the depression during both hyperventilation and exercise.[13] Jacobs[13] has noted that beta-blockade results in less S-T segment depression in these patients than under control conditions. As beta-blockade also improves a true ischemic response to exercise, response to propranolol is of no aid in differentiating a true positive from false positive result.

Diuretic usage may also cause a false positive exercise ECG test because of the frequent problem of hypokalemia and resultant metabolic alkalosis.

B. Acidosis

Acidosis causes a depression of myocardial contractility. As the ph decreases, so does the cardiac output. Moderate to severe exercise leads to the accumulation of lactic acid which results in a variable degree of metabolic acidosis. The ability to tolerate this build-up is one of the major determinants of exercise endurance. ECG alterations during acidosis include non-specific T wave abnormalities and slight prolongation of the Q-T interval.

C. Carbon Monoxide

Aronow[14] studied the effect of breathing 100 parts/million (ppm) of carbon monoxide versus compressed purified air for 1 hour during the maximal treadmill exercise ECG test. He found that the mean exercise time until exhaustion was significantly decreased after breathing carbon monoxide as compared to the controls. Carbon monoxide combines with hemoglobin to form carboxyhemoglobin, decreasing the relative amount of free hemoglobin to bind oxygen. Increased carboxyhemoglobin levels thus result in decreased oxygen delivery to the myocardium and other tissues. Increased carboxyhemoglobin levels caused by cigarette smoking and air pollution can result in a significant decrease in exercise time until onset of angina in patients with coronary heart disease. In clinically normal patients, increased carboxyhemoglobin levels would be expected to decrease exercise capacity, as Aronow clearly demonstrated.

D. Thyroid Abnormalities

Thyroid hormone in a sense acts as a false neurotransmitter, causing increased catecholamine-like effects. Excessive thyroid hormone causes an increased basal metabolic rate (BMR), tremor, tachycardia, insomnia and anxiety. It is well known that thyroid administration to the anginal patient will exacerbate the anginal syndrome. Likewise, too rapid replacement of thyroid in the initial management of hypothyroidism in the coronary patient may precipitate an accelerated anginal syndrome. The metabolically hyperactive individual with coronary heart disease, as compared to the euthyroid patient, will experience angina and ischemic S-T segment depression earlier during exercise.

The hypothyroid individual exhibits decreased ventricular contractility with a resultant decrease in exercise capacity. The ECG in the hypothyroid patient may show S-T segment sagging or depression and non-specific T wave abnormalities at rest and during exercise.[5]

Summary

The effects of commonly used drugs and metabolic abnormalities on the exercise ECG test have been reviewed. Among various factors, digitalis commonly produces a false positive exercise ECG test, whereas nitrates and propranolol frequently cause a false negative exercise ECG test. This knowledge is essential for proper interpretation of the exercise ECG test when these factors are present. This knowledge will hopefully allow the physician to increase the specificity of the exercise ECG test when used in the diagnosis and management of patients with coronary heart disease.

REFERENCES

1. Borer, J., Brensike, J., Redwood, D. et al.: Limitations of the electrocardiographic response to exercise in predicting coronary artery disease. New Engl. J. Med., 293:367, 1975.
2. Nordstrom-Ohrberg, G.: Effect of digitalis glycosides electrocardiogram and exercise test in healthy subjects. Acta Med. Scand. (Suppl. 420)176:1, 1964.
3. Goldbarg, A.: The effects of pharmacological agents on human performance, in Exercise Testing and Exercise Training in Coronary Heart Disease, edited by J. Naughton, H. Hellerstein and I. Mohler, pp. 119–128, New York, Academic Press, 1973.
4. Phillips, R.: The interaction of exercise and drugs, in Medical Aspects of Exercise Testing and Training, edited by L. Zohman and R. Phillips, pp. 104–110, New York, Intercontinental Medical Book Corp., 1973.
5. Ellestad, M.: Effects of metabolic abnormalities and drugs, in Stress Testing, Principles and Practice, pp. 249–259, Philadelphia, F. A. Davis, 1975.
6. Ganz, W. and Marcus, H.: Failure of intracoronary nitroglycerin to alleviate pacing-induced angina. Circulation, 46:880, 1972.
7. Glancy, D., Richter, M., Ellis, E. and Johnson, W.: Effect of swallowed isosorbide dinitrate on blood pressure, heart rate and exercise capacity in patients with coronary artery disease. Am. J. Med., 62:39, 1977.
8. Frishman, W., Smithen, C., Befler, B. et al.: Noninvasive assessment of clinical response to oral propranolol therapy. Am. J. Cardiol., 35:635, 1975.
9. Giles, T. and Modlin, R.: Death associated with ventricular arrhythmia and thioridazine hydrocholoride. J.A.M.A., 205:108, 1968.
10. Demers, R. and Heninger, G.: Electrocardiographic T wave changes during lithium carbonate treatment. J.A.M.A., 218:381, 1971.
11. Tengedahl, T. and Gau, G.: Myocardial irritability associated with lithium carbonate therapy. New Engl. J. Med., 287:867, 1972.
12. Tilkian, A., Schroeder, J., Kao, J. and Hultgren, H.: Effects of lithium on cardiovascular performance: report of extended ambulatory monitoring and exercise testing before and during lithium therapy. Am. J. Cardiol., 38:701, 1976.
13. Jacobs, F., Battle, W. and Ronan, J.: False-positive ST-T wave changes secondary to hyperventilation and exercise. Ann. Intern Med., 81:479, 1974.
14. Aronow, W. and Cassidy, J.: Effect of carbon monoxide on maximal treadmill exercise. Ann. Intern Med., 83:496, 1975.

7

Indications of the Exercise ECG Test

Edward K. Chung, M.D., F.A.C.P., F.A.C.C.

General Considerations[1-10]

Before the exercise ECG test is performed, the objectives of the test should be clearly delineated. The indications of the exercise ECG test are summarized in Table 7-1.

The major indication of exercise testing is, needless to say, to diagnose overt or latent coronary artery disease, particularly angina pectoris. By the same token, exercise testing provides useful information for the differential diagnosis of chest pain due to various causes. The next major indication of the exercise ECG test is to evaluate the functional capacity of cardiac patients. Exercise testing provides valuable information in evaluating medical as well as surgical treatment for cardiac patients. Functional classification by the New York Heart Association criteria of a given individual can be easily assessed by the maximal exercise workloads performed by a given patient (expressed by METs—multiples of the resting metabolic activity, see Chapters 9 and 12). The functional capacity of a given individual will change according to various factors, particularly the progress of the underlying heart disease and the efficacy of the medical and/or surgical therapy. It is also important to evaluate the functional capacity of healthy individuals by exercise testing for any occupation or sport which may exceed the ordinary levels of daily physical activity.

Another important indication of exercise testing is for rehabilitation purposes and preventive measures in cardiac as well as non-cardiac patients. Exercise testing is valuable to encourage individual motivation for cardiac patients who are engaged in exercise training programs. Even in healthy subjects, exercise testing will stimulate a physically inactive individual toward a healthier life style.

Less important indications of the exercise ECG test include research purposes (e.g., evaluation of various anti-anginal or anti-arrhythmic drugs) and screening purposes (for certain activities or occupations, and for life insurance companies, etc.).

Table 7-1. Exercise ECG Test—Indications

1. *Diagnostic Purposes*
   - Confirmation of the diagnosis of coronary artery disease
   - Assessment of a possible etiology for chest pain of unknown cause (differential diagnosis of chest pain)
   - Early detection of a latent coronary artery disease
   - Assessment of the nature of cardiac arrhythmias in relation to exercise
   - Assessment of a possible etiology for various symptoms related to exercise (e.g., fainting episode, palpitations, chest pain, etc.)
   - Early detection of labile hypertension
2. *Evaluation Purposes*
   - Evaluation of functional capacity of patients with coronary artery disease: progressive changes in a functional classification
   - Evaluation of the efficacy of medical treatment for coronary artery disease: anti-anginal drug therapy, diet therapy, weight reduction, anti-arrhythmic drug therapy, digitalis (e.g., exercise tolerance for atrial fibrillation)
   - Evaluation of the efficacy of surgical therapy: for example, coronary artery bypass surgery for intractable angina or myocardial infarction
   - Evaluation of prognosis in patients with previous myocardial infarction
   - Evaluation of cardiovascular functional capacity as a means of clearing individuals for strenuous or hazardous works (e.g., sports), rehabilitation program or exercise program
   - Evaluation of responses to conditioning and/or preventive programs
3. *Rehabilitation Purposes and Preventive Measures*
   - Rehabilitation of cardiac patients
   - Rehabilitation of non-cardiac patients
   - Encouragement of individual motivation for entering and adhering to exercise programs
4. *Research Purposes*
   - Evaluation of anti-anginal drugs
   - Evaluation of anti-arrhythmic drugs
   - Evaluation of exercise responses in various cardiovascular disorders
5. *Screening Purposes*
   - For certain activities or occupations (e.g., selection of pilots, astronauts, etc.)
   - For life insurance companies

Indications[1-10]

1. Diagnostic Purposes

Although a significant incidence of false positive and false negative exercise ECG tests is well recognized, the most important indication of exercise testing is for the diagnosis of overt and latent coronary artery disease (see Chapters 5, 6 and 12). The exercise test provides objective evidence of coronary artery disease which is suspected or diagnosed clinically. The sensitivity (the ability of the exercise ECG test to correctly identify the arteriographically documented coronary artery disease) of the exercise test varies according to the diagnostic criteria for positive exercise testing and the criteria used for the "significant" coronary artery lesions. Nevertheless, the sensitivity of the exercise test may reach near 100% (ranging from 86–100%) in 3-vessel disease, but it is only no more than 60% (ranging from 35–60%) in a single-vessel disease.[11-13] In 2-vessel coronary involvement, the sensitivity has been reported to be between 67% and 91%.[11-13]

In one study dealing with 284 apparently healthy male executives who underwent maximal stress testing, 30 individuals (11%) demonstrated ischemic S-T segment depression without chest pain.[14] Another study from the same laboratory, dealing with 1,000 patients referred for routine exercise testing, showed only 37% incidence of exercise-induced angina among those who had ischemic S-T segment changes.[5] Recently, Lindsey and Cohn[10] studied 122 consecutive, clinically stable patients with angiographically documented coronary artery disease (more than 70% stenosis) and a positive exercise ECG test. In this study, 78 patients had chest pain or angina equivalent during or after a positive exercise ECG test, whereas 44 did not, including 32 (26%) with no symptoms at all. There were no significant differences between patients with and without exercise-induced chest pain in regard to various clinical and angiographic features (e.g., age, sex, previous myocardial infarction, congestive heart failure, hypertension, extent of coronary artery disease, presence of collaterals and left ventricular ejection fraction). Thus, it was concluded that "silent" myocardial ischemia during or after exercise was not uncommon, but it was not readily attributable to any obvious clinical or catheterization findings.

It has been emphasized that typical angina pectoris exhibits its reproducibility by the exercise with the same workloads on repeated testing.[3, 4] Conversely, atypical or non-coronary chest pain is usually not reproduced by repeated testing even when exercise workloads are beyond the initial exercise testing. Thus, exercise testing provides useful information for the differential diagnosis of chest pain due to various causes, in terms of the reproducibility of the chest pain.

The reliability of the S-T segment depression for the diagnosis of coronary artery disease is significantly influenced, of course, by various factors, including the magnitude of the S-T segment depression, its onset in relation to the exercise workloads and the duration of the ischemic ECG change during the recovery period (see Chapter 12). Nevertheless, horizontal or downsloping S-T segment depression of 1 mm. or greater is generally accepted for a positive exercise ECG test to diagnose coronary artery disease providing that known factors causing false positive test (e.g., digitalis effect, left bundle branch block, WPW syndrome, mitral valve prolapse syndrome, etc.) are excluded (see Chapter 12). It can be said that the diagnosis of advanced multivessel coronary disease is certain when patients develop the diagnostic S-T segment depression (see Chapter 12) during an early phase of the exercise testing.

Various cardiac arrhythmias may be provoked by or abolished by exercise in healthy individuals as well as coronary patients. However, ventricular arrhythmias provoked by minimal exercise (below 70% of predicted maximal heart rate) are extremely unusual in healthy individuals.[3] Thus, the development of malignant ventricular arrhythmias (multifocal VPCs, grouped VPCs and ventricular tachycardia) by minimal exercise workloads (less than 70% of predicted maximal heart rate) is highly suggestive of advanced coronary artery disease and ventricular dysfunction (see Chapters 12 and 13). However, it should be emphasized that exercise-induced ventricular arrhythmias alone should not be considered confirming evidence for coronary artery disease.

When certain cardiac arrhythmias are induced by exercise testing even in apparently healthy subjects, the test can provide important information as to whether a given individual is suitable for certain hazardous activities or occupations where good coordination and alert performance are required. In addition, the proper anti-arrhythmic agent can be selected by assessing the relationship between a given cardiac arrhythmia and exercise. By and large, propranolol (Inderal) is considered to be the drug of choice for exercise-induced various tachyarrhythmias in most cases.[15]

Various symptoms such as dizziness, near-syncope, syncope, palpitations, etc. can be evaluated by relating to physical exercise. When certain symptoms are constantly provoked by exercise, the diagnostic as well as the therapeutic approach can be assisted by exercise testing.

Less well known is the value of the exercise ECG test for detection of latent or labile hypertension. It has been suggested that labile hypertension is strongly suspected when the systolic blood pressure increases beyond 220 mm. Hg. during a peak exercise period.

2. Evaluation Purposes

In addition to the diagnostic purposes, the exercise ECG test provides extremely important information for evaluation purposes. In patients with known coronary artery disease, functional capacity can be determined by exercise ECG testing. By utilizing the New York Heart Association functional classification method in conjunction with the exercise workloads performed by a given patient (with the expression of METs), each individual's functional capacity is assessed. For example, the patients with functional class I are able to perform exercise workloads of 6–10 METs, whereas functional class II patients can perform 4–6 METs exercise workloads (see Chapter 12). When the patient performs exercise workloads with 2–3 METs, functional class III is estimated, whereas the functional class IV patient is unable to perform any exercise workloads (1 MET). From the above information gained by functional classification, a given patient may be instructed to perform up to the limited daily activities comparable to the exercise workloads which a given individual was able to perform during exercise testing. In other words, the exercise testing provides objective evidence of what can be done prior to the development of significant symptoms and/or electrocardiographic evidence of myocardial ischemia (e.g., diagnostic S-T segment changes and/or serious cardiac arrhythmias). In addition to the daily activities at home, such information will be very essential in making decisions regarding a given individual's physical capability for returning to his occupation or for engaging in any type of sport. Table 7-2 summarizes the approximate metabolic cost of activities.

Furthermore, the result of the exercise ECG test provides valuable information when healthy individuals are going to engage in strenuous work or heavy competitive sports. It has been shown that healthy sedentary individuals can perform exercise workloads beyond 10–11 METs, whereas physically active subjects may be able to perform the exercise workloads beyond 16 METs (see Chapters 9 and 12). Of course, a given individual's functional capacity can be progressively increased by participating in properly designed various exercise programs.

In patients with known coronary artery disease, the functional capacity is often altered by medical and/or surgical therapy. Thus, exercise ECG testing provides useful information in evaluating medical as well as surgical therapy. It is common to observe that the functional capacity improves after coronary bypass surgery. A good example of evaluating the efficacy of digitalis therapy is the assessment of ventricular rate response to exercise testing during digitalis therapy for chronic atrial fibrillation. In many patients with chronic atrial fibrillation, the ventricular rate is ideally controlled (ventricular rate: 60–80 beats/minute) with digitalis at resting state, but the ventricular rate is often accelerated disproportionately during minimal exercise (Figures 7-1 and 2). This finding clearly indicates that digitalis therapy is inadequate in view of poor exercise tolerance. Under this circumstance, the dosage of digitalis may be increased slightly in conjunction with careful analysis of the total clinical picture and digitalis blood level by the radioimmunoassay method.[15] Alternatively, a small amount of oral propranolol (Inderal) may be added. Needless to say, none of the above therapy will be entirely satisfactory when the underlying heart disease is far advanced.

It has been clearly documented that exercise ECG testing provides useful information in assessing prognosis in the patients with known coronary artery disease.[16] A study by Margolis[16] indicates that the patients with angina who are able to perform high stages of the exercise ECG test have a favorable prognosis regardless of the S-T segment changes, extent of coronary artery involvement or medical or surgical therapy. Conversely, the

Table 7-2. Approximate Metabolic Cost of Activities (includes resting metabolic needs)†

	Occupational	*Recreational*

METS
1¹/₂–2
ml. O₂/min./kg.
4–7
Kilocalories/min.
(70 kg. person)
2–2¹/₂
	Desk work
	Auto driving*
	Typing
	Electric calculating
	  machine operation
		Standing
		Walking (strolling 1.6 km. or 1
		  m.p.h.)
		Flying,* motorcycling*
		Playing cards*
		Sewing, knitting

METS 2–3 ml. O₂/min./kg 7–11 Kilocalories/min. (70 kg. person) 2¹/₂–4	Auto repair Radio, TV repair Janitorial work Typing, manual Bartending	Level walking 3¹/₄ km. or 2 m.p.h. Level bicycling 8 km. or 5 m.p.h. Riding lawn mower Billiards, bowling Skeet,* shuffleboard Woodworking, light Power boat driving* Golf (power cart) Canoeing 4 km. or 2¹/₂ m.p.h. Horseback riding-walk Bait casting Playing piano and many musical instruments

METS
3–4
ml. O₂/min./kg.
11–14
Kilocalories/min.
(70 kg. person)
4–5
	Brick laying, plaster-
	  ing
	Wheelbarrow—45
	  kg. or 100 lb. load
	Machine assembly
	Trailer-truck in
	  traffic
	Welding-moderate
	  load
	Cleaning windows
		Walking 4 km. or 2¹/₂ m.p.h.
		Cycling 10 km or 6 m.p.h.
		Horseshoe pitching
		Volleyball, 6 man noncompeti-
		  tive
		Golf—pulling bag cart
		Archery
		Sailing (handling small boat)
		Fly fishing standing with waders
		Horseback—"sitting" to trot
		Badminton—social doubles
		Pushing light power mower
		Energetic musician

METS 4–5 ml. O₂/min./kg. 14–18 Kilocalories/min. (70 kg. person) 5–6	Painting, masonry Paperhanging Light carpentry	Walking 5 km. or 3 m.p.h. Cycling 13 km. or 8 m.p.h. Table tennis Golf (carrying clubs) Dancing, Foxtrot Badminton—singles Tennis—doubles Raking leaves Hoeing Many calisthenics

METS
5–6
ml. O₂/min./kg.
18–21
Kilocalories/min.
(70 kg. person)
6–7
	Digging garden
	Shoveling light earth
		Walking 5¹/₂ km. or 3¹/₂ m.p.h.
		Cycling 16 km. or 10 m.p.h.
		Canoeing 5 km. or 3 m.p.h.
		Horseback—"posting" to trot
		Stream fishing—walking in light
		  current in waders
		Ice or roller skating 15 km. or 9
		  m.p.h.

Table 7-2. *Continued*

	Occupational	*Recreational*
METS 6–7 ml. O_2/min./kg. 21–25 Kilocalories/min. (70 kg. person) 7–8	Shoveling 10/min.—$4^{1}/_{2}$ kg. or 10 lb.	Walking 8 km. or 5 m.p.h. Cycling $17^{1}/_{2}$ km or 11 m.p.h. Badminton—competitive Tennis—singles Splitting wood Snow shoveling Hand lawn mowing Folk (square) dancing Light downhill skiing Ski touring 4 km. or $2^{1}/_{2}$ m.p.h. (loose snow) Water skiing
METS 7–8 ml. O_2/min./kg. 25–28 Kilocalories/min. (70 kg. person) 8–10	Digging ditches Carrying 36 kg. or 80 lb. Sawing hardwood	Jogging 8 km. or 5 m.p.h. Cycling 19 km. or 12 m.p.h. Horseback—gallop Vigorous downhill skiing Basketball Mountain climbing Ice hockey Canoeing $6^{1}/_{2}$ km. or 4 m.p.h. Touch football Paddleball
METS 8–9 ml. O_2/min./kg. 28–32 Kilocalories/min. (70 kg. person) 10–11	Shoveling 10/min.—$5^{1}/_{2}$ kg. or 14 lb.	Running 9 km. or $5^{1}/_{2}$ m.p.h. Cycling 21 km. or 13 m.p.h. Ski touring $6^{1}/_{2}$ km. or 4 m.p.h. (loose snow) Squash racquets—social Handball—social Fencing Basketball—vigorous

METS
10 Plus
ml. O_2/min./kg.
32 Plus
Kilocalories/min.
(70 kg. person)
11 Plus
	Shoveling 10/min.
	$7^{1}/_{2}$ + kg. or 16 +
	  lb.
		Running 6 m.p.h. = 10 METS
		Running 7 m.p.h. = $11^{1}/_{2}$ METS
		Running 8 m.p.h. = $13^{1}/_{2}$ METS
		Running 9 m.p.h. = 15 METS
		Running 10 m.p.h. = 17 METS
		Ski touring 8+ km. or 5+ m.p.h.
		  (loose snow)
		Handball—competitive
		Squash—competitive

* A major excess metabolic increase may occur due to excitement, anxiety or impatience in some of these activities and a physician must assess his patient's psychologic reactivity.

† Reproduced with permission from S. M. Fox, J. P. Naughton, and W. L. Haskell: Physical activity and the prevention of coronary heart disease. Ann. Clin. Res., *3:*404, 1971.

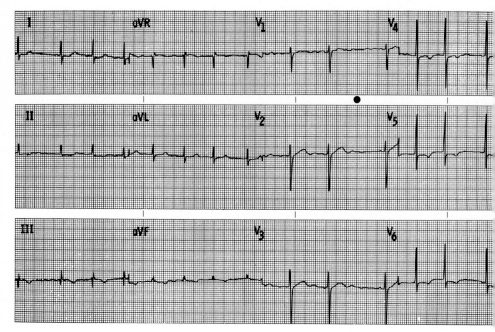

Fig. 7-1 Figures 7-1 and 2 were obtained from a 68-year-old man with chronic atrial fibrillation during maintenance digoxin therapy. His resting 12-lead ECG shown in Figure 7-1 reveals atrial fibrillation (ventricular rate: 75–90 beats/minute) with non-specific S-T, T wave abnormalities and/or digitalis effect and possible left ventricular hypertrophy.

patients who are able to perform only lower stages of exercise workloads show a poor prognosis which may be slightly improved with surgical therapy.[16]

From the electrocardiographic analysis, it can be said that the early occurrence of the diagnostic S-T segment changes (see Chapter 12) with minimal exercise workloads certainly is indicative of a grave prognosis as compared with those who develop the ischemic ECG change during near-maximal exercise. As far as the relationship between the prognosis of the coronary patients and the exercise-induced cardiac arrhythmias is concerned, serious ventricular arrhythmias induced by minimal exercise (less than 70% predicted maximal heart rate) are usually considered the greatest risk of future sudden death[3, 4] (see Chapter 13). Lown et al.[17] studied the effectiveness of exercise ECG testing for detection of ventricular arrhythmias compared with the 24-hour Holter monitor ECG. These investigators reported that ventricular arrhythmias which persisted for at least 2 hours during the Holter monitor ECG were also produced during exercise ECG testing. They concluded that these persisting ventricular arrhythmias are correlated best with severe, multivessel coronary artery disease. Exercise

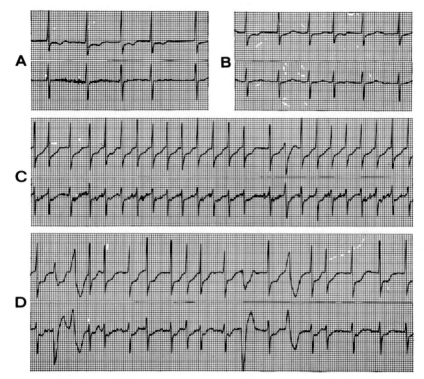

Fig. 7-2 Exercise ECG test was ordered to evaluate the efficacy of digitalis therapy because the patient complained of palpitations. The strips A and B represent resting tracings taken supine and standing, respectively. The upper strip is lead CM₅ whereas the lower strip is lead II in each rhythm strip. The strips C were recorded during exercise, while the strips D represent immediate post-exercise ECG.

The ventricular rate is markedly increased by minimal exercise (stage 1 of the exercise protocol—see Chapter 9), shown in the strips C (ventricular rate: 170–190 beats/minute). Note occasional aberrant ventricular conduction and frequent VPCs with group beats (strips C and D). In addition, the S-T segment is markedly depressed during and after exercise (strips C and D).

ECG testing also provides useful information as to the efficacy of various anti-arrhythmic drug therapy for ventricular arrhythmias.

In addition, exercise testing can be successfully utilized to evaluate the response to conditioning programs and preventive measures.

3. Rehabilitation Purposes And Preventive Measures

Exercise ECG testing is a useful tool for rehabilitation purposes and preventive measures for cardiac as well as non-cardiac patients. The functional capacity of the patients with previous myocardial infarction can be progressively improved by a properly designed exercise program. This is particularly important when strenuous physical activities are involved in certain occupations. Needless to say, post-infarction patients are not permitted to return to work when their functional capacity determined by exercise testing is not sufficient for a given individual's job.

Exercise testing can also be used to encourage individual motivation for healthy subjects as well as coronary patients who are engaged in any type of exercise program.

4. Research Purposes

When dealing with any research program to evaluate the efficacy of various anti-anginal drugs or anti-arrhythmic drugs, exercise ECG testing is always required as part of the research protocol. This is particularly true when a new anti-anginal or anti-arrhythmic agent is investigated.

In addition, exercise ECG testing is an essential tool when evaluating the exercise responses in various cardiovascular disorders. Recently, the exercise response was evaluated in 20 individuals with known Wolff-Parkinson-White syndrome to assess the incidence of ectopic tachyarrhythmias induced by exercise in our exercise laboratory.[18] It is interesting to note that none developed any ectopic tachyarrhythmia during or after submaximal exercise.[18]

5. Screening Purposes

The exercise ECG test has an important role as a screening device. For example, the exercise response, particularly the functional capacity determined by exercise testing, provides valuable information to determine whether a given individual has the physical capability to engage in strenuous activities or occupations (e.g., selection of pilots, astronauts, etc.). Such occupations require top-shape physical condition with extraordinary coordination and keen alertness. A less important role of exercise testing is the screening required by certain life insurance companies in order to estimate the life expectancy of a given individual. In addition, a pre-employment physical examination may require the exercise ECG test to determine a candidate's suitability for certain occupations, particularly in older individuals (e.g., over age 40 or 50).

Summary

1. It is essential to determine whether the exercise ECG test is definitely indicated. A physician who supervises the test must evaluate the purpose of the exercise test very carefully in a given individual.

2. It should be certain that there are no contraindications to the exercise test.

3. The major indication of the exercise ECG test is to diagnose coronary artery disease. Confirmation of the clinical diagnosis of coronary artery disease as well as differential diagnosis of chest pain of various origins can be carried out by exercise testing.

4. Assessment of the nature of cardiac arrhythmias in relation to exercise is possible by exercise testing.

5. Exercise testing may detect labile hypertension when systolic pressure rises beyond 220 mm. Hg. during peak exercise.

6. Another important role of the exercise test is to assess the functional capacity of coronary patients.

7. The functional capacity of a given individual may be altered by medical as well as surgical therapy.

8. Exercise testing provides useful information for evaluating the efficacy of various anti-anginal and anti-arrhythmic drugs.

9. The prognosis of coronary patients can be evaluated by exercise testing.

10. Another important role of the exercise ECG test is for the rehabilitation of cardiac as well as non-cardiac patients.

11. For evaluation of the efficacy of anti-anginal or anti-arrhythmic drugs, the exercise ECG test is usually included as a part of the research protocol.

12. Exercise testing is also valuable to assess the exercise responses in various cardiovascular disorders.

13. For screening purposes, the exercise test is valuable to determine the suitability of a candidate for certain strenuous activities or occupations.

14. Exercise ECG testing stimulates individual motivation for entering and adhering to various exercise programs.

15. Exercise testing is required as part of the physical examination for certain occupations or by some life insurance companies.

REFERENCES

1. Naughton, J.: Stress electrocardiography in clinical electrocardiographic correlations, *in* Cardiovascular Clinics, edited by J. C. Rios, Vol 8, pp. 127–139, Philadelphia, F. A. Davis, 1977.

2. Fortuin, J. and Weiss, J. L.: Exercise stress testing. Circulation, 56:699, 1977.

3. Faris, J. V., McHenry, P. L. and Morris, S. N.: Concepts and applications of treadmill exercise testing and the exercise electrocardiogram. Am. Heart J., 95:102, 1978.

4. McHenry, P. L. and Morris, S. N.: Exercise electrocardiography. Current state of the art, *in* Advances in Electrocardiography, edited by J. W. Hurst and R. C. Schlant, pp. 265–304, New York, Grune & Stratton, 1976.

5. Ellestad, M. H.: Stress Testing. Principles and Practice, pp. 9–13, Philadelphia, F. A. Davis, 1976.

6. Chung, E. K.: Clinical Electrocardiography (Part 9) Exercise Electrocardiography. New York, Medcom, 1978.

7. Blackburn, H.: The exercise electrocardiogram in diagnosis. Cardiology, 62:190, 1977.

8. McHenry, P. L. and Fisch, C.: Clinical applications of the treadmill exercise test. Mod. Concepts Cardiovasc. Dis., 46:21, 1977.

9. Linhart, J. W.: Stress testing in angina. Resident & Staff Physician, pp. 79–89, Feb., 1978.

10. Lindsey, H. E., Jr. and Cohn, P. F.: "Silent" myocardial ischemia during and after exercise testing in patients with coronary artery disease. Am. Heart. J., 95:441, 1978.

11. Kaplan, M. A., Harris, C. N., Aronow, W. S., Parker, D. P. and Ellestad, M. H.: Inability of the submaximal treadmill stress test to predict the location of coronary disease. Circulation, 47:250, 1973.
12. Martin, C. and McConahay, D. R.: Maximal treadmill exercise electrocardiography. Correlations with coronary arteriography and cardiac hemodynamics. Circulation, 46:956, 1972.
13. McHenry, P. L., Morris, S. N. and Jordan, J. W.: Stress testing in coronary heart disease. Heart & Lung, 3:83, 1974.
14. Kemp, G. L. and Ellestad, M. H.: The incidence of "silent" coronary heart disease. Calif. Med., 109:363, 1968.
15. Chung, E. K.: Principles of Cardiac Arrhythmias, Second Edition. Baltimore, Williams and Wilkins, 1977.
16. Margolis, J. R.: Treadmill stage as a predictor of medical and surgical survival in coronary disease. Circulation, 51 (suppl II): II–109, 1975.
17. Lown, B., Calvert, A. F., Armington, R. and Ryan, M.: Monitoring for serious arrhythmias and high risk of sudden death. Circulation, 52 (suppl.): III–189, 1975.
18. Zuckerman, G. and Chung, E. K.: Exercise responses in the Wolff-Parkinson-White syndrome (In press), 1978.

8

Contraindications of the Exercise ECG Test

Edward K. Chung, M.D., F.A.C.P., F.A.C.C.

General Considerations[1-6]

It is extremely important to consider various factors which may be possible contraindications to the exercise ECG test. This fact is as important as careful consideration of indications for the exercise ECG test (see Chapter 7). When various factors for possible contraindications to the exercise ECG test are carefully evaluated, various complications involved with the test can be markedly minimized or even prevented.

By and large, the exercise ECG test is associated with a very low morbidity or mortality rate when indications versus contraindications to exercise testing are carefully evaluated, and when the test is directly supervised by an experienced cardiologist. The mortality rate (a total of 16 deaths) was reported to be 1 in 10,000 exercise ECG tests (mostly treadmill exercise testing), according to the collected morbidity-mortality data from 73 medical institutions dealing with 170,000 tests.[7] In another 40 patients, hospitalization was required for non-fatal complications including serious cardiac arrhythmias or chest pain (morbidity rate: 2.4/10,000 tests). Exact analysis of exercise-induced myocardial infarction is not given in this study.[7]

When proper preparations and precautions (see Chapter 3) are carefully followed, even small risks of developing complications can be markedly minimized. For example, careful history taking and a good physical examination in conjunction with careful analysis of resting 12-lead ECG provide valuable information as to the indications versus contraindications to exercise ECG testing (see Chapter 3). An experienced physician who supervises the exercise ECG test can estimate the patient's physical capacity and possible risks with reasonable accuracy from the above-mentioned pre-exercise test evaluation.

The most serious complications other than death include acute myocardial infarction and ventricular tachycardia or fibrillation during and/or after exercise. The exact incidence of these complications is uncertain. These complications, of course, are likely to be observed in high risk patients such as those with multivessel involvement, previous myocardial infarction, previous history of ventricular tachyarrhythmias, etc. In this author's own experience, 2–3 patients with unexpected recent myocardial infarction (less than 48–72 hours old) have been detected annually during pre-exercise test evaluation (5,500 exercise tests over the past 5 years), and my experience seems to be similar to that of other institutions.[3]

It is not possible to clearly separate absolute versus relative contraindications to the exercise ECG test because of a significant overlap. Nevertheless, Table 8-1 summarizes absolute versus relative contraindications to exercise ECG testing. From another point of view, Table 8-2 summarizes contraindications to exercise testing in cardiac disorders, non-cardiac disorders and various drug effects or toxicity and electrolyte imbalance.

Table 8-1. Exercise ECG Test: Contraindications

Absolute
- Acute myocardial infarction
- Unstable or crescendo angina
- Serious cardiac arrhythmias (ventricular tachycardia, acquired advanced or complete A-V block)
- Acute myocarditis or pericarditis, subacute bacterial endocarditis, acute rheumatic fever
- Severe aortic stenosis
- Acute or severe congestive heart failure, cardiogenic shock
- Acute pulmonary embolism or infarction
- Any acute or serious non-cardiac disorders
- Severe physical handicaps (e.g., amputee, severe arthritis or deformity, etc.)

Relative
- Clinically significant non-cardiac disorders
- Significant physical handicaps
- Debilitated or elderly patients
- Mentally unstable or uncooperative patients
- Severe anemia or high fever
- Moderate to severe hypertension
- Pulmonary hypertension
- Moderate aortic stenosis, idiopathic hypertrophic subaortic stenosis
- Other serious heart diseases
- Clinically significant tachyarrhythmias (e.g., frequent multifocal ventricular premature contractions, grouped ventricular premature contractions, persisting supraventricular tachyarrhythmias, etc.)
- Marked bradyarrhythmias
- Various cardiac drug (e.g., digitalis) effects or toxicity and electrolyte imbalance
- Under the influence of various non-cardiac agents (e.g., alcohol, analgesics, tranquilizers, etc.)
- Fixed-rate artificial pacemaker

Table 8-2. Exercise ECG Test: Contraindications

Cardiac Disorders
- Acute myocardial infarction, unstable or crescendo angina
- Serious cardiac arrhythmias (ventricular tachycardia, acquired complete A-V block, supraventricular tachyarrhythmias)
- Myocarditis, pericarditis, subacute bacterial endocarditis, acute rheumatic fever
- Congestive heart failure, cardiogenic shock
- Severe hypertension or hypotension
- Aortic stenosis, idiopathic hypertrophic subaortic stenosis
- Pulmonary embolism and/or infarction
- Advanced heart disease—other types (e.g., cardiomyopathy, various congenital heart diseases, etc.)
- Pulmonary hypertension

Non-cardiac Disorders
- Any acute or serious illness (pulmonary, renal, hepatic, central nervous system and malignancy)
- Physical handicaps: Amputee, severe arthritis, deformity, or any neuromusculoskeletal disorders, claudication, thrombophlebitis, marked obesity
- Mentally unstable or uncooperative patients
- Extremely elderly patients
- Debilitated patients with chronic diseases
- Severe anemia
- High fever

Drugs and Electrolyte Imbalance
- Digitalis intoxication
- Overdosage of anti-arrhythmic agents: Quinidine, lidocaine (Xylocaine), procainamide (Pronestyl), propranolol (Inderal), diphenylhydantoin (Dilantin) and disopyramide (Norpace)
- Under the influence of other agents: Alcohol, sedatives, tranquilizers, anesthetics, analgesics, anti-hypertensive drugs
- Electrolyte imbalance (e.g., hypokalemia)

As repeatedly emphasized previously, it is essential to have full facilities for cardiopulmonary resuscitation in the exercise laboratory. Equipment necessary in the exercise laboratory and commonly used drugs for cardiopulmonary emergencies are listed in Tables 8-3 and 4. All medical as well as paramedical personnel working in the exercise laboratory must be capable of administering cardiopulmonary resuscitation.

In some clinical circumstances, the exercise ECG test is not exactly contraindicated, but the test provides little or no diagnostic value. In general, the exercise ECG test will provide little or no diagnostic value when there are various factors which frequently cause false positive or negative exercise ECG tests (see Chapters 5, 6 and 12). Various clinical circumstances in which the exercise ECG test provides little or no diagnostic value are summarized in Table 8-5. A typical example is that there is no diagnostic

Table 8-3. Equipment Necessary in the Exercise Laboratory

- Treadmill (motor-driven) with specially designed electrodes and cables
- 1–3 channel continuous ECG monitor and recorder
- Sphygmomanometer
- DC defibrillator
- Airways, oral and tracheal
- Oxygenator, intermittent positive-pressure capability
- Bag-valve-mask hand respirator
- Cut-down tray (sterile) with syringes and needles, intravenous sets, intravenous stand and adhesive tape
- Stethoscope
- Laryngoscope (optional)

Table 8-4. Commonly Used Drugs for Cardiopulmonary Emergencies

- Anti-arrhythmic agents:
  Lidocaine (Xylocaine), procainamide (Pronestyl), propranolol (Inderal), quinidine, diphenylhydantoin (Dilantin), disopyramide (Norpace)
- Cardiac glycosides:
  Digoxin, ouabain, deslanoside
- Atropine
- Catecholamines:
  Isoproterenol (Isuprel), epinephrine (Adrenalin), Aramine, Noradrenalin
- Nitroglycerin tablets and amyl nitrite pearls
- Morphine or Demerol
- Sodium bicarbonate solution
- Methylprednisolone sodium succinate (Solu-Medrol)
- Other agents:
  Calcium gluconate, aminophyllin, furosemide (Lasix), diazepam (Valium)
- Dextrose, 5% in wter

value when the exercise ECG test is given to patients with previously documented myocardial infarction. Similarly, the exercise ECG test provides no diagnostic value in patients with known mitral valve prolapse syndrome because of the extremely high incidence of false positive results. Another example is various pre-existing ECG abnormalities, particularly left bundle branch block, left ventricular hypertrophy and WPW syndrome in which a false positive exercise ECG test is the rule rather than the exception. In addition, the exercise ECG test has no diagnostic value in any patient during digitalis therapy, because of the high incidence of false positive exercise ECG tests.

Absolute Contraindications

Various clinical situations in which the exercise ECG test is considered to be absolutely contraindicated are summarized in Table 8-1.

Table 8-5. Little or No Diagnostic Value in the Exercise ECG Test

1. Drug Therapy and Electrolyte Imbalance
   - During digitalis therapy
   - During anti-anginal drug therapy (i.e., propranolol therapy)
   - During diuretic therapy
   - Hypokalemia

2. Cardiac Disorders
   - Previous history of proven myocardial infarction
   - Mitral valve prolapse syndrome
   - Wolff-Parkinson-White syndrome
   - Significant congenital or valvular heart disease
   - Significant cardiomyopathies

3. Pre-existing ECG Abnormalities
   - Left bundle branch block
   - Left ventricular hypertrophy
   - WPW syndrome

4. Miscellaneous
   - Serious non-cardiac disorders, marked obesity, physical handicap, etc.

1. Acute Myocardial Infarction

It is generally agreed that the exercise ECG test is hazardous in patients with recent myocardial infarction of less than 6 weeks old. In other words, the usual exercise ECG test protocol designed for diagnostic purposes (see Chapter 9) should *not* be prescribed for any patient with acute or recent myocardial infarction.

Nevertheless, there is a general trend to discharge patients with myocardial infarction early, and a modified exercise ECG test with light exercise workloads is often given 1–2 days before discharge in order to assess their functional capacity.[4-6]

Recently, the exercise ECG test was given to a 62-year-old man with diaphragmatic and extensive anterior myocardial infarction for assessment of his functional capacity in our institution. The exact duration of this patient's myocardial infarction was not certain, but it was estimated to be at least 4–6 weeks old (Figure 8-1). He developed ventricular tachycardia (Figure 8-2) with mild exercise workloads (less than 6 METs) and he became unconscious soon thereafter. Cardiopulmonary resuscitative measures, including intracardiac injection of epinephrine for cardiac standstill and 4 applications of direct current shock for ventricular fibrillation (Figure 8-3), were begun immediately. Fortunately, he recovered completely within 30 minutes and his post-cardiac arrest induced by exercise was uneventful. No evidence of new myocardial infarction was found. It is interesting to note

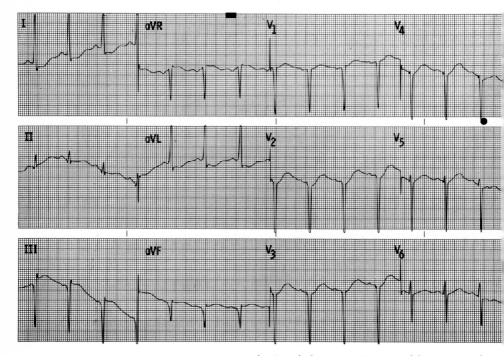

Fig. 8-1   Figures 8-1 to 4 were obtained from a 62-year-old man with myocardial infarction, age undetermined (considered to be at least 4–6 weeks old). His 12-lead ECG shown in Figure 8-1 reveals sinus rhythm (rate: 93 beats/minute) and evidence of diaphragmatic as well as extensive anterior myocardial infarction, age undetermined. In addition, left ventricular hypertrophy is suggested.

that no single ventricular premature contraction was documented on repeated 12-lead resting electrocardiograms or several Holter monitor ECGs (Figure 8-4).

From the above illustrated incident, the exercise ECG test should be carefully given to any individual with documented myocardial infarction (MI) even though the MI is considered to be not recent. Similarly, the exercise ECG test should be given with extreme caution in patients with high grade left main coronary artery disease or its equivalent. Ellestad claims that the exercise ECG test is contraindicated in patients with high grade left main coronary disease, or 90% obstruction of both the proximal left anterior descending and circumflex coronaries.[1]

2. Unstable or Crescendo Angina

The exercise ECG test should be avoided when any patient is considered to be suffering from unstable or crescendo angina. In addition to clinical

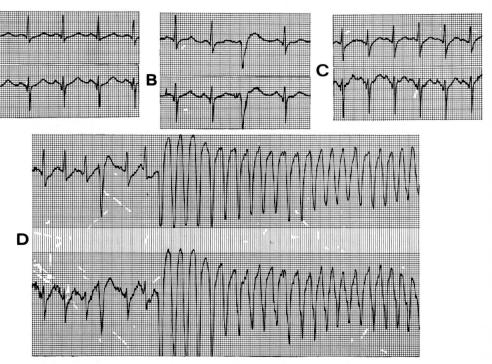

Fig. 8-2   This tracing is his exercise ECG test. The strips A and B were taken at rest, in supine and standing position, respectively. The strips C and D were recorded during exercise. The exercise was stopped immediately when he developed ventricular tachycardia (strips D). Note a VPC in strips B. (The upper strip represents lead CM_5, whereas the lower strip is lead II).

history, the patient's 12-lead resting ECG often shows deeply and symmetrically inverted T waves involving many leads (Figure 8-5). From this author's experience, 4–5 patients with unstable or crescendo angina report to our exercise laboratory for treadmill exercise testing every month. As soon as the patient is evaluated in the exercise laboratory, the exercise ECG test is cancelled accordingly. The attending physician who ordered the test is notified immediately.

3. Serious Cardiac Arrhythmias

The exercise ECG test should be contraindicated in patients with serious cardiac arrhythmias, including ventricular tachycardia or acquired advanced or complete A-V block. It should be noted, however, that the exercise ECG test is *not* contraindicated in patients with congenital complete A-V block unless there is significant coexisting congenital cardiac anomaly (see Chapter 13).

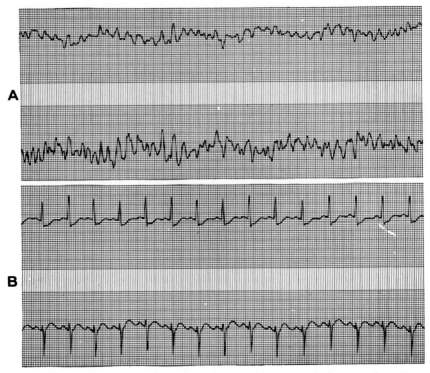

Fig. 8-3   The strips A shown in this tracing were recorded soon after Figure 8-2 was taken when he became unconscious as a result of cardiac arrest. The strips B were obtained after he was successfully resuscitated. The strips A reveal ventricular fibrillation which required 4 applications of DC shock. Sinus rhythm was restored within 30 minutes (strips B).

4. Acute Myocarditis, Pericarditis, Bacterial Endocarditis and Acute Rheumatic Fever

When there is any evidence of active heart disease such as acute myocarditis, pericarditis, bacterial endocarditis, acute rheumatic fever, etc., the exercise ECG test is definitely contraindicated.

5. Severe Aortic Stenosis

The exercise ECG test is definitely contraindicated in patients with severe aortic stenosis. Severe aortic stenosis may be defined as a gradient greater than 75 mm. Hg. at the aortic valve area, and many patients in this category have a history of fainting episodes. Loud (grade IV or more) ejection systolic murmur with palpable thrill, narrow pulse pressure and markedly diminished or absent A_2 are often recognized by physical exami-

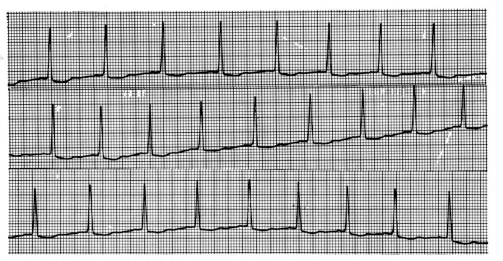

Fig. 8-4 His 24-hour Holter monitor ECG shown in this figure reveals normal sinus rhythm with no evidence of ventricular arrhythmias. The strips A, B and C are *not* continuous.

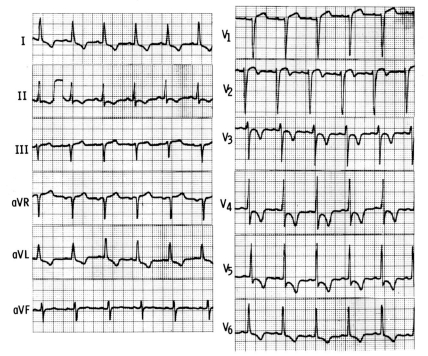

Fig. 8-5 This tracing was obtained from a 51-year-old man with crescendo angina. His 12-lead resting ECG reveals sinus rhythm with diffuse myocardial ischemia.

nation. The 12-lead electrocardiogram usually reveals typical left ventricular hypertrophy with systolic overloading pattern.[8] In advanced cases with severe aortic stenosis, inverted T waves often involve the entire precordial leads which closely resemble true myocardial ischemia.[8] When the exercise ECG test is given to the patient with severe aortic stenosis by misjudgment, there will be a great risk of developing ventricular tachyarrhythmias, fainting episodes and even sudden death.

6. Acute or Severe Congestive Heart Failure and/or Cardiogenic Shock

Needless to say, the exercise ECG test is absolutely contraindicated in patients with acute or severe congestive heart failure and/or cardiogenic shock. The exercise ECG test should be avoided when there are signs of congestive heart failure (e.g., pulmonary moist rales, gallop rhythm, etc.) in addition to the compatible clinical history (e.g., dyspnea on exertion, nocturnal dyspnea, ankle swelling, etc.), and when there is any sign suggestive of shock (e.g., hypotension, pallor, etc.).

7. Acute Pulmonary Embolism or Infarction

The exercise ECG test should be avoided when pulmonary embolism or infarction is suspected or diagnosed. Persisting sinus tachycardia is nearly always present in patients with pulmonary embolism in the resting state. In other words, the diagnosis of acute pulmonary embolism is extremely unlikely when the resting heart rate is slower than 100 beats/minute.

8. Any Acute or Serious Non-cardiac Disorders

The exercise ECG test is definitely contraindicated when there are any acute or serious non-cardiac disorders (e.g., pneumonia, advanced obstructive pulmonary disease, asthma, renal failure, hepatitis, thyrotoxicosis, malignancy, etc).

9. Severe Physical Handicaps

Any individual with marked physical handicaps (e.g., amputee, severe arthritis or deformity involving lower extremities, etc.) is unable to perform the exercise ECG testing.

Relative Contraindications

Various clinical circumstances which are considered to be relatively contraindicated for the exercise ECG test are listed in Table 8-1.

1. Clinically Significant Non-cardiac Disorders

Exercise ECG test should be avoided when there are clinically significant non-cardiac disorders (e.g., generalized skin disorders, etc.) which may interfere with the exercise ECG testing.

2. Significant Physical Handicaps

Any significant physical handicaps which may interfere with the exercise ECG testing can be considered a relative contraindication. For example, any individual with a limp due to various causes (e.g., arthritis or deformity of lower extremities), significant claudication or phlebitis of legs, is unable to perform adequate exercise. Similarly, markedly obese subjects can not perform adequate exercise testing even if the cardiac function is normal.

3. Debilitated or Elderly Patients

The exercise ECG test should be avoided in individuals debilitated by chronic illness or simple malnutrition, or very old patients (over 80 years old?). First of all, these individuals can not perform adequate exercise. Second, there is little or no value in the exercise testing in these subjects.

4. Mentally Unstable or Uncooperative Patients

It is important to emphasize that the exercise ECG test should be avoided when dealing with mentally unstable or uncooperative patients. These individuals frequently provoke various medico-legal problems, and an adequate exercise ECG test is usually difficult to expect. Unexpected accidents may occur in these patients during testing.

5. Severe Anemia or High Fever

When any individual has severe anemia, some form of systemic disease or malignancy is often present. The exercise ECG test should be avoided in this situation. In individuals with high fever, some form of infectious process is usually responsible. Thus, the exercise ECG test should be, likewise, avoided until the patient becomes afebrile and free of any infection.

6. Moderate to Severe Hypertension

As a rule, the exercise ECG test is considered to be contraindicated when the patient shows significant hypertension during the pre-exercise examination. In most exercise laboratories, the exercise ECG testing is cancelled when there is systolic blood pressure above 200 mm. Hg. and/or diastolic pressure beyond 100 mm. Hg. The reason for this is that the pre-existing hypertension may become much more exaggerated during peak exercise, and it may lead to a serious outcome. Exercise testing is usually terminated prematurely when any individual develops systolic blood pressure above 220 mm. Hg. regardless of the resting blood pressure (see Chapter 9).

7. Pulmonary Hypertension

When there is significant pulmonary hypertension, serious underlying heart disease (e.g., valvular or congenital lesions) other than coronary heart disease often exists. Accordingly, most patients with significant pulmonary hypertension may not perform the exercise testing adequately. In addition, the diagnostic value of the exercise ECG test will be limited under these circumstances; various drugs and/or ventricular hypertrophy cause a high incidence of false positive results.

8. Moderate Aortic Stenosis and Idiopathic Hypertrophic Subaortic Stenosis (IHSS)

Exercise ECG tests should be avoided in patients with moderate aortic stenosis (gradient less than 75 mm. Hg.) or IHSS because of the possible danger of provoking ventricular tachyarrhythmias, syncope and even sudden death. Aside from the possible risks, the diagnostic value of the exercise ECG test will be markedly limited; false positive results are often caused by left ventricular hypertrophy, which is very common in these individuals.

9. Other Serious Heart Disease

The exercise ECG test provides little or no diagnostic value for coronary heart disease when there is any known or suspected coexisting non-coronary heart disease (e.g., valvular or congenital lesions, cardiomyopathies, etc.). The reason for this is that the exercise capacity in these individuals is often significantly compromised by the coexisting non-coronary heart disease. As a result, adequate exercise ECG testing is difficult to expect under these circumstances. In addition, a high incidence of false positive exercise ECG tests is expected because of various drug effects, ventricular hypertrophy and bundle branch block (see Chapters 5, 6 and 12).

10. Clinically Significant Tachyarrhythmias

As described previously, the exercise ECG test is absolutely contraindicated in the presence of ventricular tachycardia and acquired advanced or complete A-V block. In addition to these serious cardiac arrhythmias, the exercise ECG test should be avoided when any patient exhibits clinically significant ectopic tachyarrhythmias such as frequent multifocal and/or grouped ventricular premature contractions (VPCs), or persisting supraventricular tachyarrhythmias (e.g., paroxysmal atrial tachycardia, flutter or fibrillation with rapid ventricular response, etc.).

Multifocal atrial tachycardia (MAT) deserves a special comment. The exercise ECG test should be avoided in patients showing MAT, because chronic obstructive pulmonary disease is the most common underlying disease.[10] In addition, hypoxia due to various causes, pulmonary embolism or pneumonia may be responsible for the development of MAT. In my experience, MAT has never been encountered in healthy individuals.[10] Therefore, most patients with MAT are unable to perform a proper exercise ECG test and, as a result, the test provides little or no diagnostic value.

The exercise ECG test provides little or no diagnostic value for coronary artery disease in individuals with known Wolff-Parkinson-White syndrome because of almost 100% incidence of false positive results.[9] Furthermore, there is always a danger of provoking ectopic tachyarrhythmias by exercise in patients with WPW syndrome (see Chapter 13). Thus, the exercise ECG test should be given with extreme caution to any individual with known WPW syndrome, especially when a history of frequent development of ectopic tachyarrhythmias is obtained. Thus, the exercise ECG test is justified only when the functional capacity is to be assessed in individuals with known WPW syndrome.

11. Marked Bradyarrhythmias

When a resting ECG demonstrates markedly slow rhythm (a rate below 45 beats/ minute), each patient should be carefully evaluated. Some athletes may show marked sinus bradycardia as a physiologic phenomenon. Otherwise, marked sinus bradycardia may be a sign of sick sinus syndrome (SSS), especially in elderly individuals.[11] The exercise ECG test is hazardous in patients with SSS because the diseased sinus node is unable to produce sufficient cardiac impulses during exercise. The exercise ECG test should also be avoided in the presence of other forms of bradyarrhythmias such as Wenckebach A-V block, Mobitz type II A-V block, sino-atrial block, etc., because the pre-existing bradyarrhythmias may become worse during exercise. In addition, an adequate exercise ECG test is difficult to expect in these individuals.

12. Various Cardiac Drug Effects or Toxicity and Electrolyte Imbalance

The exercise ECG test is contraindicated in any individual with possible cardiac drug toxicity, particularly digitalis intoxication. It should be reemphasized that the exercise ECG test provides little or no diagnostic value during digitalis therapy because of the extremely high incidence of false positive results (see Chapters 6 and 12). It is recommended that digoxin or similar cardiac glycoside be discontinued for at least 2 weeks prior to the exercise test for diagnostic purposes. Similarly, hypokalemia should be corrected before exercise testing is ordered since a false positive result is very common in hypokalemia (see Chapter 6). On the other hand, propranolol (Inderal) frequently causes a false negative exercise ECG test (see Chapter 6). When the exercise ECG test is ordered for diagnostic purposes, the test should be postponed until at least 1 week after discontinuation of the drug as clinical circumstances permit.

13. Under the Influence of Various Non-cardiac Agents

Needless to say, an adquate exercise ECG test is impossible to expect when any individual is under the influence of various agents, including alcohol, sedatives, tranquilizers, anesthetics and analgesics. Therefore, the exercise ECG test is contraindicated under these circumstances. Various anti-hypertensive agents often produce false positive exercise ECG tests. Thus, the test should be postponed until at least 1 week after discontinuation of anti-hypertensive agents, if possible. Remember that significant hypertension is considered a contraindication to the exercise ECG test.

14. Fixed-rate Artificial Pacemaker

By the unique feature of the fixed-rate artificial pacemaker, the pacing rate will remain constant regardless of the clinical circumstances. In other words, the ventricular rate can not be altered in patients with a fixed-rate artificial pacemaker during exercise, although the atrial rate may be increased when the sinus mechanism is present in the atria. Therefore , the exercise ECG test is contraindicated in patients with a fixed-rate pacemaker. In addition, the result of the exercise ECG test is difficult to evaluate when the cardiac rhythm is under the control of an artificial pacemaker.

Summary

1. In many clinical circumstances, the exercise ECG test is either absolutely or relatively contraindicated (see Tables 8-1 and 2).

2. Morbidity and mortality related to the exercise ECG test can be markedly minimized when indications versus contraindications are carefully evaluated.

3. The exercise ECG test is absolutely contraindicated in patients with acute myocardial infarction or crescendo angina.

4. In the presence of serious cardiac arrhythmias such as ventricular tachycardia or acquired complete A-V block, the exercise ECG test is absolutely contraindicated.

5. In patients with infectious heart disease, significant valvular or congenital heart disease, the exercise ECG test is, likewise, contraindicated.

6. The exercise ECG test is definitely contraindicated in the presence of significant congestive heart failure, cardiogenic shock, severe aortic stenosis, acute or serious non-cardiac disorders (e.g., renal failure, hepatitis, malignancy, etc.), and severe physical handicaps (e.g., amputee, severe arthritis or deformity of the lower extremities).

7. In mentally disturbed or uncooperative individuals, the exercise ECG test should be avoided.

8. The exercise ECG test should be avoided in patients with significant hypertension.

9. When the patient is under the influence of various cardiac as well as non-cardiac agents, the exercise ECG test should be postponed.

10. When the resting ECG shows persisting ectopic tachyarrhythmias such as paroxysmal atrial tachycardia, flutter or fibrillation with rapid ventricular response, or frequent multifocal or grouped VPCs, the exercise ECG test should be cancelled.

11. The exercise ECG test is definitely contraindicated in digitalis toxicity and/or significant hypokalemia.

12. When the resting ECG exhibits marked sinus bradycardia, a possibility of SSS should be raised unless it is drug-induced. The exercise ECG test is hazardous in patients with SSS.

13. The exercise ECG test is contraindicated in patients with a fixed-rate artificial pacemaker.

14. Cardiopulmonary resuscitative equipment with commonly used drugs must be available in the exercise laboratory (see Tables 8-3 and 4).

15. All medical as well as paramedical personnel working in the exercise laboratory must be capable of administering cardiopulmonary resuscitative measures.

REFERENCES

1. Ellestad, M. H.: Stress Testing. Principles and Practice, pp. 15–23, Philadelphia, F. A. Davis, 1976.
2. Linhart, J. W.: Stress testing in angina. Resident & Staff Physician, pp. 79–89, Feb., 1978.
3. McHenry, P. L. and Morris, S. N.: Exercise electrocardiography. Current state of the art, *in* Advances in Electrocardiography, edited by J. W. Hurst and R. C. Schlant, pp. 265–304, New York, Grune & Stratton, 1976.
4. Markiewicz, W., Houston, N. and DeBusk, R. F.: Exercise testing soon after myocardial infarction. Circulation, *56*:26, 1977.
5. Sivarajan, E. S., Syndsman, A., Smith, B. et al.: Low-level treadmill testing of 41 patients with acute myocardial infarction prior to discharge from the Hospital. Heart & Lung, *6*:975, 1977.
6. Simoons, M. L. Van den Brand, M. and Hugenholtz, P. G.: Quantitative analysis of exercise electrocardiograms and left ventricular angiocardiograms in patients with abnormal QRS complexes at rest. Circulation, *55*:55, 1977.
7. Rochmis, P. and Blackburn, H.: Exercise tests: A survey of procedures, safety, and litigation experience in approximately 170,000 tests. J.A.M.A., *216*:1061, 1971.

8. Chung, E. K.: Electrocardiography: Practical Applications with Vectorial Principles. Hagerstown, Md., Harper & Row, 1974.

9. Zuckerman, G. and Chung, E. K.: The exercise responses in the Wolff-Parkinson-White syndrom (In press), 1978.

10. Chung, E. K.: Principles of Cardiac Arrhythmias, Second Edition, Baltimore, Williams & Wilkins, 1977.

11. Chung, E. K.: Sick sinus syndrome and brady-tachyarrhythmias, *in* Artificial Cardiac Pacing: Practical Approach, edited by Edward K. Chung, Baltimore, Williams & Wilkins, 1979.

9

Protocols for the Exercise ECG Test

Edward K. Chung, M.D. F.A.C.P., F.A.C.C.

General Considerations[1-11]

It is extremely important to use a proper protocol for the exercise ECG test because the sensitivity (the ability of the exercise ECG test to identify correctly the arteriographically documented coronary artery disease) is directly influenced by the exercise protocol used. There are many protocols available for the exercise (treadmill) ECG test, and many investigators have modified different protocols suitable for their special needs and purposes.

Other than the treadmill exercise ECG test, there are many types of exercise testing, including the Master's two-step test (see Chapter 2), the Harvard step test, bicycle test and atrial pacing, etc. (see Chapters 1 and 4). These tests will not be described in detail because the treadmill exercise ECG test is the most popular and practical method of exercise testing, particularly in the United States of America.

There is some controversy among physicians regarding the practical value of maximal versus submaximal exercise testing, but there seems to be no significant difference between these two methods. On the other hand, the possible risks associated with the maximal exercise ECG test are reported to be *not* statistically higher than those associated with submaximal exercise testing.

In some medical institutions, the exercise ECG test is continued until significant symptoms, particularly chest pain, are provoked by exercise. On the other hand, others are satisfied with a heart rate-limited exercise ECG test when the submaximal heart rate (85–90% of the predicted maximal heart rate) is reached regardless of the presence or absence of exercise-induced symptoms or ECG abnormalities. Naturally, the risks involved with symptom-limited exercise ECG test will be greater than the heart rate-limited exercise test. A chance of producing a positive exercise ECG test, however, will be higher when the symptom-limited exercise ECG test is utilized.

Instructions to Patients on How to Prepare for the Exercise (Treadmill) ECG Test

When any individual is scheduled for the exercise ECG test, brief instructions should be given to the patient before the actual test. At our exercise laboratory, a small booklet explaining the purpose of the exercise ECG test, necessary preparations for the test and possible risks involved with the test is available for patients, physicians and nursing stations. A portion of the booklet on how to prepare for the exercise (treadmill) ECG test is reproduced in Table 9-1.

Various Parameters to be Observed and Assessed

There are various parameters to be observed and assessed during and after exercise (see Table 9-2). Various ECG changes, particularly S-T segment alteration, and blood pressure and heart rate changes must be carefully monitored in conjunction with an assessment of a variety of symptoms, particularly chest pain, and physical findings. One can assess the functional capacity of a given patient judging from the amount of exercise workloads; one can also evaluate the efficacy of medical and/or surgical therapy.

End Points to Terminate the Exercise ECG Test

It is essential to set up a guideline as to when to stop the exercise ECG test. Many individuals may be able to perform the full course of the exercise

Table 9-1. Preparations for the Exercise (Treadmill) ECG Test Instructions to Patients

1. Plan to be in the Exercise Laboratory (Heart Station) for approximately 1 to 1½ hours.
2. Do not eat for at least 2 hours before the test.
3. The preceding (last) meal should be light, without butter or cream, coffee, tea or alcohol.
4. You should be free of any acute or serious symptoms. Consult your doctor if you have any questions.
5. Continue to take your medications as prescribed by your doctor.
6. Some drugs such as digitalis ("heart pill"), nitroglycerine, propranolol (Inderal) and diuretics ("water pills") will interfere with the test. Please consult your doctor.
7. Wear or bring appropriate clothing. Comfortable shoes such as sneakers (tennis shoes); soft flat shoes are needed. Slippers are *not* acceptable and neither are bare feet.
8. Men should bring gym shorts, bermuda shorts or a pair of loose-fitting, light trousers.
9. Women should bring or wear a bra, short-sleeved, loose-fitting blouse that buttons in the front, and slacks, shorts or even pajama pants. No one-piece undergarments or pantyhose are to be worn.

Table 9-2. Exercise ECG Test: Various Parameters to be Observed and Assessed

1. ECG Changes
   - S-T segment alterations
     Elevation or depression
     Type and magnitude of depression
     Exercise time and heart rate at onset
     Post-exercise duration
   - Cardiac arrhythmias:
     Mechanisms (origin, type, frequency, etc.)
     Relationship to exercise, heart rate, S-T segment change, and symptoms
   - Other findings:
     Inverted U waves
     R-wave amplitude
2. Hemodynamic Responses
   - Blood pressure and heart rate changes
3. Symptoms and Signs
   - Onset of symptoms
   - Character of symptoms
   - Relationship to exercise
   - Reproducibility
   - Relationship to other findings (e.g., S-T segment or blood pressure change)
   - S_3, S_4, heart murmurs, rales
4. Miscellaneous
   - Assessment of functional capacity and efficacy of medical or surgical therapy

protocol and reach the predicted submaximal or maximal heart rate without any symptom of ECG abnormality. Nevertheless, it is often necessary to terminate the test prematurely before the predicted heart rate is reached because of significant symptoms, particularly chest pain, abnormal hemodynamic responses, the diagnostic S-T segment alterations and/or significant cardiac arrhythmias (see Chapters 12 and 13).

Table 9-3 summarizes the end points to terminate the exercise ECG test—absolute versus relative indications.

A. Absolute Indications

When the patient requests a premature termination of the exercise test, usually because of significant symptoms, the supervising physician must stop the test immediately. In some situations, however, less than enthusiastic individuals may ask to stop the test simply because of a lack of motivation and *not* because of any significant symptom. Under this circumstance, a decision should be made carefully by the supervising physician whether the given individual should be encouraged to continue the exercise testing or to stop the test. Whenever the patient requests a premature termination of

Table 9-3. End Points to Terminate Exercise ECG Test

A. Absolute Indications
  • Patient's request
  • Reduction of blood pressure and/or heart rate during increasing workloads
  • Significant symptoms or signs: severe chest pain, ataxia, vertigo, visual or gait disturbance, confusion, pallor, cyanosis
  • Serious arrhythmias: grouped (3 or more) ventricular premature contractions, ventricular tachycardia, ventricular fibrillation
  • Acute myocardial infarction
  • Malfunctioning equipment in the exercise laboratory (e.g., treadmill, ECG monitor and recorder, etc.)

B. Relative Indications
  • Less serious symptoms: Significant chest pain, dizziness, marked fatigue or dyspnea, severe anxiety, leg cramp, intermittent claudication
  • Marked (2 mm. or more) horizontal or downsloping S-T segment depression or marked (2 mm. or more) horizontal or upsloping S-T segment elevation
  • Marked hypertension (systolic blood pressure above 220 mm. Hg., or diastolic pressure above 110 mm. Hg.)
  • Failure of blood pressure to rise during increasing workloads (systolic blood pressure rise less than 20 mm. Hg. during the first 3 stages)
  • Frequent ventricular premature contractions or multifocal ventricular premature contractions
  • Persisting supraventricular tachyarrhythmias

the test, various parameters listed in Table 9-2 should be carefully and immediately evaluated in order to reach the correct decision.

The exercise ECG test should be stopped immediately when definitely abnormal hemodynamic responses to exercise (e.g., reduction of systolic blood pressure or heart rate) are observed. Similarly, the exercise ECG test should be terminated when the patient develops significant symptoms or signs (e.g., severe chest pain, pallor, cyanosis, visual or gait disturbances, etc.). Another absolute indication of the premature termination of the exercise ECG test is the production of serious cardiac arrhythmias (e.g., 3 or more grouped ventricular premature contractions, ventricular tachycardia or fibrillation) during exercise. The exercise test must be stopped immediately, of course, when the clinical picture and/or ECG finding strongly suggest acute myocardial infarction. In addition, the exercise test has to be stopped immediately when any equipment used for the test shows malfunction.

B. Relative Indications

When any patient develops significant symptoms, the supervising physician has to determine whether the exercise test should be continued or it should be stopped. Among various symptoms, leg weakness, fatigue and dyspnea are the most common causes for the premature termination of exercise testing. Significant chest pain induced by exercise is not too common reason to stop the test prematurely.

There are different views among physicians regarding the magnitude of the S-T segment alteration which is necessary for the premature termination of the exercise test. Ellestad states that the S-T segment depression of 6.0–7.0 mm. or more is an indication for stopping,[1] whereas Linhart uses the S-T segment depression or elevation of 5 mm. for an indication of premature termination of exercise testing.[5] In this author's viewpoint, however, it is not necessary to push the exercise test until the patient develops severe S-T segment alteration of 5 mm. or more when the test is performed for diagnostic purposes. In our laboratory, the S-T segment depression (horizontal or downsloping) or elevation (horizontal or upsloping) of 2 mm. or greater is considered sufficient reason to stop the test unless a false positive result is strongly suspected in certain cases. The reason for this is that the diagnostic S-T segment alteration of 2 mm. or greater is more than enough evidence for a positive test (see Chapter 12) providing that the resting ECG shows no S-T segment abnormality. The same S-T segment alteration criterion is not applicable, of course, when there are any known factors to cause a false positive test (e.g., left bundle branch block, WPW syndrome, digitalis effect, etc.). On the other hand, the exercise ECG test may be pushed further (up to 4–5 mm. S-T segment alteration) even after the recognition of S-T segment alteration of 2 mm. when the test is performed primarily for the assessment of functional capacity. It should be pointed out, however, that there will always be a greater risk when the exercise ECG test is excessively pushed beyond the acceptable limit in a given patient.

In our exercise laboratory, I consider the development of systolic blood pressure above 220 mm. Hg. to be an indication of premature stopping of the exercise ECG test. Some other institutions use the cutline at 230 mm. Hg. or even 250 mm. Hg. of systolic pressure for an indication of premature termination of the test. Similarly, it is recommended that the test be stopped when the diastolic pressure rises beyond 110 mm. Hg.

Perhaps a more important sign for stopping the exercise ECG test prematurely is a failure of systolic blood pressure to rise during a progressive increment of workloads. In general, the test may be stopped when the systolic blood pressure rises less than 20 mm. Hg. during the first 3 stages of the exercise protocol unless there is a known reason for the unusual blood pressure response (e.g., athletes, during propranolol therapy, extremely anxious individuals, etc.). Whenever unusual blood pressure response is observed, other parameters should be evaluated simultaneously (see Table 9-2).

The development of frequent unifocal VPCs alone during exercise is *not* sufficient to stop the test. However, the exercise test should be stopped when VPCs occur together with significant chest pain, hypotension and/or diagnostic S-T segment alteration. By and large, it is recommended that the test be stopped when frequent multifocal (particularly originating from 3 or more foci) VPCs are provoked by exercise.

Exercise-induced various supraventricular tachyarrhythmias are not serious clinically. However, the exercise ECG test must be stopped when the supraventricular tachyarrhythmias (e.g., atrial tachycardia, flutter or fibrillation with rapid ventricular response, etc.) persist during exercise. Transient supraventricular arrhythmias alone provoked by exercise are *not* sufficient reason to stop the test prematurely. Various exercise-induced cardiac arrhythmias are discussed in detail elsewhere in this book (see Chapter 13).

Exercise Protocols

There are many exercise protocols available for the clinical exercise laboratory,[1-4] but none will be ideal for every clinical situation. The suitability of the exercise protocol also varies according to the objectives of the exercise test. For example, a vigorous exercise protocol may be suitable for the screening of relatively healthy individuals. On the other hand, a milder exercise protocol may be adequate primarily for the evaluation of the functional capacity in patients with known cardiac disease. An exercise protocol of modified light workloads is required for patients with relatively recent myocardial infarction when the assessment of functional capacity is desired before discharge or before returning to their previous occupations.

The ideal exercise protocol should be as follows:

(a) The initial workload should be well within a given individual's anticipated physical working capacity.

(b) The workloads should be increased gradually and *not* abruptly, and maintained for a sufficient length of time to achieve a near physiologic steady-state.

(c) The exercise protocol should not cause any excessive mental or physical stress beyond tolerable workloads.

(d) Continuous monitoring ECG (at least a 2-channel recorder) with periodic (usually with 1-minute interval) recording of the rhythm strips throughout the entire exercise period and at least 6–8 minutes during the post-exercise period is essential. In addition, periodic (1–3 minute intervals) measurement of blood pressure before, during and after exercise (at least 6–8 minutes post-exercise period) should be done in conjunction with continuous evaluation of symptoms and signs.

(e) The exercise should be terminated prematurely when abnormal symptoms, signs, blood pressure responses, heart rate responses, serious cardiac arrhythmias and/or the diagnostic S-T segment alterations are produced (see Table 9-3). Otherwise, the exercise ECG test is terminated when the predicted heart rate is reached.

Table 9-4 shows my protocol which has been used in our exercise laboratory for the past 10 years with satisfactory results. The sensitivity and the specificity of the test by using my protocol seem to be as good as any other exercise protocol used in various institutions,[1-4] and most individuals—both coronary patients and healthy subjects performed the test satisfactorily without any significant untoward complications. In my protocol, the initial speed is 1.7 m.p.h. with 0% grade for 3-minutes during the warming-up period. The grade is increased with 4% at each stage with 3-minute intervals, and the speed (3.0 m.p.h.) remains constant. The protocol includes 7 full stages, and an extra 8 and 9 stages are designed only for physically active individuals. Each stage is expressed as METs to explain the estimation of the workloads (1 "MET"—Metabolic equivalent—means the basal metabolic oxygen requirement, and "METs" are multiples of the basal metabolic rates).

Most of the patients with significant coronary heart disease do not require the workloads beyond 8 METs (stage 4), whereas sedentary healthy subjects can seldom exercise the workloads above 10–11 METs (stage 6 or 7). Only physically active people such as athletes may be able to perform the exercise workloads beyond 16 METs (stage 9). By evaluating the amounts of the exercise workloads in terms of METs, a functional capacity of a given individual can be easily assessed (see Chapter 12). Functional class-I patients may be able to perform the workloads with 6–10 METs, whereas functional class-IV patients are unable to do any exercise (1 MET). Functional class-II patients can perform the exercise workloads with 4–6 METs, whereas the functional class-III patients may be able to perform the exercise with only 2–3 METs. The target heart rate, which is estimated to be 85–90% of the maximal heart rates in different age groups, is shown in Table 9-5.

Table 9-4. Chung's Protocol for Exercise (Treadmill) ECG Test

Stage	Speed (m.p.h.)	Grade (%)	Duration (min.)	METs (units)	Total Time Elapsed (min.)
1	1.7	0	3	2	3
2	3.0	4	3	4–5	6
3	3.0	8	3	6	9
4	3.0	12	3	8	12
5	3.0	16	3	9	15
6	3.0	20	3	10	18
7	3.0	24	3	12–13	21
8*	3.0	28	3	14	24
9*	3.0	32	3	16	27

* Optional for physically active individuals.

One of the most popular protocols is the Bruce protocol (see Table 9-6) in which both speed and grade are increased every 3 minutes in each of 7 stages.[4] His protocol has the advantage of being relatively short in duration, but the disadvantages include (1) overly vigorous exercise workloads for most cardiac patients or elderly individuals with high grade (10%) from the beginning of the test; and (2) the fact that the protocol is more anaerobic in design. In practice, many patients may have to run as workloads progress beyond stage 3 of the Bruce protocol. In the Ellestad protocol, the speed is increased progressively every 3 minutes from 1.7 m.p.h. to 6.0 m.p.h. during 6 stages with constant grade (10%) for the first 4 stages and 15% grade in stages 5 and 6 (see Table 9-7).[1] It has been said that more ischemic S-T segment changes may be expected by using the Bruce or Ellestad protocol, but the incidence of false positive results may be increased due to the anaerobic nature of their protocols. In general, when any exercise protocol

Table 9-5. Target Heart Rate for Exercise ECG Test

Age	85–90% of Maximal Heart Rates
20–29	175–180
30–39	170–175
40–49	165–170
50–59	160–165
60–69	155–160
70 and above	150–155

Table 9-6. Bruce Protocol for Exercise (Treadmill) ECG Test[4]

Stage	Speed (m.p.h.)	Grade (%)	Duration (min.)	METs (units)	Total Time Elapsed (min.)
1	1.7	10	3	4	3
2	2.5	12	3	6–7	6
3	3.4	14	3	8–9	9
4	4.2	16	3	15–16	12
5	5.0	18	3	21	15
6	5.5	20	3	—	18
7	6.0	22	3	—	21

Table 9-7. Ellestad Protocol for Exercise (Treadmill) ECG Test[1]

Stage	Speed (m.p.h.)	Grade (%)	Duration (min.)	METs (units)	Total Time Elapsed (min.)
1	1.7	10	3	4	3
2	3.0	10	2	6–7	5
3	4.0	10	2	8–9	7
4	5.0	10	3	10–12	10
5	5.0	15	2	13–15	12
6	6.0	15	3	16–20	15

requires speeds beyond 3.4 m.p.h., many patients with shorter stature have to run or jog in order to keep pace. This may result in various problems, including very awkward physical posture with excessive mental stress to the patients and frequent production of excessive artifacts due to deterioration of the ECG signal.

Table 9-8 shows the Naughton protocol[2] in which 3 different methods are included. The 3 different workloads are designed according to the objectives of the test and the populations studied—different age groups from adolescence to 80 years, different status in health, physical fitness and body statures, etc. Obviously, more vigorous protocol using 3.4 m.p.h. speed may be utilized for younger and healthier populations, whereas less intense workloads with 2.0 m.p.h. speed may be required for older individuals or coronary patients (see Table 9-8). The workloads in the Naughton protocol are increased in each stage every 2 minutes for clinical exercise laboratory, whereas the workload increment is every 3 minutes for most research purposes.[12] A similar approach regarding the exercise protocol with various workloads requirements, depending upon the objectives of the test and different clinical circumstances rather than the use of any fixed exercise protocol, is also recommended by Fox.[13]

The exercise protocol designed by McHenry[3] is similar to my protocol (see Table 9-9). In his protocol,[3] after a warming-up period with 2.0 m.p.h. speed and 3% grade for 3 minutes, 3% grade is increased every 3 minutes with a constant speed of 3.3 m.p.h. during 7 stages.

Table 9-8. Naughton Protocol for Exercise (Treadmill) ECG Test[2]

Stage	2.0 m.p.h. Grade (%)	3.0 m.p.h. Grade (%)	3.4 m.p.h. Grade (%)	Duration* (min.)	METs (units)	Total Time Elapsed (min.)
1	—	—	—	2	1.0	2
2	0.0	—	—	2	2.0	4
3	3.5	0.0	—	2	3.0	6
4	7.0	2.5	2.0	2	4.0	8
5	10.5	5.0	4.0	2	5.0	10
6	14.0	7.5	6.0	2	6.0	12
7	17.5	10.0	8.0	2	7.0	14
8	—	12.5	10.0	2	8.0	16
9	—	15.0	12.0	2	9.0	18
10	—	17.5	14.0	2	10.0	20
11	—	20.0	16.0	2	11.0	22
12	—	22.5	18.0	2	12.0	24
13	—	25.0	20.0	2	13.0	26
14	—	27.5	22.0	2	14.0	28
15	—	30.0	24.0	2	15.0	30
16	—	32.5	26.0	2	16.0	32

* 3 minutes in duration for research purposes in each stage.

Table 9-9. McHenry Protocol for Exercise (Treadmill) ECG Test[3]

Stage	Speed (m.p.h.)	Grade (%)	Duration (min.)	Total Time Elapsed (min.)
1	2.0	3	3	3
2	3.3	6	3	6
3	3.3	9	3	9
4	3.3	12	3	12
5	3.3	15	3	15
6	3.3	18	3	18
7	3.3	21	3	21

Summary

1. It is extremely important to use the proper protocol for the exercise ECG test. Otherwise, the acceptable sensitivity and specificity can not be expected.

2. Nevertheless, there is no single protocol which is ideal for every clinical circumstance. Thus, the most effective and suitable protocol for a given medical institution should be carefully selected or specially designed for the expected objectives.

3. My exercise protocol consists of 7 stages in which 4% grade is increased every 3 minutes with a constant speed (3.0 m.p.h.) following the initial warming-up period with 1.7 m.p.h. and 0% grade for 3 minutes. Physically active individuals may perform further up to stage 8 or 9 as shown in Table 9-4.

4. Some investigators use different protocols requiring different workloads according to the objectives of the test and different clinical situations rather than any single fixed protocol.

5. Various parameters which should be observed and assessed during and/or after exercise include ECG changes (e.g., S-T segment alterations, cardiac arrhythmias), hemodynamic responses (blood pressure and heart rate responses), and various symptoms and signs.

6. End points to terminate the exercise ECG test should be clearly known to the physician who supervises the test. Absolute versus relative indications for the premature termination of the exercise test are listed in Table 9-3.

7. Any exercise protocol requiring speed faster than 3.4 m.p.h. often creates various untoward problems because individuals with short stature practically have to run in order to keep up the required pace. This results in a very awkward feeling for many individuals mentally or physically, and excessive artifacts are often produced on the exercise ECG tracings.

8. It is ideal to make a small booklet explaining briefly the objectives of the test, preparations for the test, and possible risks, etc., available to patients, physicians and nursing stations (see Table 9-1), so that each individual can prepare properly for the forthcoming exercise ECG test.

9. The functional capacity of a given individual can be assessed with relative accuracy judging from the exercise workloads performed in the expression of METs (see Table 9-4).

10. It is essential that properly functioning equipment be available for the exercise ECG test. Otherwise, the acceptable results from the exercise test—useful for clinical practice—can not be expected regardless of what exercise protocol is utilized.

11. The use of proper protocol will minimize or prevent possible risks involved with exercise testing.

REFERENCES

1. Ellestad, M. H.: Stress Testing. Principles and Practice, pp. 47–84, Philadelphia, F. A. Davis, 1976.
2. Naughton, J.: Stress electrocardiography in clinical electrocardiographic correlations, in Cardiovascular Clinics, edited by J. C. Rios, Vol. 8, pp. 127–139, Philadelphia, F. A. Davis, 1977.
3. McHenry, P. L. and Morris, S. N.: Exercise electrocardiography. Current state of the art, in Advances in Electrocardiography, edited by J. W. Hurst and R. C. Schlant, pp. 265–304, New York, Grune & Stratton, 1977.
4. Bruce, R. A., Blackmon, J. R., Jones, J. W. and Strait, G.: Exercise testing in adult normal subjects and cardiac patients. Pediatrics, 32:742, 1963.
5. Linhart, J. W.: Stress testing in angina. Resident & Staff Physician, pp. 79–89, Feb. 1978.
6. Fortuin, N. J. and Weiss, J. L.: Exercise stress testing. Circulation, 56:699, 1977.
7. Blackburn, H.: The exercise electrocardiogram in diagnosis. Cardiology, 62:190, 1977.
8. Faris, J. V., McHenry, P. L. and Morris, S. N.: Concepts and applications of treadmill exercise testing and the exercise electrocardiogram. Am. Heart J., 95:102, 1978.
9. Pollock, M. L., Bohannon, R. L., Cooper, K. H. et al.: A comparative analysis of four protocols for maximal treadmill stress testing. Am. Heart J., 92:39, 1976.
10. Chaitman, B. R., Bourassa, M. G., Wagniart, P. et al.: Improved efficacy of treadmill exercise testing using a multiple lead ECG system and basic hemodynamic exercise response. Circulation, 57:71, 1978.
11. Åström, H. and Jonsson, B.: Design of exercise test, with special reference to heart patients. Br. Heart J., 38:289, 1976.
12. Naughton, J.: Personal communication, 1978.
13. Fox, S. M.: Personal communication, 1978.

10

Exercise ECG Test in Children

Frederick W. James, M.D., F.A.C.C.

General Considerations

The exercise ECG test is a useful procedure in the evaluation of young subjects with cardiovascular diseases. Myocardial ischemia and cardiac arrhythmias occur in children with cardiovascular abnormalities and are often recorded on the exercise electrocardiogram. The results from this measurement have been used in the assessment of the severity and progression of cardiac disease and the evaluation of the effectiveness of medical and surgical treatment in certain patients. Although the electrocardiogram is an important variable to obtain during stress, it must be emphasized that measurements of blood pressure, systolic time intervals, cardiac output, ventilation and working capacity are also important in determining the functional impairment in a patient with a specific cardiac lesion.

This report contains illustrations of exercise electrocardiograms from different populations of children with and without clinical cardiac disease. The methods of performing an exercise ECG test and obtaining readable electrocardiographic tracings in young subjects are briefly discussed.

There is no attempt to provide a comprehensive discussion of such relevant subjects as cardiac electrophysiology, cardiac metabolism or the pathophysiologic effects of cardiac hypertrophy and/or dilatation. Furthermore, the anatomical description and clinical manifestations of specific congenital heart lesions are only briefly discussed. For any of these subject areas, the reader is referred to other available texts for appropriate discussions. The purpose of this Chapter is to demonstrate the usefulness of the exercise method and to increase the level of awareness for the abnormal electrocardiographic changes that may influence the management of cardiac disease in children.

Indications

To date, the established indications for the exercise ECG test in children are:

(1) Left or systemic ventricular outflow obstructions (i.e., subvalvar, valvar, supravalvar or coarctation of the aorta).

(2) Chronic left or right ventricular volume overload (i.e. atrioventricular or semilunar valve incompetence or left to right shunts).

(3) Cardiac rhythm and conduction disturbances (i.e., post-operative ventriculotomy, bradytachyarrhythmia syndrome or other cardiac arrhythmias in patients with or without symptoms or cardiac disease).

Further information is needed to establish the contribution of the exercise ECG test in other areas such as premature atherosclerosis, elevated resting blood pressure or in the screening of young patients with signs or symptoms suggestive of cardiovascular disease (e.g., chest pain, palpitations, fainting spells or exercise intolerance).

Preparations and Methods

The skin is cleansed with alcohol or acetone and slightly abraided with a dental burr attached to a high speed drill (Figure 10-1). This procedure is painless and, when gently applied, does not produce fluid or blood at the abraided site. The skin resistance is lowered with dental burr, and the fluid-column electrodes with electrode gel are attached to the prepared skin surface with adhesive-coated discs. These techniques facilitate obtaining electrocardiographic tracings of high fidelity and are well accepted by children.

Fourteen electrodes are attached to each subject in order to record the conventional 12-lead electrocardiogram and Frank orthogonal leads (X, Y, Z, Figures 10-2A and 2B). We have found this lead system to be very useful in detecting electrocardiographic abnormalities in subjects within the pediatric age group. Three electrocardiographic leads (usually V_1, V_5, V_6) are simultaneously recorded and the other leads are rapidly scanned for significant changes. The left precordial (V_{4-6}) leads are reviewed in left heart lesions, and the right precordial and augmented leads in right heart lesions. In both right and left heart lesions, the inferior leads are also recorded. This 15-lead system is very simple to set up and use for routine exercise testing in children (Figure 10-2A). We advocate multilead electrocardiography with perhaps a minimum of three leads (V_1 or V_2, V_5, aVF or X, Y, Z) for proper detection and analysis of cardiac arrhythmia and S-T segment displacement in children with or without clinical cardiac disease.

Exercise ECG Test in Various Clinical Circumstances

A continuous graded bicycle[1] and steady-state exercise ECG tests with a 20-minute interval rest period between each test are routinely performed in our laboratory. There are three work schedules which are based upon body surface area in the continuous graded exercise test protocol. The details of the work schedules are given in Table 10-1. The challenge in each work schedule is designed for the majority of subjects to reach their maximal voluntary capacity in less than 9 minutes in schedule I, less than 12 minutes

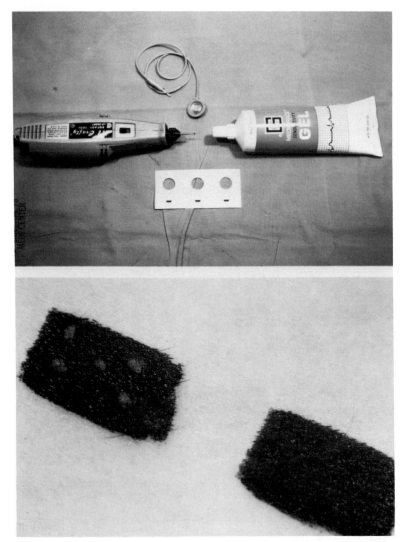

Fig. 10-1   (Upper panel) The skin is abraided with a dental burr attached to a high speed drill. The fluid-column electrodes with electrode gel are attached to the skin with adhesive-coated discs. (Lower panel) A marking pencil is used at each electrode site. The drill is gently applied five times at each site. There is no discomfort, fluid or blood produced when the technique is gently applied.

in II, less than 15 minutes for untrained subjects and less than 30 minutes for highly trained subjects in III. The goals of this continuous graded exercise test are:

(1) to reach the maximal voluntary capacity level (exhaustion) or to provoke significantly abnormal cardiovascular responses in a subject;

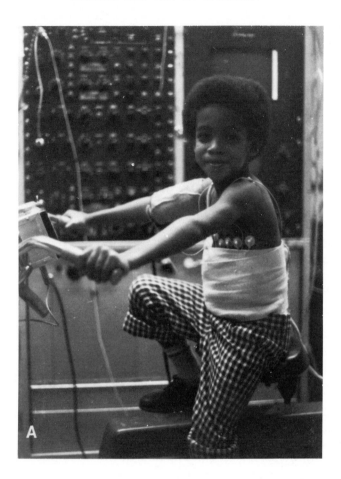

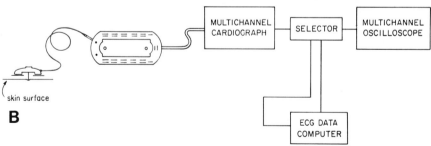

Fig. 10-2 (A) This 5-year-old normal child has 14 electrodes attached to the chest and back. The upper limb leads are attached over the acromion of each shoulder and the lower limb leads are placed at the umbilical area (left leg lead) and right hip (right leg lead). (B) This schematic diagram reveals the components of the recording system. All electrodes are connected to a 14-wire flexible cable. The electrocardiographic leads are displayed on an oscilloscope. Any lead can be analyzed manually or by the data computer.

Table 10-1. Continuous Graded Bicycle Exercise Protocol Work Schedules (I, II, III)*

BSA	I	II	III
	<1M²†	1–1.19 M²	≥1.2 M²
Level 1	200	200	200
Level 2	300	400	500
Level 3	500	600	800
Increments	100	100	200

* Three exercise programs are used for three ranges of body surface areas (BSA). If three exercise levels are completed, the workload is increased at 100 or 200 kilogram-meters/min. increments until the maximal voluntary capacity is reached (rpm = revolutions/min.; adapted from James et al. Circulation, 54: 671, 1976, by permission of the American Heart Association, Inc.)

† M^2 = meters², body surface area; pedal speed = 60–70 rpm; workload = kilogram-meters/min.; workload duration = 3 min.

(2) to assess the process of adaptation to a given stress level by the non-invasive measurement of multiple variables (i.e., heart rate, electrocardiogram, blood pressure, etc.); and

(3) to obtain the highest steady-state workload for the estimation of maximal oxygen consumption.

A steady-state exercise ECG test usually follows the continuous graded exercise after a 20-minute interval rest period. The steady-state exercise ECG test is an addition to the pre-operative and longitudinal post-operative assessment of patients with congenital heart disease. Both exercise procedures are well tolerated by children and have been successfully performed in many subjects as young as 5 or 6 years old.

A. Exercise Electrocardiogram in Normal Children

In the normal child, a major change on the exercise electrocardiogram is a decrease in the R-R interval, which is commensurate with the level of exercise. The decrease in the duration of the R-R interval is primarily due to shortening of the T-P and Q-T intervals (Figure 10-3). The amplitude of the QRS complex may vary considerably with respiration, especially in the left precordial leads in adolescent subjects during high levels of exercise. The morphology of T waves in the left precordial and inferior leads is often influenced by position, respiration and heart rate.

In 40 normal subjects (20 males and 20 females) ages 5 to 22 years with normal blood lipids, the average decrease in R-R interval from rest to the

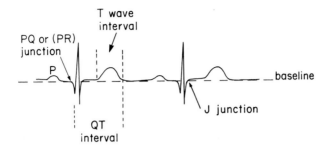

PRE EXERCISE

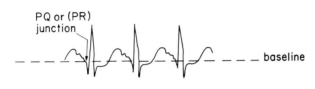

DURING EXERCISE

Fig. 10.3 Schematic diagram of typical changes of the electrocardiogram from rest to exercise. The baseline is established by connecting the P-Q (or P-R) junction of consecutive QRS complexes. The P-Q (or P-R) segment coincides with this baseline at rest but is often deviated upward by the terminal portion of the T wave. The T-P, Q-T intervals and T wave duration decrease with shortening of the R-R interval. The S-T segment displacement during exercise is analyzed in relation to the baseline of connecting P-Q or P-R junctions.

maximal voluntary capacity level was approximately 56%. The major change in the R-R interval was due to the shortening of the T-P interval with a 33% decrease in the Q-T interval (Table 10-2). The duration of the T wave decreased by 18% in the males and 48% in the females. The QRS interval remained fairly constant in each group at rest and during exercise. Frequently, the apex of the P wave was recorded on the terminal portion of the T wave, affecting satisfactory estimates of the P-R interval.

The S-T segment also decreased in duration during exercise and was occasionally encroached upon by the initial portion of the T wave. During strenuous exercise, the baseline for measuring S-T segment displacement was established by connecting the P-R or P-Q junctions of 5 consecutive QRS complexes (Figure 10-3). The criteria for a positive exercise electrocardiogram were S-T segment depression greater than or equal to 1 mm. extending for at least 0.06 second after the J-point below the baseline with

Table 10-2. Analysis of Exercise Electrocardiogram in Normal Male and Female Children

No.			Levels (mm)			Intervals (Sec)			
			J Point	S-T Seg-ment	S-T* Slope	R-R	Q-T	T-wave Duration (sec)	Age (yrs)
Males	R	X̄	+0.59	+0.68	+0.79	0.72	0.35	0.17	15.3
(20)		±SE	0.09	0.09	0.17	0.03	0.00	0.00	1.6
	E	X̄	−0.75	−0.30	+5.7	0.31	0.23	0.14	
		±SE	0.16	0.07	0.5	0.00	0.00	0.00	
Females	R	X̄	+0.32	+0.37	+0.35	0.76	0.36	0.21	14.5
(20)		±SE	0.06	0.07	0.10	0.03	0.00	0.00	1.2
	E	X̄	−1.2	−0.62	+2.8	0.33	0.24	0.11	
		±SE	0.12	0.08	0.3	0.00	0.00	0.00	

† (Slope = millivolts/second; mm = millimeter; sec = seconds; yrs = years; X̄ ± SE = mean ± standard error of mean).

a horizontal, upward or downward sloping S-T segment or the induction or aggravation of cardiac arrhythmia. We have reported the electrocardiographic results of 103 (55 males and 48 females) asymptomatic children, ages 5 to 21 years, with normal blood lipids, resting supine blood pressures, cardiac examinations and without documented cardiac arrhythmias at rest using the above criteria.[2] Seven percent of normal males and 14% of normal females had 1 to 2 mm. S-T segment depression on the exercise electrocardiogram. The magnitude and distribution of the S-T segment depression are illustrated in Table 10-3. Eleven children had significant depression of the S-T segment with 8/11 (73%) recorded in lead V_5 only and 1/11 (10%) in the inferior leads (Y, II, III and aVF). Isolated depression of the J-junction (i.e., without S-T segment depression) did not exceed 2 mm. in any normal subject. Cardiac arrhythmias were not recorded pre-exercise, during or within 20 minutes post-exercise in any of the normal children. The significance of the S-T segment depression in this normal pediatric population is uncertain at this present time. Interestingly, the higher percentage of normal female children with S-T segment depression than normal male children is similar to the occurrence in the normal adult female as compared to the normal adult male.[3] We have used these observations in this asymptomatic population as a reference in identifying the normal exercise electrocardiographic changes in children.

B. Abnormal S-T Segmental Depression

(1) Pressure Overload of the Left Ventricle

Congenital aortic stenosis is reported in up to 5% of pediatric cardiac patients with most frequent site of obstruction located at the valvar and

Table 10-3. Segmental S-T Depression (in Millimeters) According to Electrocardiographic Leads During Maximal Voluntary Exercise in Normal Children

		V_5	V_6	X	Y, II, III or aVF
			Leads		
Males					
	1.)	2			
	2.)	1			
	3.)	1			
	4.)	1	1		
Females					
	5.)	1			
	6.)	1			
	7.)	1.5			
	8.)				1
	9.)	2			
	10.)	1			
	11.)			1	

subvalvar areas.[4] Many patients with significant valvar or subvalvar obstruction may have normal resting electrocardiograms (ECG) and normal heart sizes on routine chest radiographs. On the other hand, the exercise electrocardiogram is frequently abnormal in this cardiac lesion and appears to be more sensitive to the effect of significant obstruction to the left ventricle than the resting electrocardiogram.[5] The frequency of significant depression of S-T segment on the exercise electrocardiogram increases with a rising resting peak left ventricular to aortic (LV-Ao) systolic pressure gradient.[5, 6] The magnitude of the S-T segment depression is usually greatest in those patients with peak LV-Ao systolic pressure gradient at or above 70 mm. Hg. In 52 patients with valvar or discrete subvalvar aortic stenosis, significant S-T segment depression occurred during exercise in 46% of patients with resting LV-Ao systolic pressure gradient of less than 30 mm. Hg., 58% with resting gradients between 30 and 69 mm. Hg. and 87% with resting gradients at or above 70 mm. Hg. There were no episodes of syncope, dizziness or pallor in this patient group during the exercise procedure. However, two patients with LV-Ao gradients of 75 and 235 mm. Hg. developed mild chest pain during the exercise test. Figure 10-4 illustrates depression of the S-T segment in a 12-year-old patient with a resting LV-Ao systolic pressure gradient of 110 mm. Hg. This degree of S-T depression occurred at 85% of the patient's estimated maximal working capacity with an oxygen consumption approximately 5 times normal. The S-T segment depression regressed immediately after exercise with almost a complete return to the pre-exercise level at 5 minutes. In this patient, the ischemic S-T segment regressed towards normal after adequate surgical relief of obstruction although com-

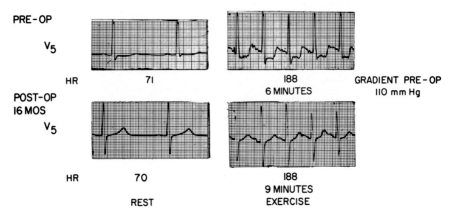

Fig. 10-4 Exercise electrocardiograms in a 12-year-old boy with valvar aortic stenosis before and after valvotomy. Pre-operative (Pre-op), horizontal S-T segment depression was recorded without symptoms of chest pain. Sixteen months (MOS) post-operative (Post-op), S-T segments are normal with a significant increase in working capacity (exercise time). (HR—heart rate, paper speed—50 mm/second). (From F. W. James,[18] with permission.)

plete resolution did not occur until the late post-operative period (Figure 10-4).

Significant obstruction at the supravalvar area (supravalvar aortic stenosis) also produces S-T depression on the exercise electrocardiogram. Figure 10-5 depicts depression and resolution of the S-T segment in the same patient before and after adequate relief of an aortic gradient of 66 mm. Hg.

In our laboratory, exercise studies have been performed on 5 patients with *idiopathic hypertrophic subaortic stenosis* and resting peak left ventricular to aortic systolic pressure gradient greater than or equal to 50 mm. Hg. Significant S-T segment depression occurred in each patient with an inappropriate rise in heart rate for the specific level of exercise. Figure 10-6 illustrates the heart rate and S-T segment displacement in a 10-year-old girl during exercise before and during propranolol therapy. The resting LV-Ao systolic pressure gradient was 65 mm. Hg. with a normal cardiac output. Prior to drug therapy, the elevated heart rate with significant S-T segment depression occurred during the early phase of the exercise test (2.5 minutes). During propranolol therapy, exercise tolerance increased with an appropriate response in heart rate. However, significant S-T segment depression was also recorded when the heart rate reached 140 beats/minute. Further studies are needed to determine the usefulness of exercise testing in the medical management of patients with cardiomyopathy with or without obstruction.

The frequency of S-T segment depression during exercise is increased in

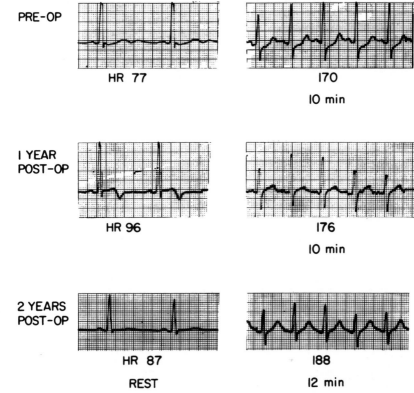

Fig. 10-5 Serial exercise electrocardiograms in a patient with subvalvar aortic stenosis. Pre-operatively (pre-op), the resting aortic gradient was 66 mm. Hg. Upper panel, S-T segment depression with upward sloping segment occurred at heart rate (HR) of 170 beats/minute. One year post-operatively (Post-op), T waves are inverted at rest and upright during exercise. S-T segments are normal. Two years post-op, resting T waves are improved and exercise electrocardiogram is normal (paper speed—50 mm./second; lead V₅).

patients with *coarctation of the aorta* before or after resection of coarctation of the aorta.[7] The S-T segment depression occurs in the absence of significant aortic valve disease or residual obstruction across the site of surgical resection (Figure 10-7). In 21 patients who had pre-operative exercise studies, 5 of 12 (42%) males and 6 of 9 (67%) females had S-T segment depression between 1 and 3 mm. during exercise. Similarly, increased frequency of S-T segment depression between 1 to 5 mm. was recorded in

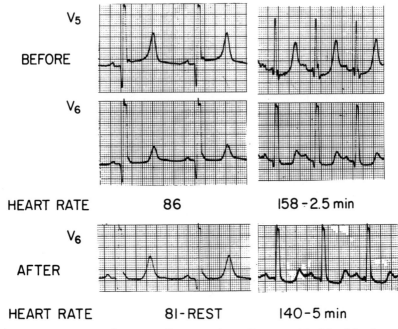

Fig. 10-6. Exercise electrocardiograms in a 10-year-old girl with obstructive cardiomyopathy before and after propranolol therapy. Upper panel, the depression of the S-T segment occurs with an inappropriately elevated heart rate for the exercise level. Lower panel, although the S-T segment is depressed, after propranolol therapy, the exercise time has doubled and the heart rate is appropriate for the exercise level (paper speed—50 mm./second).

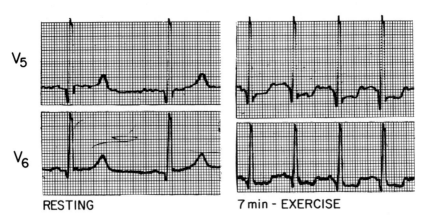

Fig. 10-7 Significant depression of the S-T segment in a 15-year-old boy, 6 years after coarctectomy. The aortic valve was functioning normally and a 25 mm. Hg. gradient was measured across the site of resection (paper speed—50 mm./second). (From F. W. James,[18] with permission.)

48 patients (28% of 29 males and 63% of 19 females) after coarctectomy. In several pre-operative or post-operative patients, the exercise test was stopped because of exertional dyspnea and/or systolic hypertension. Although these responses may precede the electrocardiographic changes, often the abnormal S-T segment depression in part may be related to residual left ventricular hypertrophy due to chronic hypertension[7, 8] or atheromatous changes in the coronary arteries.[9]

It is important to realize that significant S-T segment depression may not always appear on the electrocardiogram in a few patients with severe left ventricular outflow tract obstruction. Figure 10-8 depicts the exercise electrocardiogram in a 7-year-old boy who has severe valvar aortic stenosis (resting gradient 235 mm. Hg.) and 2 years after resection of coarctation of the aorta. During exercise, the heart rate increased to 176 beats/minute without any significant depression of the S-T segment. Despite these findings, it is uncommon to have normal S-T segment on the exercise electrocardiogram in subjects with isolated significant aortic stenosis.[5, 6] The severity of the obstruction in this patient was demonstrated by additional measurements of blood pressure, systolic time intervals and working capacity.[6]

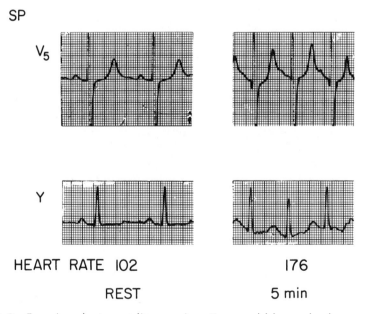

SP

V₅

Y

HEART RATE 102   176

REST   5 min

Fig. 10-8 Exercise electrocardiogram in a 7-year-old boy who has a resting left ventricular to aortic peak systolic gradient of 235 mm. Hg., 2 years after a successful coarctectomy. There is no significant depression of the S-T segment during exercise (paper speed—50 mm./second).

(2) Volume Overload of the Left Ventricle

Isolated *aortic valve incompetence* with significant left ventricular dilatation may be associated with ischemic-like S-T segment.[10] The frequency appears to increase with progressive enlargement of the left ventricle. Figure 10-9 illustrates S-T segment depression in a 15-year-old patient with aortic valve incompetence, left ventricular hypertrophy on resting electrocardiogram and mild to moderate cardiac enlargement on chest radiograph. Since the timing of surgical treatment is difficult in patients with aortic valve

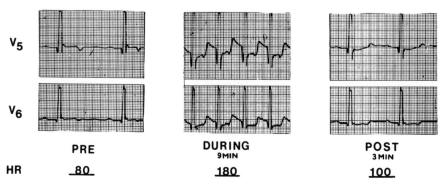

PRE	DURING 9MIN	POST 3MIN
HR 80	180	100

Fig. 10-9 Marked depression of the S-T segment during exercise in a 15-year-old adolescent with aortic insufficiency. There is a rapid regression towards pre-exercise level of the S-T segment within 3 minutes after exercise. T waves are affected by position and heart rate (paper speed—50 mm./second). (Adapted from F. W. James.[18])

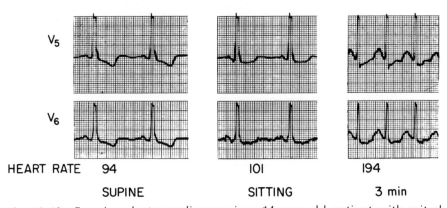

HEART RATE 94	101	194
SUPINE	SITTING	3 min

Fig. 10-10 Exercise electrocardiogram in a 14-year-old patient with mitral incompetence due to a past episode of rheumatic fever. Significant S-T segment depression and an inappropriately elevated heart rate for the exercise level are recorded (paper speed—50 mm./second).

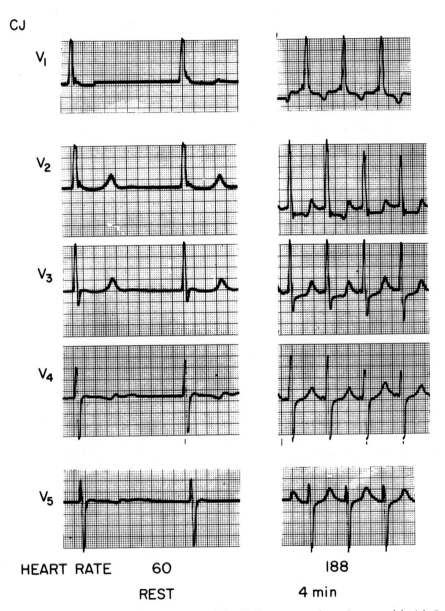

Fig. 10-11 Significant depression of the S-T segment in a 9-year-old girl, 5 years after Mustard operation for transposition of the great vessels. The abnormal S-T segments are primarily recorded in leads V_2 and V_3 (paper speed—50 mm./second).

incompetence, these results are of clinical importance because of the potential benefit of detecting early dysfunction of the myocardium.

Patients with *mitral valve incompetence* and cardiac enlargement may have an abnormal electrocardiogram at rest and more progressive changes during stress. Depression of the S-T segment is seen during exercise in a 14-year-old patient with moderate to severe mitral incompetence due to a previous episode of rheumatic fever (Figure 10-10). At cardiac catheterization, the left ventricular end diastolic pressure was 11 mm. Hg. with pulmonary arterial pressure of 60/41 mm. Hg. Left ventricular end diastolic and left atrial dimensions were 67% (7 cm.) and 300% (6.7 cm.) of predicted normal. It appears that the frequency of S-T segment depression increases in young patients with progressive enlargement of the left ventricle from valvular incompetence.

Mitral valve prolapse is often present without any significant cardiac enlargement. However, ventricular arrhythmia and exercise-induced S-T segment depression[11] occur more frequently in this disease than in normal children. These electrocardiographic abnormalities occurred in 16% of 30 young patients (average age 13.9 years) with mitral valve prolapse. During

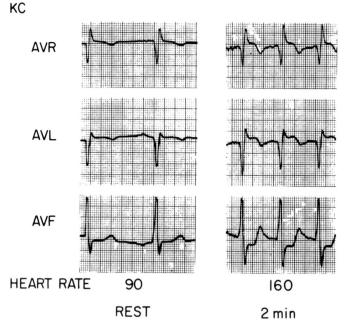

Fig. 10-12 Significant S-T segment displacement in a 13-year-old girl with tetralogy of Fallot, significant pressure and volume overloads of the right ventricle. The S-T segments are elevated in leads aVR, aVL and depressed in aVF (paper speed—50 mm./second).

exercise, S-T segment depression of 1 to 3 mm. occurred in 12 patients (3 of 10 males and 9 of 20 females). Chest pain did not occur in any of the 30 patients. Although the degree of mitral incompetence varies in this disease, the S-T segment depression is probably not related to cardiac enlargement in these patients.

(3) Pressure Overload of the Right Ventricle

In *transposition of the great vessels* and after a Mustard procedure, the systemic arterial chamber is now the morphologic right ventricle and the systemic venous chamber is the morphologic left ventricle. There is much

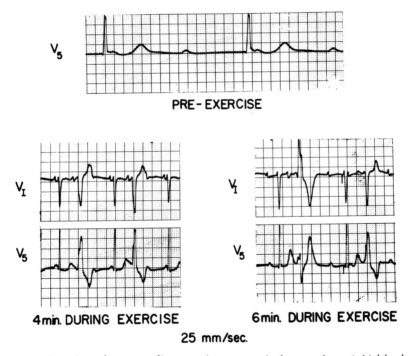

Fig. 10-13 Exercise electrocardiogram in congenital complete A-V block. Atrial rates were 75 beats/minute at rest and 136 at 6 minutes of exercise. Multifocal ventricular premature contractions with left or right bundle branch block patterns in bigeminal rhythm were recorded. This arrhythmia persisted until 10 minutes after exercise. The spike before the third QRS complex in the 6-minute tracing is an artifact (Upper panel: paper speed—50 mm./second). (From F. W. James: Postgrad. Med., 56:53, 1974, with permission.)

concern as to whether the right ventricle is capable of sustaining a systemic pressure load for the expected life span of the child.

Jarmakani et al.[12] reported abnormally low right ventricular ejection fractions in infants with complete transposition of the great vessels and intact ventricular septum before and after Mustard procedure. These results suggested the presence of right ventricular dysfunction. On the other hand, Godman et al.[13] assessed the contractility of the right ventricle by measuring the peak velocity of the contractile element in 13 of 14 patients 4 to 10 years after a Mustard operation. These authors concluded that the right ventricle is capable of functioning as a sytemic arterial ventricle. It is obvious that further clinical studies are needed before any firm conclusion can be drawn on this important subject.

An evaluation of these patients under stress is potentially beneficial in detecting right ventricular dysfunction and conduction or rhythm disturbances. In Figure 10-11, ischemic S-T segment depression occurred selectively in leads V_2 and V_3 with minimal or no changes in remaining precordial or inferior leads. There is also an absence of normal sinus node function in this patient 5 years after the Mustard operation.

In *tetralogy of Fallot* pre-operatively, the exercise response is characterized by early exertional dyspnea and cyanosis due to increased right to left intracardiac shunting and decreased pulmonary blood flow. The right ventricle is under an increased pressure load because of the severe obstruction in the right ventricular outflow tract. When the pulmonary valve is absent and the outflow tract is hypoplastic, the right ventricle is exposed to pressure and volume overloads. Figure 10-12 illustrates the superior and inferior lead S-T segment changes in a patient with tetralogy of Fallot with absent pulmonary valve and left pulmonary artery. In patients with right ventricular hypertrophy with or without dilatation, the S-T segment changes are

KB

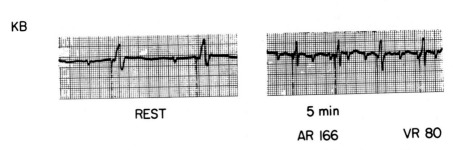

REST   5 min

                        AR 166   VR 80

Fig. 10-14 Exercise electrocardiogram in a 13-year-old patient with complete A-V block after closure of a ventricular septal defect (left panel: paper speed—25 mm./second). At 5 minutes of exercise, atrial rate (AR) increased normally with no change in the ventricular rate (VR). An artificial pacemaker spike is seen before each ventricular complex (right panel: paper speed—50 mm./second; lead V_1).

mostly recorded in the mid- to right precordial, inferior and superior leads on the electrocardiogram.

C. Cardiac Arrhythmias

(1) With Congential Heart Lesions

Patients with congenital *complete atrioventricular (A-V) block* often have near normal physical activity. The exercise capacity, in part, is related to an increased stroke volume and a moderate rise in ventricular rate. The ventricular rate may rise up to 160 beats/minute with a normal increase in atrial rate commensurate with the level of exercise. Ventricular arrhythmias

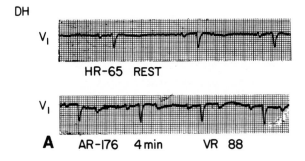

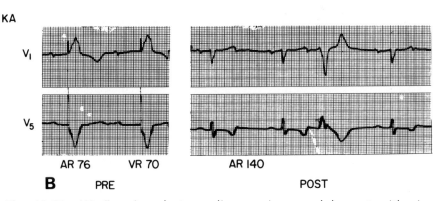

Fig. 10-15 (A) Exercise electrocardiogram in an adolescent with sinus bradycardia with first degree A-V block at rest and 2:1 A-V block during exercise one year after closure of secundum atrial defect (paper speed—50 mm./second). (B) Second degree (2:1) A-V block and unifocal ventricular premature contractions during exercise in a 7-year-old patient after surgical closure of secundum atrial septal defect. The artificial pacemaker spikes are not seen because of the shorter R-R intervals (paper speed—50 mm./second).

have been induced by exercise in patients with congenital complete A-V block.[14] In Figure 10-13 the electrocardiogram shows a normal atrial and increased ventricular rates with ventricular arrhythmia during exercise in a 19-year-old patient with congenital complete A-V block. In nine patients with complete A-V block five developed frequent unifocal or multifocal ventricular premature contractions during exercise which persisted after exercise in three. Further studies are needed to determine the clinical significance of these arrhythmias in this congenital lesion.

Complete A-V block is a well recognized complication after open heart surgery for congenital heart disease. Figure 10-14 illustrated an expected exercise response in the atrial rate while the ventricle is being artificially paced in a patient after surgically induced complete A-V block. Ventricular arrhythmias may also occur during exercise in these patients with acquired complete A-V block.

Serious rhythm or conduction disturbances have occurred after surgical repair of *atrial septal defect*. Figures 10-15A and 15B represent two patients with conduction abnormalities following surgical closure of secundum atrial septal defect. Figure 10-15A contains electrocardiographic tracings in a patient who had normal atrioventricular conduction at rest. At 3 minutes of exercise, the heart rate was 140 beats/minute. One minute later, a Wenckebach A-V block occurred with further progression to 2:1 A-V block and a decrease in the ventricular rate to 88 beats/minute. The second patient

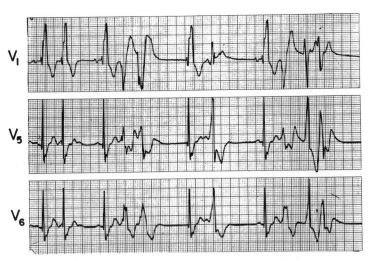

Fig. 10-16   Post-exercise electrocardiogram in a patient after intracardiac repair for tetralogy of Fallot. Short "bursts" of ventricular tachycardia were recorded (paper speed—50 mm./second). (From F. W. James and S. Kaplan: Circulation, 52:691, 1975, with permission of the American Heart Association, Inc.)

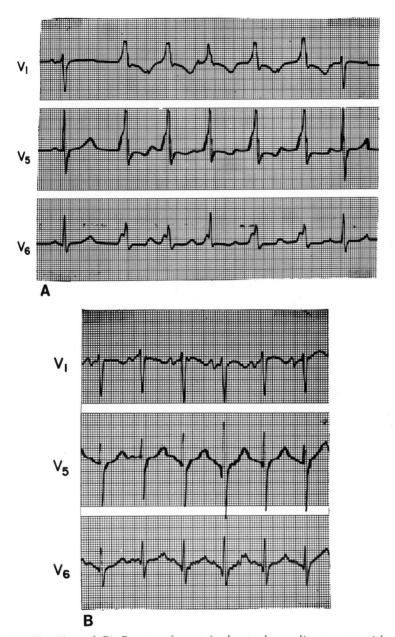

Fig. 10-17 (A and B) Bursts of ventricular tachycardia at rest with sinus suppression during exercise in a 13-year-old male with a "normal" heart (paper speed—50 mm./second). (From F. W. James,[18] with permission.)

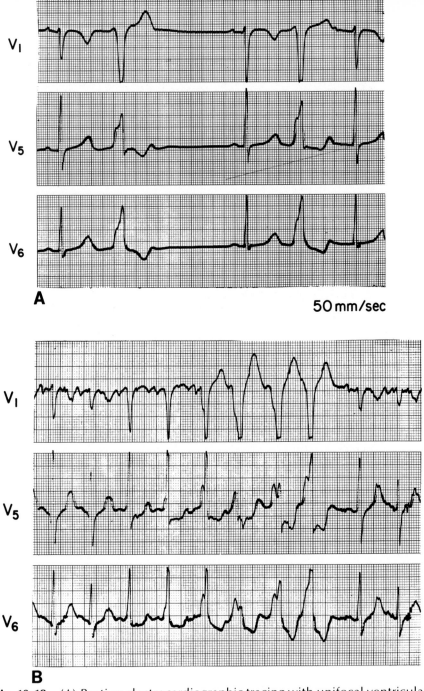

Fig. 10-18 (A) Resting electrocardiographic tracing with unifocal ventricular premature contractions in a 10-year-old girl with a "normal" heart. (B) Burst of ventricular tachycardia during exercise in the same patient with a "normal" heart. A series of fusion beats are seen after two normal QRS complexes (Paper speed—50 mm./second). (From F. W. James and S. Kaplan, Primary Cardiology, *3*:34, 1977, with permission.)

(Figure 10-15B) required an artificial pacemaker after surgical repair of the atrial septal defect because of symptoms due to a slow ventricular rate (40 beats/minute). During exercise, the ventricular rate increased with 2:1 atrioventricular conduction.

Conduction disturbances are common in patients after intracardiac repair of *tetralogy of Fallot.* Unexpected cardiac arrest has occurred several years after adequate surgical repair of the defects in patients without bifascicular or trifascicular block immediately following surgery.[15] Exercise can be used to detect serious ventricular arrhythmias in patients after intracardiac surgery. Atrial or ventricular premature contractions have been recorded in up to 23% of patients after surgery for Fallot's tetralogy.[1] Patients who developed multifocal ventricular premature contractions also had short bursts of ventricular tachycardia after exercise (Figure 10-16). It is hypothesized that the sudden cardiac arrest in these patients was preceded by ventricular tachyarrhythmias. Our current approach is to perform the Holter monitor ECG and exercise ECG test in patients who have ventricular premature contractions at rest. If frequent ventricular premature contractions or bursts of ventricular tachycardia are documented, we recommend antiarrhythmic therapy in an attempt to prevent ventricular tachyarrhythmias. The effectiveness of the drug therapy is determined by repeated Holter monitor ECG and/or exercise ECG test.

(2) Without Congenital Heart Lesions

Ventricular ectopy probably occurs more frequently in children without overt cardiac abnormalities than is currently appreciated. Although many children are asymptomatic, some may have symptoms which necessitate

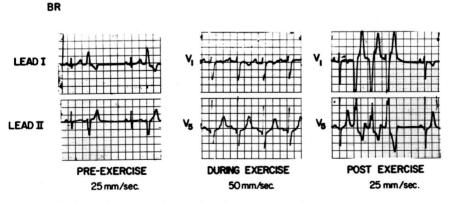

Fig. 10-19 Ventricular tachycardia after exercise in a 13-year-old patient with a "normal" heart. (From F. W. James, Postgrad. Med., *56:*53, 1974, with permission.)

drug therapy in an attempt to control the ventricular arrhythmias.[16] Figures 10-17A and B, 18A and B and 19 are exercise electrocardiograms of three patients which describe the pattern of response of three subgroups in the pediatric population with ventricular ectopy. Ventricular tachycardia is recorded in each patient. In Figures 10-17A and B, ventricular tachycardia is recorded at rest and suppressed during exercise in a 13-year-old boy. In Figures 10-18A and B and 19, ventricular tachycardia is recorded only during exercise or after exercise in the remaining two patients. Each of these patients had ventricular ectopy at rest. Although exercise may suppress ventricular arrhythmias, it is unclear as to whether this procedure can be used to determine the prognosis of ventricular ectopy in children.

D. Coronary Artery Disease

Overt coronary occlusive disease occurs in a small percentage of patients within the pediatric age group. The clinical picture of patients with *homozygous familial hypercholesterolemia* is characterized by angina pectoris, myocardial infarction (usually prior to age 20) and aortic stenosis due to aortic ring atheromata.[17] Figure 10-20 demonstrates the progressive change in S-T segments on the exercise electrocardiogram with only a modest increase in the heart rate. This patient died suddenly 2 months after the exercise study at the age of 17.

Summary

(1) Significant depression of the S-T segment and serious cardiac arrhythmias may occur in a variety of cardiac lesions which are clinically significant in the pediatric patients.

(2) The exercise ECG test is useful in unmasking these electrocardiographic abnormalities which are important in the clinical management of cardiovascular disease.

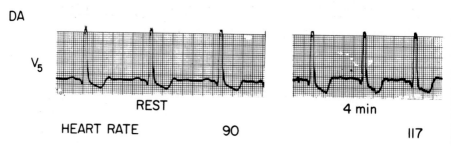

DA

V₅

REST   4 min

HEART RATE   90   117

Fig. 10-20 Progressive depression of the S-T segment on exercise electrocardiogram with minimal elevation of heart rate in a patient with familial homozygous hypercholesterolemia (paper speed 50 mm./second).

(3) The S-T segment depression and serious cardiac arrhythmias relate to the severity of a cardiac lesion, and the resolution of these findings may be an index of the adequacy of medical and surgical treatments.

(4) It has been demonstrated that multilead electrocardiography yields more information than single-lead electrocardiography and perhaps should be the basic monitoring system during the exercise ECG test in children.

REFERENCES

1. James, F. W., Kaplan, S., Schwartz, D. C., Chou, T. C., Sandker, M. J. and Naylor, V.: Response to exercise in patients after total surgical correction of tetralogy of Fallot. Circulation, 54:671, 1976.
2. James, F. W., Glueck, C. J., Fallat, R. W., Millett, F. and Kaplan, S.: Maximal exercise stress testing in normal and hyperlipidemic children. Atherosclerosis, 25:85, 1976.
3. Cumming, G. R., Dufresne, C., Kich, L. and Samm, J.: Exercise electrocardiogram patterns in normal women. Br. Heart J. 35:1055, 1973.
4. Lambert, E. C., Colombi, M., Wagner, H. R. and Vlad, P.: The clinical outlook of congenital aortic stenosis (valvar and discrete subvalvar) prior to surgery, In The Natural History and Progress in Treatment of Congenital Heart Defect, edited by B. S. L. Kidd and J. D. Keith, p. 205, Springfield, Ill., Charles C Thomas, 1971.
5. Halloren, H. H.: The telemetered exercise electrocardiogram in congenital aortic stenosis. Pediatrics, 47:31, 1971.
6. James, F. W. and Kaplan, S.: Spectrum of exercise responses in children with aortic stenosis. Pediatr. Res., 11:393, 1977.
7. James, F. W., Kaplan, S. and Schwartz, D. C.: Ischemic ST segments during exercise in children after coarctectomy. (Abstr.) Am. J. Cardiol., 37:145, 1976.
8. James, F. W. and Kaplan, S.: Systolic hypertension during submaximal exercise after correction of coarctation of aorta. Circulation (Suppl. II), 50:11–27, 1974.
9. Vlodaver, Z. and Newfeld, H. N.: Coronary arteries in coarctation of the aorta. Circulation, 37:449, 1968.
10. James, F. W. and Kaplan, S.: ST depression and systolic hypertension during exercise in aortic insufficiency. Proceeding: American Academy of Pediatrics, San Francisco, Oct. 1974.
11. Schwartz, D. C., James, F. W. and Kaplan, S.: Exercise induced ST segment depression in children with mitral valve prolapse. Circulation (Suppl. II), 52:11–67, 1975.
12. Jarmakani, J. M. M. and Canent, R. V., Jr.: Preoperative and postoperative right ventricular function in children with transposition of the great vessels. Circulation (Suppl. II), 50:11–39, 1974.
13. Godman, M. J., Friedli, B., Pasternac, A., Kidd, B. S. L., Trusler, G. A. and Mustard, W. T.: Hemodynamic studies in children four to ten years after the Mustard operation for transposition of the great arteries. Circulation, 53:532, 1976.
14. Holmgren, A., Karlberg, P. and Pernow, B.: Circulatory adaptation at rest and during muscular work in patients with complete heart block. Acta Med. Scand., 164:119, 1959.
15. James, F. W. and Kaplan, S.: Unexpected cardiac arrest in patients after surgical correction of tetralogy of Fallot. Circulation, 52:691, 1975.
16. Hernandez, A., Strauss, A., Kleiger, R. E. and Goldring, D.: Idiopathic paroxysmal ventricular tachycardia in infants and children. J. Pediatr., 86:182, 1975.
17. Goldstein, J. L., Schrott, H. R., Hazzard, W. R., Bierman, E. L. and Motulsky, A. G.: Hyperlipidemia in coronary heart disease, Part 2 (Genetic analysis of lipid levels in 176 families and delineation of new inherited disorder, combined hyperlipidemia). J. Clin. Invest., 52:1544, 1973.
18. James, F. W.: Exercise testing in children and young adults: An overview. In Cardiovascular Clinics, Exercise and the Heart, edited by N. K. Wenger, p. 187, Philadelphia, F. A. Davis, 1978.

11

Physiologic Versus Abnormal Responses to Exercise

John P. Naughton, M.D., F.A.C.P., F.A.C.C.

General Considerations

Physical activity or exercise is an action in which all forms of animal life participate regardless of age or health status. By definition, exercise requires movement, and as such, increases the metabolic rate of the body over that of normal resting demands. Many forms of physical activity place no greater stress on the body than do various forms of emotional stress. Examples of such activity include sitting, standing, typewriting and playing a game of cards. However, activities customarily performed such as stair climbing, fast walking, gardening and sailing, to name but a few, can place relatively heavy demands on the body and require an integral set of adaptations in order to cope in an efficient and safe manner. Some of the normal and abnormal adaptations to physical stress with which all physicians participating in cardiac care should be familiar will be discussed in this Chapter.

Physiologic Responses to Exercise

I. Oxygen Metabolism

Physical activity places a stress on the body which requires multiple adaptations. This activity by necessity increases the body's metabolic rate; therefore, the required oxygen (O_2) intake that satisfies an aerobic performance is increased. Oxygen is the fuel which makes it possible to use the substances provided by fat and carbohydrate to supply the required energy of metabolism. In a normal aerobic form of activity the body responds to the increased stress by increasing the O_2 intake. Although the level of metabolic rate increases immediately with the onset of activity, there is a lag from the onset to the time at which the body consumes the level of O_2 required for the effort. The lag time is related to the intensity of the effort in relation to the individual's performance capacity. Thus, at a low level of exercise stress, the time from the onset of activity to equilibration is short, and at a high level of exercise stress it can be as long as several minutes. Several terms are used to define the O_2 intake curve:

1. O_2 intake—the O_2 consumed/unit time.
2. O_2 deficit—the amount of deficit which occurs from the time an activity begins until the proper level of O_2 is consumed. During this period of time, energy is being supplied from other, non-O_2 sources, and the deficit must be repaid at the end of the performance.
3. Steady state—that point at which the O_2 intake remains constant and is ample to meet the metabolic requirements of the task.
4. O_2 debt—the O_2 requirement which exists above the resting requirements during recovery. Its value should approximate all of the anaerobic requirements of the exercise, and it might take several hours to satisfy the effort, particularly if it was maximal or near maximal.

In the performance of aerobic exercise, the goal is to work within the range of an individual's maximal O_2 threshold and to attain a steady state performance. In all but minimal efforts the time required to achieve a steady state level of O_2 intake ranges from as low as 3 to as high as 6 minutes. As a general rule, the shorter and more taxing the task, the greater the degree of anaerobic work, whereas the longer the task, the more likely that it is performed aerobically.

Man's capacity for O_2 intake varies considerably depending on factors such as age, sex, muscle mass, body weight and composition, physical conditions and health status. World champion athletes capable of Olympic pentathalon competition may have maximal O_2 intakes of 6.0 liters/minute or approximately 80 ml. O_2/Kg./min. Healthy human subjects who are regularly active, but not competitive, may have maximal O_2 intakes in the range of 3.4 liters or 45 ml. O_2/kg./min., whereas cardiovascular patients of functional class II status (NYHA) may be limited to less than 1.0 liter of maximal O_2 intake or from 10.5–14.0 ml. O_2/kg./min.

In every activity, there is an element of anaerobiosis. However, if the activity is adjusted to the individual's particular capacity and maintained for a prolonged period of time, the anaerobic requirements can be minimized. As an individual approaches his aerobic limitations the degree of anaerobic metabolism increases. This is best reflected in the blood lactate and pH levels. When a subject works at an energy requirement which exceeds his aerobic capacity, he is performing anaerobic work, a type of effort that the physically unconditioned can tolerate for a very brief period of time and the well conditioned athlete for 4–6 minutes. The point at which a person begins working at an energy requirement to which he cannot increase his O_2 intake is that individual's maximal O_2 intake.

II. Cardiovascular Adaptation

The cardiovascular system senses the need for increased O_2 intake almost immediately. Proper accommodation requires an increase in cardiac output commensurate with the degree of exercise stress. Cardiac output is increased through three basic adaptations, namely, increased heart rate, increased stroke volume and increased arteriovenous O_2 difference (A-V O_2 difference). In order to accommodate the increased volume and increased rate of blood flow, the vascular bed makes a series of adaptations. Included among them are vasodilatation of the arterial and venous systems, and the opening up of large capillary beds in the exercising muscles. These alterations result in a decrease in peripheral vascular resistance in both the systemic and the pulmonary beds. The myocardium itself adapts by increasing its contractile rate and by reducing its heart wall tension. Despite the fact that systolic stroke volume is increasing with exercise and the volume of blood pumped/minute is greater, the size of the normal, healthy heart becomes smaller during exercise when compared to the resting state. Conversely, in patients with severe myocardial limitations or congestive cardiac failure, the heart size becomes larger during exercise.

The multiple changes in the cardiovascular system during exercise stress are reflected by many indirect, non-invasive measurements. Some of these are as follows:

1. Heart Rate

This is the first adaptation to occur. The effects of exercise stress on heart rate are accurately obtained in a number of ways, including palpation, ECG recording or cardiotachometry. The resting heart rate in healthy subjects usually indicates the state of physical conditioning. As a general rule, the lower the resting heart rate, the better the physical condition. Well trained athletes may have heart rates as low as 40 beats/minute (b.p.m), and almost never above 70 b.p.m. The peak heart rates that are achievable vary according to a subject's age, health and physical condition. Peak heart rates of 200–210 b.p.m are common in the late teens and early twenties. The level of peak heart rate that can be achieved decreases gradually with age and at age 65, approximates 145 b.p.m. For subjects from ages 20 through 55, a correlation between level of effort and heart rate exists. Subjects working at heart rates of 120 b.p.m. or less are usually performing light physical effort; 121–140 b.p.m., moderate; 141–160, moderately severe; 161–175, severe; and above 175, exhaustive.

2. Systolic Blood Pressure (SBP)

This parameter increases in a linear manner with exercise stress. The level of resting SBP and peak SBP vary with age, the lowest values recorded in younger subjects, and the highest values in older subjects. Thus, the mean peak SBP for subjects in their third decade, 20–29 years of age, approximates 190 mm. Hg, and for subjects 50–55, approximates 230 mm. Hg. Theoretically, the peak SBP can approach 300 mm. Hg, but to this author's knowledge, such pressures have been observed during exercise only in exceptionally well trained, highly motivated athletes during an all-out effort. When subjects attain their threshold for maximal O_2 intake, there is often a decrease in the level of SBP. This is thought to reflect a decrease in the stroke volume and cardiac output which often accompanies the onset of anaerobic work. Should such a situation occur, this is an indication that the test should be terminated. An increasing level of SBP signifies two physiologic adaptations, namely, the increasing volume of cardiac output and of systolic stroke volume. Unlike heart rate, the adjustments in stroke volume do not occur immediately with the onset of exercise, but only as it becomes moderately heavy.

3. A-V O_2 Difference

These parameters can be measured indirectly and non-invasively using such techniques for measuring cardiac output as the CO_2 rebreathing method. However, this is not usually done in the routine clinical situation. Systemic or O_2 difference is usually 4.0 ml. O_2/100 ml. blood flow in the resting state. During exercise the rate of O_2 extraction increases in relation to the severity of the stress and can increase by as much as 4.0–4.5-fold or to values of 16.0–18.0 ml O_2/100 ml. blood flow. Since the myocardium uses an O_2 extraction to minimize its requirements for coronary blood flow, there is virtually no change in this value during any level of exercise stress. Thus, myocardial O_2 requirements during exercise stress are met principally through the mechanism of increased coronary blood flow.

4. Diastolic Blood Pressure (DBP)

This parameter usually decreases slightly in the healthy sedentary individual or markedly in the trained athlete. This decrease is thought to reflect the decrease in systemic vascular resistance which occurs during exercise.

5. Cardiac Output

This measurement can be determined by non-invasive or invasive techniques. Increases of up to six times the usual resting values are possible at peak exercise. It is apparent that the decreased peripheral resistance that accommodates exercise stress is accomplished in order to handle this tremendous increase in cardiac output. At peak exercise, peripheral vascular resistance approaches 50% of the resting value.

6. Electrocardiogram

The most often evaluated clinical tool for the assessment of exercise stress is the ECG. The normal changes in the ECG complex are those known to occur in relationship to an increased heart rate, namely, the P-R interval decreases as does the Q-T interval. Depending on the lead selection, the T-P baseline will shift upwards from its original baseline, and reciprocal J-junction displacements will occur. These changes reflect the alterations in atrial repolarization, and again, depending upon lead selection, a long P-Q segment might be recorded. Athletes, in particular, develop peaking and late spiking of the T wave. Whether this is due to release of intracellular myocardial potassium or not has not been clarified.

III. Pulmonary Adaptation

Several adaptations occur in the respiratory system analogous to those of the cardiovascular system. In order to transport greater volumes of O_2, the respiratory rate, tidal volume and diffusion rate for O_2 all must increase. Healthy subjects can tolerate peak respiratory rates of 40/minute, and at near-maximal levels of work the tidal volume will approximate the subject's 1-second vital capacity. Thus, peak respiratory volume/minute can reach values of from 120–200 liters/minute. Since there is a critical time for contact of oxygenated air with alveolar blood the lung accommodates by increasing the number of alveoli to be ventilated as well as the diffusion rate for O_2.

IV. Metabolic Adaptations

A large number of metabolic changes are required for the performance of exercise. Since glucose provides the basic substance for the provision of energy, its mobilization is increased. If the exercise is of short duration glucose will probably fuel most of it. However, in endurance events fat metabolism plays an important role. The degree of aerobiosis or anaerobiosis is reflected by monitoring such parameters as blood lactate, pH or ketones. In aerobic efforts these parameters will not vary significantly from those measured during the resting state, whereas in anaerobic efforts blood lactate can rise to values 10-fold those at rest, arterial blood pH can fall to levels as low as 6.8 and ketone bodies can appear in the blood.

Since the body must protect itself against harm, it develops an integral set of vascular adaptations. Blood flow to the myocardium, brain, working muscles and skin is increased to attain the desired results and to dissipate heat. However, splanchnic blood flow to the liver and kidneys decreases markedly during exercise. At peak exercise, blood flow to the splanchnic organs may be virtually non-existent.

Limitation of Performance Capacity

Since exercise requires virtually the mobilization of all systems in the body, investigators have examined the factors which limit man's performance capacity for physical effort. It is now a well accepted fact that for a healthy, well conditioned man the primary limitation is related to the capacity of the cardiovascular system. At maximal effort, it is this system that reaches its limits of adaptation, whereas other systems still have some reserve capacity. Thus, physical conditioning is designed to maximize the capacity of the cardiovascular system and to make it as efficient as possible at rest and during submaximal efforts.

Abnormal Responses to Exercise

Subjects may respond to exercise stress with a variety of abnormal responses. These may occur as singular expressions or in some individuals, a number of abnormal responses may occur simultaneously.

1. Symptoms

In most subjects, their ability to perform exercise is determined by the presence or absence of symptoms. For the healthy subject, exercise performance is limited by exhaustion. However, for the ill patient, it can be limited by chest pain or discomfort, leg pain or discomfort, dyspnea or fatigue. A report for the National Exercise and Heart Disease Project (NEHDP) indicated that in 651 patients with healed myocardial infarctions, chest pain and leg discomfort accounted for the largest number of symptoms which resulted in the termination of their exercise stress tests. On the other hand, a significant number terminated exercise stress because of subjective need which was not well defined.

2. Signs

It has long been suggested that exercise can be accompanied by such abnormal signs as ataxia, cyanosis, pallor or cold sweat. If such abnormal events occur, they are indicative of an existing underlying abnormality. However, it should be emphasized that other abnormalities usually precede those of abnormal signs.

Systolic Blood Pressure

Systolic blood pressure response to exercise indicates indirectly the ability of the myocardium to generate sufficient contractile energy to increase cardiac output and stroke volume. A failure to increase SBP, or a decrease in its level as the threshold for external work is increased, are considered abnormal responses. Although sufficient data are not yet available, there is evidence that SBP increases from 10–14 mm. Hg/increase in MET load.* Thus, at an O_2 intake 3–4 times that of the resting metabolic state at SBP of 160–180 mm. Hg is probably normal. Bruce has reported that an inability to generate a peak SBP of 130 mm. Hg or greater during exercise stress carries with it a serious prognostic outcome, and that, of all abnormalities recorded during exercise stress, its predictive value was greatest.

4. Diastolic Blood Pressure

DBP should decrease during exercise. Some investigators have identified subjects whose DBP increases during exercise stress, and today, most clinical exercise physiologists consider an increase of 20 mm. Hg or greater above the value recorded at rest as abnormal. However, to this author's knowledge, there has not been a study which confirms the significance of this abnormality nor its predictive value.

5. Electrocardiogram

Aside from the presence or absence of symptoms, the ECG response to exercise is the most reliable indicator of abnormality. In general, any change not recorded in the resting tracing and not related to change in heart rate level should be considered an abnormal response. This includes significant, prolonged displacement of the S-T segment, upward or downward, onset of intraventricular blocks, multiform ventricular extrasystoles and ventricular fibrillation.

The response of the S-T segment to exercise stress has received the greatest emphasis by investigators in recent years because of its relationship to the clinical manifestations of coronary heart disease.[4] It is now well accepted that the original observations of Feil and Siegel[5] were correct. Namely, significant displacement of the S-T segment in association with exercise stress carries with it a high likelihood of the presence of underlying coronary artery disease. At issue is the sensitivity and specificity of this finding. It now appears that the sensitivity is quite good if the following conditions are met (see Chapter 12):

1. The S-T displacement exceeds 1.0 mm.
2. The prolongation of the displacement exceeds 0.08 msec.
3. Chest pain characteristic of the patient's presenting complaint occurs in association with the onset of the ECG changes.
4. The chest discomfort and ECG abnormality occur at relatively low thresholds of effort, preferably less than 7 METs.

---

* MET represents the approximated value of required O_2 intake in the relaxed resting metabolic state. It is assumed to be 3.5 ml. O_2/Kg. An oxygen requirement of 7.0 ml. O_2/kg./min. is 2 METs; one of 35 ml. O_2/kg./min. is 10 METs, etc.

Should a patient experience ECG abnormality in the absence of chest pain or discomfort and at a relatively high level of exercise tolerance, the sensitivity decreases markedly and the specificity increases.

A perplexing situation for those engaged in the administration of exercise stress testing is the finding of ischemic ECG responses in a large number of asymptomatic subjects, especially young and early middle-aged women. There is little doubt, from the prospective data available,[6, 7] that such a finding in an asymptomatic individual portends a greater likelihood of manifesting some aspect of coronary heart disease in later years. These subjects have from 6–16 times the incidence of heart disease that is documented in their colleagues with normal stress ECG's. However, if the subject is asymptomatic and has a reasonable level of physical performance capacity, the likelihood of finding significant, operable coronary arterial disease is not great. Thus, in this author's opinion, this ECG finding in a healthy, asymptomatic subject should be treated in the same manner as are the risk factors of cigarette smoking, hypertension and elevated plasma cholesterol levels (see also Chapter 12).

Every clinician should remember that coronary occlusive disease is but one cause of ischemic S-T, T wave change. At least 18 other causes have been identified. These include hypertension, anaerobic exercise, digitalis administration, cardiomyopathy, hypokalemia and the performance of exercise in close association either with cigarette smoking or eating (see Chapters 5, 6 and 12).

The significance of dysrhythmias is more complicated. Few would question the relationship of multiform ventricular extrasystoles, ventricular tachycardia and ventricular fibrillation precipitated or aggravated by exercise stress as usually signifying evidence of an underlying cardiovascular abnormality. However, such findings need not be specific for coronary heart disease. When it comes to other dysrhythmias, they need to be documented, may or may not reflect serious underlying cardiovascular disease and certainly carry little sensitivity. Whether each should be intervened with pharmacologically requires independent evaluation on the merits of the patient's case history and the physician's judgment (see Chapter 13).

6. Performance Capacity

Few investigators have elaborated on the concept of a normal or abnormal performance capacity. Theoretically, a normal capacity or level of physical fitness is defined as that level of maximal O_2 intake which is required to perform one's routine activity effortlessly and without adverse symptoms. As more and more measurements of exercise stress are determined, this author believes it is possible to describe normal and abnormal limits of performance capacity. For instance, subjects with peak O_2 intakes of 6.0 METs or less should have histories which indicate that their functional cardiovascular status (NYHA) is Class II or worse. In an earlier study[8] it was observed that subjects with a capacity of 7.0 METs or greater had few symptoms associated with exercise stress, and when they did appear they were usually of non-cardiac origin.

It appears that for healthy subjects a performance capacity of 7.0 METs or less is undesirable and unnecessary. Physical fitness studies on healthy subjects indicate that middle-aged sedentary men have peak O_2 intakes of from 33.0–37.0 ml./kg./min. (9–11 METs). Studies on the reconditioning of middle-aged men indicate that capacities of 11–14 METs can be achieved and maintained. Similar O_2 intake levels have been experienced in programs of rehabilitation for cardiac patients. With rare exceptions, it is unusual to maintain thresholds above 14 METs unless the subject is physically active in exceptionally rigorous training programs on a daily basis. Thus, a normal level of performance capacity ranges from a low of 9 to a high of 14 METs. Levels below 7.0 METs should be considered abnormal. To date the highest levels measured range from 20–21 METs.

Summary

The foregoing discussion should make it apparent that in the field of exercise testing and fitness evaluation, the physician should avoid confusing the concepts of health and fitness. It is possible to be healthy, yet unfit; conversely, it is possible to be unhealthy, yet very physically fit. Subjects with healed myocardial infarctions who participate in jogging programs or marathon events are examples of the latter. Many individuals who are apparently disease-free are unable to participate comfortably in a hard tennis game, calisthenics or other events.

An adequate appraisal designed to evaluate a subject's overall capacity for work or sport should include performance of a standardized, multistage exercise test. During the test, blood pressure, heart rate, at least a single-lead ECG and the presence or absence of abnormal symptoms and physical signs are monitored simultaneously during each workload. The physician's summation should characterize each normal and abnormal response, integrate the information and provide adequate guidance for both the patient and the referring physician.

REFERENCES

1. Clausen, J. P., Larsen, O. A. and Trap-Jense, J.: Cardiac output in middle-aged patients with CO_2 rebreathing method. J. Appl. Physiol., 28:337, 1970.
2. Naughton, J. P., Barry, A., Gilbert, C. et al.: The national exercise and heart disease project: Development, recruitment, implementation, in Exercise And The Heart, Cardiovascular Clinics, edited by N. K. Wenger, Vol. 9, Philadelphia, F. A. Davis, 1978.
3. Irving, J. B., Bruce, R. A. and DeRowen, T. A.: Variations in and significance of systolic pressure during maximal exercise (treadmill) testing. Am. J. Cardiol., 39:841, 1977.
4. Naughton, J.: Stress electrocardiography in clinical electrocardiographic correlations, in

Cardiovascular Clinics, edited by J. C. Rios, Vol. 8, pp. 127–139, Philadelphia, F. A. Davis, 1977.

5. Feil, H. and Siegel, M. L.: Electrocardiographic changes during attacks of angina pectoris. Am. J. Med. Sci., *175:*255, 1978.

6. Doyle, J. T. and Kirsch, S.: The prognosis of an electrocardiographic stress test. Circulation, *41:*545, 1970.

7. Robb, G. P. and Marks, H. H.: Latent coronary artery disease: determination of its presence and severity by the exercise electrocardiogram. Am. J. Cardiol., *13:*603, 1964.

8. Patterson, J. A., Naughton, J., Pietras, R. J. and Gunnar, R. M.: Treadmill exercise in the assessment of functional capacity of patients with cardiovascular disease. Am. J. Cardiol., *30:*757, 1972.

12

Interpretation of the Exercise ECG Test

Edward K. Chung, M.D., F.A.C.P., F.A.C.C.

General Considerations[1-19]

There are 3 major myocardial ischemic responses to the exercise ECG test. They include:

(1) Electric events: electrocardiographic changes (e.g., S-T segment and T wave alterations and various cardiac arrhythmias)
(2) Hemodynamic events: alterations in blood pressure and heart rate, and
(3) Symptomatic manifestations: chest pain, dyspnea, etc.

Among these ischemic responses, the electric events (electrocardiographic changes) are considered the most reliable criteria for the diagnosis of coronary artery disease. In particular, the S-T segment alteration (horizontal or downsloping S-T segment depression) is the most reliable finding to diagnose positive exercise ECG test. Nevertheless, there is no uniform agreement regarding the precise diagnostic criteria for positive or negative exercise ECG tests. The main reason for this is that numerous factors influence the result of the exercise ECG test (see Table 12-1). Namely, the result will be clearly influenced by the test method, the interpreter's ability, medical knowledge and experience, population studied, purpose of the test and the presence or absence of various factors which may cause a false positive or negative exercise ECG test. For example, the incidence of true positive exercise ECG tests will be greater when dealing with an older age group with a high prevalence of coronary artery disease. Conversely, the majority of young subjects (e.g., Air Force personnel) without clinical manifestation of heart disease will show true negative exercise ECG tests. Another example is that the criteria to terminate the exercise ECG test significantly influences the test result. Obviously, premature termination of the exercise judging from mild chest pain or ECG changes will reduce the incidence of positive exercise ECG tests (see Chapter 9). In addition, the physician's knowledge certainly influences the result of the exercise ECG test.

Table 12-1. Factors Influencing Result of Exercise ECG Test

1. *Methods:* Protocol, lead system, selection of patient group, criteria to terminate, etc.
2. *Interpreter's ability, knowledge and experience:*
   - Diagnostic criteria of positive vs. negative test
   - Correct diagnosis of arrhythmias
3. *Population studied and purpose of test:*
   - Young healthy groups vs. older patients with coronary heart disease
   - Diagnostic purpose
   - Insurance purpose
   - Research purpose
4. *Various factors for false positive vs. false negative test*

Among various factors, digitalis most commonly produces a false positive exercise ECG test whereas propranolol (Inderal) most commonly causes a false negative test. Factors which may cause false positive and false negative tests will be discussed later in this Chapter.

The terms sensitivity,* specificity** and predictive value*** are frequently used in the literature dealing with the exercise ECG test. A high degree of sensitivity and specificity for the Master's two-step test had been reported initially,[20-22] but various recent studies using coronary angiographic correlations have indicated its sensitivity to be in the range of 43–66 per cent.[23-26] Initially, Master et al. claimed that a negative Master's test virtually ruled out the presence of coronary artery disease.[20-22] It is clearly proven, however, that the Master's two-step test fails to provide sufficient exercise workloads, leading to a high incidence of false negative tests. Recent studies using multistage exercise ECG tests indicate that sensitivity approaches 100%, especially when dealing with multivessel disease.[3, 16, 19] It has been shown recently that computer analysis of the S-T segment alteration further enhances the sensitivity and specificity.

---

* *Sensitivity* indicates the percentage of patients with a positive exercise ECG test out of all patients studied with arteriographically documented coronary artery disease (the ability of a positive exercise ECG test to correctly identify patients with documented coronary artery disease).

$$\frac{\text{true positives}}{\text{true positives} + \text{false negatives}}$$

** *Specificity* indicates the percentage of subjects with a negative exercise ECG test out of all subjects studied with normal coronary arteriograms (the ability of a negative exercise ECG test to correctly identify healthy subjects).

$$\frac{\text{true negatives}}{\text{false positives} + \text{true negatives}}$$

*** *Predictive Value* of abnormal test indicates the percentage of patients with abnormal exercise ECG tests, indicating coronary artery disease.

$$\frac{\text{true positives}}{\text{true positives} + \text{false positives}}$$

It is interesting to note that a false positive exercise ECG test is higher in women than men, and many middle-aged women (between the ages of 40 and 60) often demonstrate "borderline" ("equivocal") exercise ECG tests. The fundamental reason for this phenomenon is uncertain.

It is well documented that the exercise ECG test has great value in the diagnosis of coronary artery disease when it is used as a clinical tool in conjunction with other information obtained from the history, physical examination, resting 12-lead electrocardiogram and other basic laboratory findings. It is extremely important to apply the result of the exercise ECG test properly on an individual basis. It should be reemphasized that the S-T segment alteration is *not* necessarily indicative of coronary artery disease, whereas a negative exercise ECG test does *not* exclude the possibility of coronary artery disease.

Physiologic Responses[1-10, 15, 16]

Various physiologic responses to exercise are expected in normal individuals (see Table 12-2), but certain findings, particularly S-T segment alteration, are often difficult to interpret accurately.

1. Blood Pressure and Heart Rate Changes

As expected, there will be a progressive increment of blood pressure and heart rate during exercise in healthy individuals. As far as the precise analysis of blood pressure is concerned, the systolic blood pressure often decreases slightly during the first 3 minutes following the initial rise. Systolic blood pressure progressively rises thereafter, up to a point of near-maximal

Table 12-2. Exercise ECG Test—Physiologic Responses

1. Progressive increment of blood pressure and heart rate during exercise
2. Shortening of Q-T interval with increased Q-T:R-R ratio
3. Physiologic S-T segment alteration:
   - Functional (J-point) S-T segment depression 2 mm. with duration < 0.06 sec.
   - Vasoregulatory asthenia
   - Orthostatic ECG changes
   - Labile T wave change
   - Reynolds syndrome
   - S-T segment depression only in the post-exercise period(?)
4. Alteration of T wave direction or morphology
5. Slight reduction of R wave amplitude
6. Shortening of P-R interval or varying P-R intervals
7. Downward displacement of P-R segment due to prominent T-a wave amplitude
8. Peaking and tall P wave during very rapid heart rate
9. Minor symptoms: Dyspnea, fatigue, sweating, etc.

exercise capacity and then declines rather sharply. Then, blood pressure increases again approximately 1 minute after the termination of exercise. Within another 1–2 minutes during the post-exercise period, it begins to decline as the cardiac output decreases during recovery period. It is not certain whether the temporary reduction of systolic blood pressure during the early post-exercise period is due to a sudden change in peripheral resistance, or to a reduction of cardiac output, or both. In most subjects, the peak systolic blood pressure is not more than 160–170 mm. Hg. Elevation of systolic blood pressure beyond 220 mm. Hg (particularly above 250 mm. Hg) during exercise is considered abnormal. Under this circumstance, the diagnosis of labile hypertension should be considered.

As far as the diastolic blood pressure is concerned, there is no significant alteration during exercise. Many healthy subjects may develop slight elevation (not more than 10 mm. Hg) during the first 2 minutes followed by a progressive reduction toward the maximal exercise period. There is often a slight elevation of diastolic pressure again immediately following termination of exercise until gradual reduction takes place thereafter during the recovery period. At any rate, the fluctuation of diastolic blood pressure during and after exercise is minimal (10–15 mm. Hg) compared with systolic blood pressure change.

Heart rate increases progressively during exercise, and the degree of heart rate acceleration is greater in younger individuals than older people. The predicted maximal heart rate acceleration during exercise among different age groups is shown in Chapter 9.

It should be noted that physically active healthy individuals such as athletes may not show a significant rise in blood pressure or heart rate because of excellent (possibly supernormal) physical condition. In addition, anxious individuals also may show paradoxical blood pressure or heart rate change during the first 1–2 minutes of the exercise period. Otherwise, organic heart disease, particularly coronary heart disease, is strongly suspected when the expected elevation of systolic blood pressure or heart rate is not observed during exercise testing. Sick sinus syndrome is a good possibility when there is only insignificant acceleration of sinus rate (less than 120 beats/minute), especially in older individuals in spite of near-maximal or maximal exercise.[27]

2. Alteration of Q-T Interval

During the multistage exercise ECG test, a shortening of the Q-T interval with increased Q-T:R-R ratio is observed as the heart rate is accelerated. In 1950, Yu et al.,[28] reported that there is a definite prolongation in corrected Q-T intervals in patients with coronary and hypertensive heart disease. However, from the practical viewpoint, it is extremely difficult to measure the Q-T interval accurately during rapid heart rate provoked by exercise.

Thus, the usefulness of the Q-T interval value is limited. In addition, the significance of Q-X*:Q-T ratio had been studied in 1965 by Roman and Bellet.[29] They claimed that Q-X:Q-T ratio more than 1:2 is highly suggestive of a positive exercise ECG test. However, its practical value is found to be limited.

3. Physiologic S-T Segment Alteration

Slight functional (junctional or J-point) S-T segment depression (less than 2 mm. with less than 0.06 second in duration) is expected in healthy individuals as the heart rate is accelerated by the exercise (Figure 12-1). However, it should be noted that the precise assessment of so-called "functional S-T segment depression" is difficult because of the relatively wide range of variations in healthy population as well as in patients with coronary artery disease. In addition, although the functional S-T segment depression may be as innocuous as it seems in most cases, the horizontal or downsloping S-T segment depression is often preceded by the former in patients with documented coronary heart disease (Figures 12-2 and 3). If this fact is kept in mind in evaluating the S-T segment alteration, an erroneous diagnosis of the exercise ECG test can be minimized.

Many healthy individuals show non-specific S-T segment and T wave abnormalities on their resting electrocardiograms, and these ECG changes become pronounced on standing or during hyperventilation. This phenomenon has been termed "vasoregulatory asthenia" by different authors.[30-34] Vasoregulatory asthenia may be observed in both sexes at any age, but it is most commonly seen in young to middle-aged women who are often hyperactive emotionally. They may complain of chest pain suggestive of angina pectoris. The S-T, T wave changes recorded at rest often become pronounced during the early period of exercise, and the normalization of these changes may be observed with more vigorous exercise and immediately following termination of exercise (Figures 12-4 and 5). Non-specific S-T, T wave abnormalities usually reappear within 3–6 minutes during the post-exercise period upon resting (Figure 12-5). In other cases of vasoregulatory asthenia, the resting 12-lead ECG may be completely normal, but the S-T segment depression begins to appear when the individual stands up, and it becomes pronounced during exercise (Figures 12-6 and 7). The S-T segment usually returns to normal upon termination of exercise (Figure 12-7). The term "Reynolds syndrome" has been used by Ellestad et al. to describe a similar phenomenon.[5] They reported that most individuals with the Reynolds syndrome show increased sympathetic drive but normal coronary arteriographic findings. These orthostatic S-T, T wave changes are usually augmented by upright posture or hyperventilation, and may improve during

---

* *Q-X interval:* Interval from the onset of the QRS complex to the crossing point of the isoelectric line extended from the P-R segment and the S-T segment.

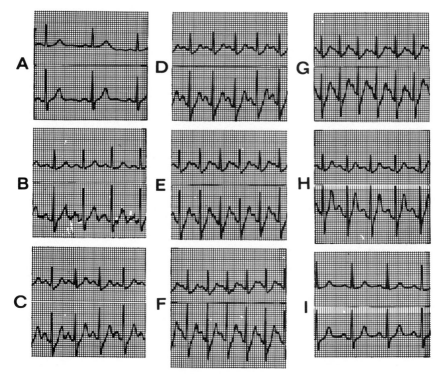

Fig. 12-1   This exercise ECG was taken on a 54-year-old man because of atypical chest pain. He had exercised all the way through a 7-stage course without any difficulty. The maximal heart rate reached 174 beats/minute. The rhythm strips A represent a control tracing. The strips B to G are taken during exercise, whereas the strips H and I represent post-exercise tracings. The exercise ECG test is negative. Note a slight functional (J-point) S-T segment depression. In addition, the T waves are tall in strips E to H. In each rhythm strip, the top strip represents a modified lead V_5 (CM$_5$). The bottom strip is lead II in this tracing and all subsequent figures when a 2-channel recorder is used, unless otherwise indicated. When a single-channel recorder is used in subsequent figures, a modified lead V_5 (CM$_5$) is recorded.

a Valsalva maneuver. These individuals often demonstrate heart rate lability with inappropriate sinus tachycardia on standing or with mild exercise. The S-T, T wave changes due to vasoregulatory asthenia are usually observed on multiple leads. It has been shown on cardiac catheterization that these individuals reveal a rapid heart rate, reduced blood volume and higher than normal cardiac output with a very small arteriovenous difference in their O_2 saturation.[5] During S-T segment depression, the T wave is either biphasic or inverted (Figures 12-5 and 7), and some authors used the term "labile T wave change" under this circumstance.

In some individuals, S-T segment depression only occurs 3–8 minutes

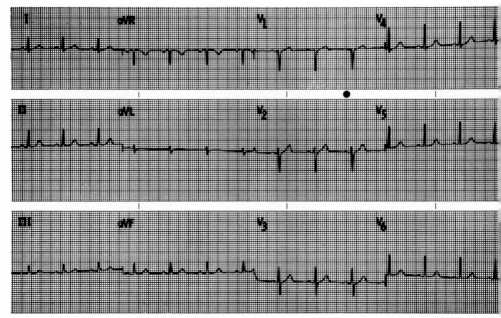

Fig. 12-2 Figures 12-2 and 3 were obtained from a 55-year-old man with occasional chest pain of several weeks' duration. Figure 12-2 represents a resting 12-lead ECG, whereas Figure 12-3 is his exercise ECG. His control (resting) 12-lead ECG shows normal sinus rhythm and within normal limits.

after the termination of exercise, and the S-T segment remains isoelectric during exercise and/or immediately after exercise (Figures 12-8 and 9). The resting 12-lead ECG is usually normal. This type of S-T segment alteration is difficult to evaluate, but this author observed this finding in apparently healthy individuals. Under this circumstance, the S-T segment usually shows downsloping depression with biphasic T wave (Figure 12-9). On the other hand, isolated post-exercise *horizontal* S-T segment depression is probably indicative of a positive exercise ECG test.

4. Alteration of T Wave Direction or Morphology

Although tall T waves during exercise or immediately after exercise were considered indicative of inferior wall myocardial ischemia in the early days of exercise ECG test,[35, 36] the finding is no longer considered abnormal. In practice, many healthy and young individuals show tall and peaked T waves during near-maximal exercise or early post-exercise period (Figure 12-10). This finding is a physiologic phenomenon secondary due to an increased stroke volume. The progressive increment of the T wave amplitude is shown to be well correlated with the increasing stroke volume.

Similarly, the development of isolated T wave inversion or flattening of T waves during or after exercise is considered insignificant clinically. These T wave alterations may occur in apparently healthy individuals. It is of interest that the T wave alteration during exercise was traditionally considered an important indicator of myocardial ischemia in the early days of the exercise ECG test.[37] The T wave inversion is commonly observed during exercise in patients with left ventricular dysfunction due to hypertension or other organic heart diseases. It has been suggested that inversion or flattening of T waves may be due to increased catecholamines in the blood as well as various non-cardiac factors. It should be noted, however, that inverted or biphasic T waves are often associated with downsloping S-T segment depression in patients with proven coronary artery disease (Figure 12-11). In this case, the exercise ECG test is, of course, positive.

In the early days of the exercise ECG test, myocardial ischemia was diagnosed when the inverted T waves become upright during or after exercise.[38, 39] Again, at present, this T wave change is considered non-specific and has no clinical significance. It has been shown that many individuals with inverted T waves due to metabolic abnormalities show upright T waves during exercise, and this finding seems to be more common in females.

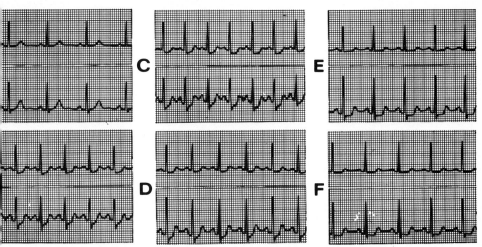

Fig. 12-3   His resting rhythm strips A are entirely within normal limits. The strips B and C taken during exercise show initial functional (J-point) S-T segment depression followed by upsloping S-T segment depression until horizontal and downsloping S-T segment depression develops during post-exercise period (the strips D to F). It is interesting to note that the S-T segment depression is more pronounced in lead II than in lead CM$_5$. His maximal heart rate reached was 145 beats/minute. The test was terminated prematurely because of angina associated with S-T segment change. Thus, his exercise ECG test is interpreted as a positive (incomplete) test.

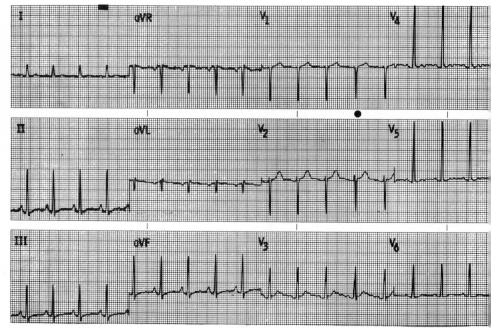

Fig. 12-4   Figures 12-4 and 5 were obtained from a 25-year-old intern as part of the exercise research program. Figure 12-4 is a 12-lead ECG taken at rest, and it shows an atypical juvenile T wave pattern (flat or biphasic T waves in many leads), otherwise within normal limits. He is found to be an athletic individual and perfectly healthy.

In sum, isolated T wave alterations in direction or morphology during or after exercise are considered to be of no diagnostic importance. Thus, most exercise laboratories pay no attention to alterations in T waves for the diagnosis of coronary artery disease.

5. Alterations in the R Wave Amplitude

It is difficult to assess the QRS amplitude alterations precisely during exercise because of significant variations due to postural or respiratory changes. Nevertheless, it is generally agreed that the total amplitude of the QRS complex is reduced slightly during near-maximal exercise or early post-exercise period (Figure 12-12). This R wave amplitude reduction seems to be more marked in healthy individuals than in coronary patients. The reduced R wave amplitude following maximal exercise is probably due to a reduced stroke volume, which often occurs after maximal cardiac output is reached. The reduction of the R wave amplitude may be associated with simultaneous T wave amplitude reduction (Figure 12-12), but tall and

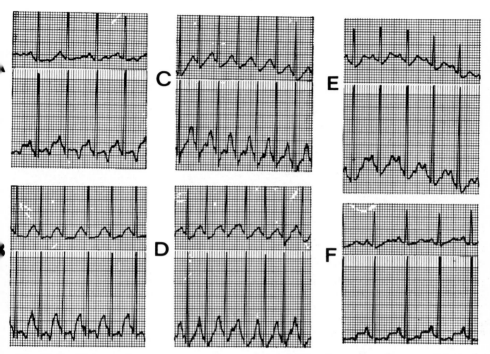

Fig. 12-5 This tracing represents the exercise ECG taken on a 25-year-old intern without any heart disease. The strips A are taken at rest and they show inverted T waves (juvenile T wave pattern). The strips B to D are obtained during exercise; the strips E and F represent post-exercise tracings. He has exercised a complete 7-stage course plus an additional stage 8 without any difficulty. The maximal heart rate reached 195 beats/minute. The exercise ECG test is negative. Note alteration of the T wave direction as well as morphology.

peaked T waves may occur when the reduced R wave amplitude is observed (Figure 12-10).

The diagnostic value of the R wave amplitude as a predictor of coronary artery disease in exercise ECG tests has been studied recently in 108 selected cases by Christison et al.[40] They concluded that increment or no change in R wave amplitude during treadmill stress testing is a more reliable indicator of significant coronary artery disease than S-T segment changes. Another study using a group of 159 patients from the same laboratory indicated that recognition of the increased R wave amplitude can significantly reduce the incidence of false positive and false negative tests during treadmill exercise testing.[41] These investigators concluded that S-T segment depression with reduction of R wave amplitude is suggestive of a false positive test or single-vessel disease, whereas increased R wave amplitude without significant S-T

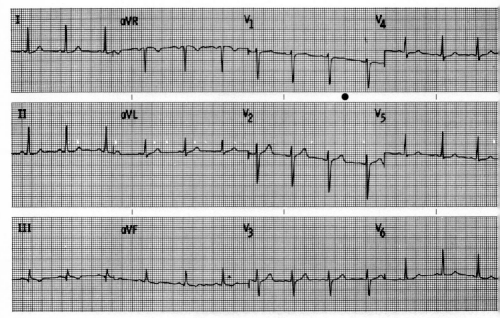

Fig. 12-6   Figures 12-6 and 7 were obtained from a 30-year-old anxious man with non-specific chest discomfort. His resting 12-lead ECG shown in this figure is within normal limits.

segment depression is suggestive of a false negative exercise ECG test. However, these R wave amplitude alterations in exercise ECG tests require further investigation for more definitive diagnostic implications.

6. Alterations of the P-R Intervals

The P-R interval is often shortened soon after the initiation of the exercise as a physiologic phenomenon.[42] In addition, some variations of the P-R intervals may occur during or after exercise in healthy individuals. Recently, marked prolongation of the P-R interval was observed during the post-exercise period in a healthy young woman, and the P-R interval returned to normal value 5–6 minutes after the termination of exercise (see Chapter 13).

7. Downward Displacement of P-R Segment

Downward displacement of the P-R segment may occur during exercise as the P wave becomes taller and the T-a wave (atrial repolarization wave) becomes prominent as a physiologic phenomenon.[43] Under this circumstance, the T-a wave tends to extend through the QRS complex and it may alter the junction between the S-T segment and the T wave leading to false appearance of S-T segment abnormality.

8. Peaking and Tall P Waves

It is extremely common to observe peaking and tall P waves during exercise as the heart rate is accelerated (pseudo P-pulmonale). When the

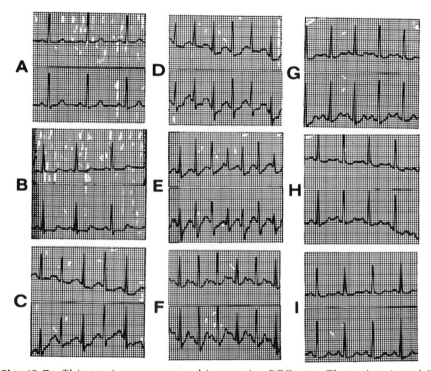

Fig. 12-7 This tracing represents his exercise ECG test. The strips A and B were taken at rest while supine and standing, respectively. The strips C to E were taken during exercise, whereas the strips F to I represent the post-exercise tracings. It is noteworthy that the S-T segment becomes depressed on standing (strip B) and the S-T segment becomes more depressed during exercise (the strips C and D). However, the S-T segment depression becomes progressively less pronounced during peak exercise (strip E) and post-exercise period (the strips F to I). This type of S-T segment alteration is not uncommonly found in healthy and anxious young individuals. The term "Reynold's syndrome" has been used to describe this normal S-T segment variation, which is a form of vasoregulatory asthenia. His maximal heart rate reached was 200 beats/minute, and he was able to complete stage 9 of Chung's exercise protocol (see Chapter 9). Thus, his exercise tolerance is excellent.

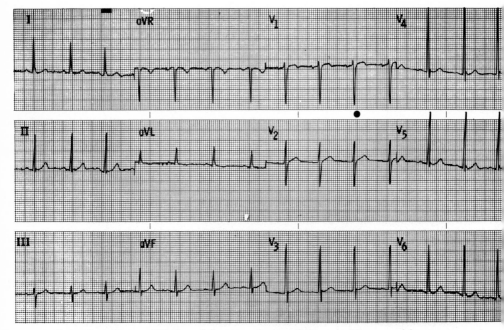

Fig. 12-8   Figures 12-8 and 9 were obtained from a 49-year-old man as part of his annual check-up. His resting 12-lead ECG shown in this figure is within normal limits other than high left ventricular voltage (no chamber enlargement was shown in his chest X-ray).

heart rate is extremely rapid, the P wave and T wave often partially or totally fuse, leading to one large wave (Figures 12-5 and 10). This P wave change is a physiologic phenomenon.

9. Minor Symptoms

As expected, any individual will experience the usual minor symptoms such as slight dyspnea, fatigue, sweating, feeling of hot sensation, etc. during vigorous exercise as a physiologic phenomenon.

Physiologic versus abnormal responses to exercise are discussed in detail elsewhere (see Chapter 11).

Abnormal Responses to Exercise[1-10, 14-20]

Various abnormal responses to exercise may be observed in patients with coronary heart diseases, but myocardial ischemic responses to exercise can be categorized under 3 subheadings. They include: (1) Electrocardiographic changes, (2) Hemodynamic changes, and (3) Symptoms and signs (see Table 12-3). Among these ischemic responses, alterations of the S-T segment are probably the most important and useful criteria to diagnose coronary heart disease. The S-T segment horizontal depression is the traditional diagnostic criterion for a positive exercise ECG test. Although some investigators suggested that the increased R wave amplitude and the development of typical angina by exercise are more reliable findings to diagnose coronary heart disease, this view is not uniformly accepted. However, it should be emphasized that the accuracy of the diagnosis of coronary heart disease will be markedly enhanced when the S-T segment alterations are interpreted in conjunction with other ischemic responses, particularly typical chest pain, significant cardiac arrhythmias (see Chapter 13) and abnormal blood pressure response, etc.

As described previously, there are numerous factors which may influence

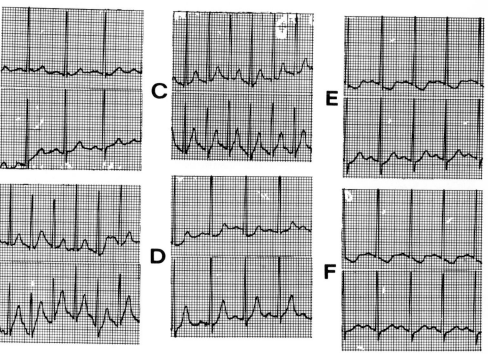

Fig. 12-9   This tracing shows the exercise ECG test on this 49-year-old man. The strips A are a resting ECG, while the strips B and C are taken during exercise. The strips D to F represent post-exercise ECG. It is interesting to note that downsloping S-T segment depression with biphasic T wave appears only during post-exercise period (the strips E and F only in lead CM_5—top strips). This type of isolated downsloping S-T segment depression is probably insignificant clinically—a negative exercise ECG test. He was able to complete the 7-stage exercise protocol and his maximal heart rate was 170 beats/minute.

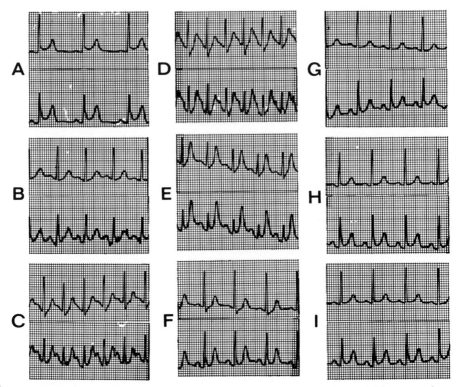

Fig. 12-10 This exercise ECG was obtained from a 36-year-old man who complained of non-specific chest discomfort. He has completed a 7-stage course without any complaint and the maximal heart rate reached to 176 beats/minute. The rhythm strips A represent a control (resting) tracing. The strips B to D are the tracings taken during exercise, whereas the strips E to I represent post-exercise tracings. The exercise ECG test is negative. Note peaking and tall T waves during rapid heart rate, associated with reduction of the R wave amplitude during exercise and immediate post-exercise period (strips C to E).

the results of the exercise ECG test (see Table 12-1). Many factors may produce false positive (see Table 12-4) or false negative exercise ECG tests (see Table 12-5). A higher incidence of false positive exercise ECG tests in females has been emphasized repeatedly. In addition, many young to middle-aged women demonstrate a borderline or equivocal exercise ECG test (not exactly positive nor exactly negative result). Its reason is not clearly understood.

The sensitivity of the exercise ECG test (definition described previously in this Chapter) varies markedly depending upon numerous factors, but it is particularly influenced by the number of coronary vessels involved. As expected, sensitivity for a single-vessel coronary artery disease is relatively low (between 37 and 60%), whereas it is nearly 100% (ranging from 86–100%) when triple vessels are involved.[44-47] In 2-vessel disease, sensitivity is between 67 and 91%.[44-47]

1. Electrocardiographic Changes

Among various electrocardiographic changes induced by exercise, the most reliable diagnostic finding is the horizontal or downsloping S-T seg-

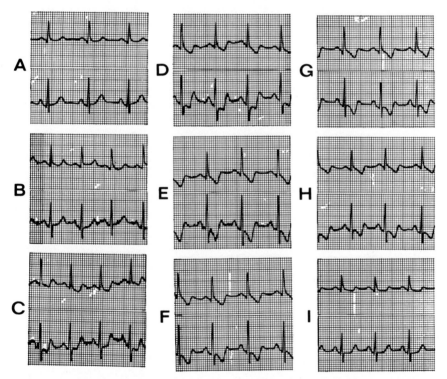

Fig. 12-11 This exercise ECG test was obtained from a 60-year-old man with a history of angina for several years. He was unable to complete the scheduled exercise because he developed significant chest pain. He has exercised only up to stage 2, and the maximal heart rate reached to 108 beats/minute. His resting 12-lead ECG was within normal limits (not shown here). The strips A represent a resting rhythm tracing. The strips B and C are taken during exercise, whereas the strips D to I represent post-exercise ECG. The exercise ECG test is positive (incomplete). Note horizontal to downsloping S-T segment depression with biphasic to inverted T waves during and after exercise. The ECG returns to normal within 10 minutes after the termination of exercise.

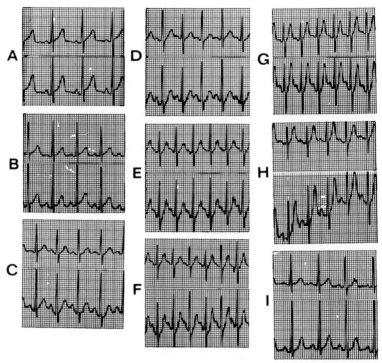

Fig. 12-12 This exercise ECG was obtained from a 29-year-old healthy male. He has completed a 7-stage course without any difficulty. The maximal heart rate is 175 beats/minute. The strips A represent a control (resting) tracing, whereas the strips B to G are recorded during exercise with 2–3 minutes apart. The strips H and I are post-exercise ECG tracings with a few minutes' interval. The exercise ECG test is negative (typical negative exercise ECG test). Note some reduction of the R wave amplitude during the peak exercise period and immediate post-exercise period (the strips E to H) associated with peaking T waves.

ment depression of 1 mm. or more. Certain cardiac arrhythmias induced by exercise such as unifocal ventricular premature contractions (VPCs) and various supraventricular tachyarrhythmias have no diagnostic value for coronary artery disease, whereas exercise-induced multifocal VPCs, grouped (particularly 3 or more) VPCs and ventricular tachycardia are highly suggestive of coronary heart disease, especially when these arrhythmias are provoked by minimal (less than 70% of the maximal workloads) exercise (see Chapter 13). Other findings, such as inverted U waves or increased amplitude of R wave by exercise, strongly suggestive of positive exercise ECG tests are summarized in Table 12-6.

(A) Diagnostic S-T Segment Alterations

1) S-T Segment Depression. Traditionally, the horizontal (square-wave) S-T segment depression during or after exercise has been considered the single most reliable diagnostic criterion for a positive exercise ECG test. Although there is a controversy regarding the amount of the horizontal S-T segment depression, 1 mm. or more depression is generally accepted for a definite positive exercise ECG test (see Table 12-7, Figure 12-13). An almost equally reliable criterion for a positive exercise ECG test is a downsloping S-T segment depression of 1 mm. or more (see Table 12-7, Figure 12-11).

Table 12-3. Exercise ECG Test—Abnormal Responses

1. Electrocardiographic changes
   - (A) Diagnostic S-T segment alterations
     - 1) S-T segment depression
     - 2) S-T segment elevation
     - 3) S-T segment change with pre-existing ECG abnormalities
   - (B) Cardiac arrhythmias
   - (C) Inversion of U waves
   - (D) Intraventricular blocks
   - (E) Increased R wave amplitude
   - (F) Acute myocardial infarction
   - (G) Miscellaneous findings:
     Q-X:Q-T ratio, Q-T interval change, P wave change, T wave change, etc.
2. Hemodynamic changes
   - (A) Hypotension
   - (B) Slowing of heart rate
   - (C) Marked hypertension
3. Symptoms and signs
   - (A) Symptoms: Severe chest pain, dyspnea, pallor, cyanosis, fainting, etc.
   - (B) Signs: 3rd or 4th heart sounds, heart murmurs, precordial bulging, double cardiac impulse, pulsus alternans, etc.

Table 12-4. Factors Which May Cause False Positive Exercise ECG Test

1. *Drugs:* Digitalis, diuretics, anti-depressant drugs, sedatives, estrogen
2. *Cardiac disorders:* Mitral valve prolapse syndrome, Wolff-Parkinson-White syndrome, cardiomyopathy, idiopathic hypertrophic subaortic stenosis, myocarditis, pericarditis, rheumatic heart disease, hypertensive heart disease
3. *Electrolyte imbalance:* Hypokalemia
4. *Pre-existing ECG abnormalities:* Left ventricular hypertrophy, left bundle branch block, non-specific abnormality of S-T, T waves, right ventricular hypertrophy, right bundle branch block, Wolff-Parkinson-White syndrome
5. *Miscellaneous:* Healthy persons, women, hyperventilation, food-glucose intake, pectus excavatum

Table 12-5. Factors Which May Cause False Negative Exercise ECG Test

1. *Drugs:* Propranolol, nitroglycerin and other anti-anginal drugs, procain-amide, quinidine, phenothiazines
2. *Coronary heart disease:* Old myocardial infarction, proven angina pectoris (especially single-vessel disease)
3. *Inadequate exercise:* Premature termination of the test, physical training
4. *Improper lead system*
5. *Miscellaneous:* Left axis deviation, left anterior hemiblock

Table 12-6. Criteria—Strongly Suggestive of Positive Exercise ECG Test

1. Horizontal or downsloping S-T segment depression < 1 mm.
2. Upsloping S-T segment depression ≥ 2 mm. beyond 0.08 second from J-point
3. Hypotension
4. Inverted U wave
5. Frequent ventricular premature contractions, multifocal ventricular premature contractions, grouped ventricular premature contractions, ventricular tachycardia provoked by mild exercise (≤ 70% of maximal heart rate)
6. Increased R wave amplitude (?)
7. Exercise-induced typical angina
8. Third or fourth heart sound, or heart murmur

Table 12-7. Criteria—Positive Exercise ECG Test

1. Horizontal or downsloping S-T segment depression ≥ 1 mm.
2. Horizontal or upsloping S-T segment elevation ≥ 1 mm.

Recently, the term, "upsloping" S-T segment depression has been introduced.[48, 49] It has been suggested that upsloping S-T segment depression of 2 mm. or more beyond 0.08 second in duration from J-point is a reliable finding for a positive exercise ECG test (see Table 12-6). It is common to observe upsloping S-T segment depression initially, and it is followed by the horizontal or downsloping S-T segment depression (Figure 12-14). Other investigators used different names such as slow-rising or slow-ascending S-T segment depression, but the ECG findings appear to be almost identical to those showing upsloping S-T segment depression.[2,48] Various types of S-T segment responses to exercise are summarized in Table 12-8.

An isolated functional (junctional or J-point) S-T segment depression is usually considered non-diagnostic in exercise electrocardiography, but in occasional cases, functional S-T segment depression may be followed by the diagnostic horizontal or downsloping S-T segment depression in proven coronary patients (Figure 12-3). Various non-diagnostic ECG findings for coronary artery disease are summarized in Table 12-9.

It has been suggested, based on existing knowledge and experience of the pathophysiology of myocardial oxygen supply and demand, that patients with more advanced coronary heart disease should develop the diagnostic S-T segment depression at a lower heart rate induced by minimal exercise.[16] Namely, significant horizontal or downsloping S-T segment depression at an exercise heart rate less than 70% of the predicted maximal heart rate (Figures 12-11, 13 and 14) should represent more diagnostic value than similar degrees of S-T segment depression at near-maximal exercise heart rates (Figure 12-15) to identify individuals with greater risk of symptomatic coronary artery disease.

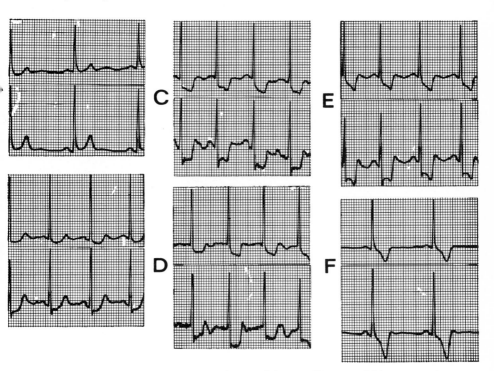

Fig. 12-13 This exercise ECG was obtained from a 50-year-old hypertensive woman who has been suffering from angina for 6–8 months. She was unable to finish the scheduled exercise because of significant chest pain associated with marked S-T segment depression. The exercise was stopped in the middle of stage 2, and the maximal heart rate reached to only 102 beats/minute. Her resting 12-lead ECG was within normal limits other than high left ventricular voltage (not shown here). The rhythm strips A represent a resting ECG. The strips B to D are recorded during exercise, whereas the remaining strips (E and F) represent post-exercise ECG. Her ECG returns to normal 15 minutes after the termination of exercise. The exercise ECG test is markedly positive (incomplete). Note marked horizontal to downsloping S-T segment depression with biphasic to inverted T waves. She underwent aortocoronary bypass surgery with excellent results.

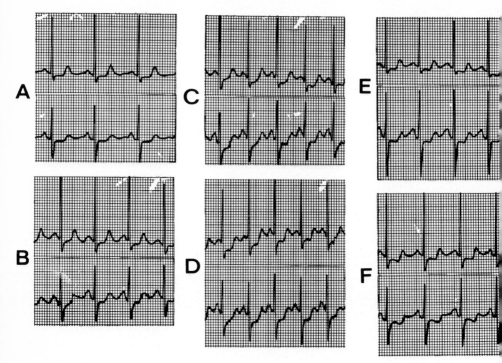

Fig. 12-14 This exercise ECG was taken on a 58-year-old woman with occasional mild angina on exertion. She was not taking any drug. She was unable to complete the scheduled exercise because of chest pain during stage 5. The maximal heart rate reached to 148 beats/minute. The resting 12-lead ECG shows non-specific S-T, T wave changes (not shown here). The same ECG finding is shown in the strips A taken at rest. The strips B to D are taken during exercise, whereas the remaining strips E and F represent post-exercise ECG. The exercise ECG test is positive (incomplete). Note horizontal to downsloping S-T segment depression with biphasic T waves during and after exercise preceded by upsloping S-T segment depression. It took 10 minutes until the ECG finding returned to the resting ECG finding.

Table 12-8. Various Types of S-T Segment Responses to Exercise ECG Test

1. *S-T Segment depression:*
   - Horizontal (square-wave)
   - Functional (junctional or J-point)
   - Downsloping
   - Upsloping
   - Slow-rising (slow-ascending)
   - Sagging
2. *S-T Segment elevation:*
   - Horizontal
   - Upsloping

Table 12-9. ECG Findings with Equivocal or No Value for Diagnosis

1. Development of insignificant cardiac arrhythmias:
   - Occasional unifocal ventricular premature contractions
   - Atrial or junctional tachyarrhythmias
   - First degree or Wenckebach A-V block (?)
2. Development of intraventricular block:
   - Bundle branch block, hemiblocks, bifascicular block, etc.
3. Changing A-V conduction
4. Alteration of T wave morphology
5. Alteration of P wave morphology
6. Functional S-T segment depression < 2 mm.
7. Miscellaneous findings:
   - Q-X:Q-T ratio
   - Q-T interval change
   - Prominent U waves

For a similar reason, an isolated S-T segment depression (mostly down-sloping depression) diagnostic of a positive exercise ECG test only during the post-exercise period in asymptomatic individuals (Figure 12-9) probably represents a false positive exercise ECG test. McHenry and Morris[45] emphasized recently that the appearance of horizontal or downsloping S-T segment depression during the post-exercise period without accompanying horizontal or slowly upsloping S-T segment depression during exercise may prove to be a false positive exercise ECG test in asymptomatic subjects. Their findings are in keeping with this author's experience in our exercise laboratory.

On the other hand, coronary heart disease should be strongly suggested when *horizontal* S-T segment depression of 1 mm. or more occurs, even if only during the post-exercise period, especially when it is associated with other ischemic responses such as chest pain or hypotension. It has been postulated that myocardial ischemia is produced by an inordinate reduction of coronary blood flow as the cardiac output suddenly decreases because of venous pooling.[50] The long-term prognosis of these patients compared with subjects who develop S-T segment change during exercise is not certain.

When the diagnostic S-T segment depression is associated with frequent VPCs, multifocal VPCs, grouped VPCs (Figure 12-16), or a marked slowing of the heart rate during the post-exercise period with or without hypotension (Figures 12-17 and 18), advanced coronary artery disease with multivessel involvement is most likely present.

On rare occasions, electrical alternans may involve only S-T segment and T waves leading to alternating S-T segment depression on every other beat during or after exercise. This finding is invariably associated with severe myocardial ischemia.[5] In general, the prognosis of electrical alternans is grave.[51]

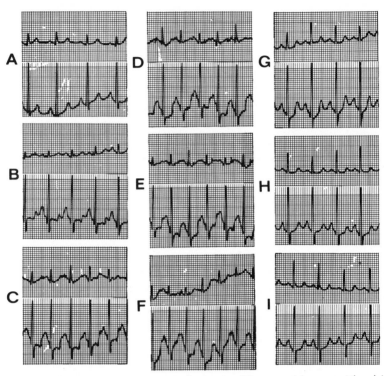

Fig. 12-15   This exercise ECG was taken on a 50-year-old man with a history of atypical chest pain of several months' duration. He had completed a 7-stage course with slight chest discomfort. The maximal heart rate reached to 170 beats/minute. The resting 12-lead ECG was within normal limits (not shown here). The strips A show a resting ECG. The strips B to F are recorded during exercise, whereas the remaining strips (G to I) represent post-exercise ECG. The exercise ECG test is positive. Note horizontal S-T segment depression with biphasic T waves, particularly during exercise. The ECG returns to normal 8 minutes after termination of the exercise.

Computer analysis of the S-T segment depression has gained increasing popularity in recent years, and the sensitivity of the exercise ECG test is said to be markedly enhanced by this means.[12-15, 45] The concept of the "S-T Index" has been utilized recently for the computer analysis of exercise ECG tests.[45] The S-T Index is said to be abnormal when the S-T segment depression is 1 mm. or more, and the sum of the S-T segment depression (in mm.) and the S-T slope (in mv./sec.) = 0 or less.[45] McHenry and Morris[45] stressed that the S-T Index criteria are valid only during exercise or in the immediate recovery period. However, most physicians are satisfied with a visual inspection of the exercise electrocardiogram for the interpretation by using standard diagnostic criteria (see Table 12-7).

The fundamental electrophysiologic mechanisms responsible for the production of the S-T segment depression or elevation in coronary artery disease will be omitted here since an exhaustive description of the subject is beyond the scope of this Chapter (see Chapter 1). Physiologic versus abnormal responses to exercise are described in detail elsewhere in this book (see Chapter 11).

2) S-T Segment Elevation. On occasion, horizontal or upsloping S-T segment elevation may occur during or after exercise. When the S-T segment elevation is 1 mm. or greater, the finding is definitely considered a positive exercise ECG test (see Table 12-7). The S-T segment elevation is most commonly encountered in patients with previous myocardial infarctions

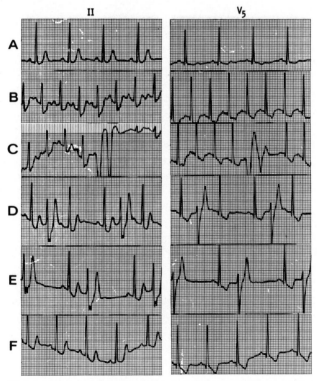

Fig. 12-16 This exercise ECG was obtained from a 50-year-old man with exertional angina associated with palpitations. His resting 12-lead ECG (not shown here) revealed tall T waves in leads V_{1-3} suggestive of posterior myocardial ischemia, and within normal limits otherwise. The strips A are a resting ECG, whereas the strips B and C were taken during exercise. The strips D to F represent post-exercise ECG. His maximal heart rate was 143 beats/minute. The exercise test was prematurely terminated because of significant chest pain associated with frequent VPCs and S-T segment depression. The exercise ECG test is, of course, positive (incomplete).

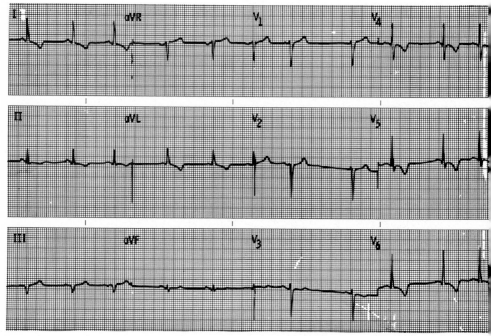

Fig. 12-17   Figures 12-17 and 18 were obtained from a 57-year-old man with myocardial infarction 3 months previously. His resting 12-lead ECG shown in this figure reveals sinus rhythm with occasional atrial premature contractions and old diaphragmatic myocardial infarction with postero-lateral myocardial ischemia.

(particularly anterior wall involvement) associated with areas of akinesis or dyskinesis[5, 45] (Figures 12-19 and 20). Many of these patients reveal ventricular aneurysm. The S-T segment elevation may involve diffusely many leads (Figures 12-21 and 22), but more commonly reciprocal S-T segment depression is observed in the lead facing the uninfarcted zone (Figure 12-20).

Recently, Chahine et al.[52] reviewed the treadmill tests of 840 consecutive patients, and 29 of them (3.5%) showed exercise-induced S-T segment elevation. Anterior myocardial infarction was found on the resting ECG in 25 (85%). Angiographic studies on 21 patients demonstrated critical lesions of the left anterior descending artery in 19 (90%) and left ventricular aneurysm in 18 (86%). They concluded that exercise-induced S-T segment elevation reflects the presence of severe coronary artery disease commonly associated with ventricular aneurysm, and it may be related more to the abnormal ventricular wall motion than to the myocardial ischemia per se.

Exercise-induced S-T segment elevation is extremely rare in patients with normal resting ECG. Recently, Widlansky et al.[53] reported a case with variant angina and arteriographically documented coronary artery spasm. The patient developed angina associated with exercise-induced S-T segment elevation. In general, the patients with atypical angina or Prinzmetal's angina, characterized by the S-T segment elevation during spontaneous

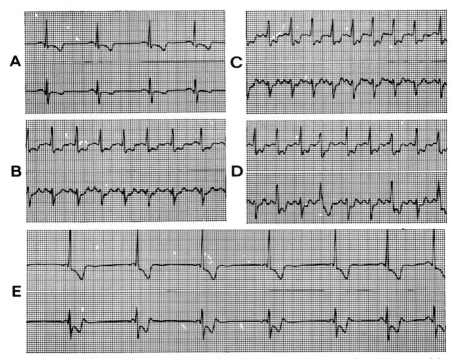

Fig. 12-18 This tracing is an exercise ECG test taken on this 57-year-old man with previous myocardial infarction. An exercise ECG test was performed in order to assess his functional capacity. The strips A are his resting ECG, whereas the strips B and C were taken during exercise. The strips D and E represent the post-exercise ECG. Note the progressive increment of downsloping S-T segment depression with biphasic to inverted T waves during and after exercise. He developed frequent VPCs causing ventricular bigeminy immediately following the termination of exercise (strips D). Within 1-2 minutes, he developed a marked slowing of his heart rate (area of A-V junctional escape rhythm and sinus bradycardia—rate: 43–52 beats/minute) associated with hypotension. His exercise ECG test was prematurely terminated because of chest discomfort and extreme fatigue associated with significant S-T segment depression. His maximal heart rate was 140 beats/minute. His exercise capacity was estimated to be functional class II because he was unable to complete stage 2 of the exercise protocol. His exercise ECG test is, of course, positive (incomplete).

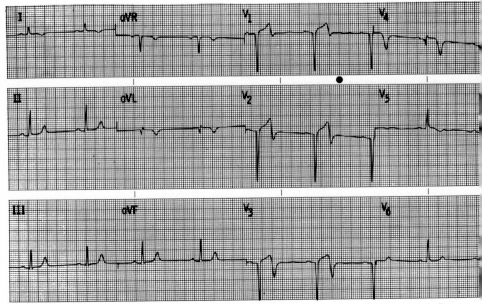

Fig. 12-19 Figures 12-19 and 20 are taken on a 45-year-old man who had suffered from myocardial infarction 1½ years earlier. His 12-lead ECG shown in this figure represents sinus bradycardia with a rate of 52 beats/minute and the evidence of old antero-septal myocardial infarction. He has been taking Isordil 10 mg. 3 times daily for chest pain following his heart attack.

episodes of angina due to coronary artery spasm, often show negative exercise ECG tests.[54, 55] Ellestad[5] occasionally observed patients who initially developed the S-T segment depression during exercise and it was followed by S-T segment elevation if exercise was continued.

It should be noted that some patients with previous myocardial infarction may develop diagnostic horizontal or downsloping S-T segment depression (Figures 12-17 and 18) rather than the above-mentioned S-T segment elevation. In addition, small numbers of patients with documented previous myocardial infarction (either anterior or diaphragmatic) may reveal negative exercise ECG tests (Figures 12-23 to 26).

In healthy young individuals (most commonly young black males) with so-called "early repolarization pattern" (J-point S-T segment elevation at rest), S-T segment usually returns to isoelectric as the exercise is continued, and the S-T segment elevation reappears during recovery period. This finding, of course, is a physiologic phenomenon.

3) S-T Segment Change with Pre-existing ECG Abnormalities. As emphasized previously, there are numerous factors which influence the result of the exercise ECG test (see Table 12-1). Consequently, many cardiac as well as non-cardiac factors cause false positive (see Table 12-4) and false negative (see Table 12-5) exercise ECG tests.

When the resting ECG shows non-specific S-T segment and T wave abnormality due to various causes, the exercise ECG test is extremely difficult to interpret. Nevertheless, Linhart[9] suggested that additional 1 mm. or more S-T segment depression is diagnostic of a positive exercise ECG test in patients with pre-existing abnormal S-T, T wave change on resting ECG (Figure 12-27) as long as they are not taking cardiac drugs, particularly digitalis or tranquilizing drugs. Recently, Kansal et al.[56] studied near-maxi-

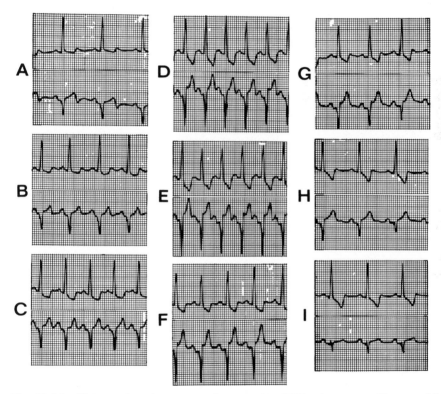

Fig. 12-20   This tracing represents the exercise ECG taken on a 45-year-old man with previous myocardial infarction 1½ years ago. Each rhythm strip contains lead II (top) and CM₅ (bottom). The strips A are a resting tracing. The strips B to E are taken during exercise while the remaining strips (F to I) represent post-exercise tracings. He was unable to complete the scheduled exercise because of chest pain with S-T segment alteration during stage 5. His maximal heart rate reached to 152 beats/minute. The exercise ECG test is positive (incomplete). Note marked S-T segment depression in leads II with S-T segment elevation in lead CM₅. Aorto-coronary bypass surgery was performed with a good result.

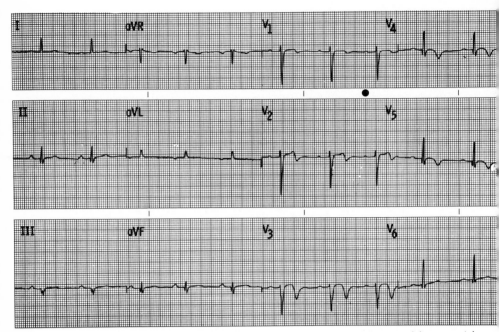

Fig. 12-21   Figures 12-21 and 22 were obtained from a 42-year-old man with myocardial infarction 2 months previously. His resting 12-lead ECG shown in this figure reveals sinus rhythm and old diaphragmatic myocardial infarction associated with anterior myocardial ischemia.

mal graded exercise tests on 37 patients with a history of chest pain and with S-T segment depression at rest. They observed additional S-T segment depression of 1 mm. or greater with exercise in 26 patients, and 23 of these patients had obstruction of one or more coronary arteries. Eleven patients demonstrated no additional S-T segment depression wth exercise, and 9 of these had normal coronary arteriograms.

Abnormal S-T, T wave change is often due to left ventricular hypertrophy (LVH) or left bundle branch block (LBBB). When the resting ECG reveals LVH, the exercise ECG test is unreliable in most cases. In some cases with LVH, the patient may develop LBBB during exercise as the heart rate is accelerated. Then, the exercise ECG test is unreliable because the secondary S-T, T wave change due to LBBB becomes exaggerated by the exercise regardless of the presence or absence of coronary heart disease (Figures 12-28 and 29) leading to a false positive exercise ECG test.[57] For the same reason, the exercise ECG test is unreliable when the resting ECG shows LBBB[57] (Figures 12-30 and 31). Similarly, a false positive exercise ECG test is the rule rather than the exception when a resting ECG reveals LVH because the secondary S-T, T wave change due to LVH is exaggerated by the exercise.

When the resting ECG demonstrates right bundle branch block (RBBB), it does not seem to alter the interpretation of the exercise ECG test in any significant degree. In other words, one can not predict the outcome of the exercise ECG test in individuals with pre-existing RBBB. The diagnostic S-T segment depression may be observed in patients with RBBB when ischemic response is produced by exercise (Figures 12-32 and 33). On the other hand, the exercise ECG test may be negative in healthy individuals with pre-existing RBBB (Figures 12-34 and 35). Recently, Whinnery et al.[58] studied maximal treadmill testing in 40 asymptomatic, apparently healthy men with acquired RBBB. Eight had significant angiographic coronary artery disease, and 6 of the 8 had single-vessel disease. None of the men developed abnormal S-T segment changes in response to maximal treadmill testing. They concluded that the sensitivity of exercise testing for coronary artery disease in men with RBBB is uncertain.

Left anterior hemiblock (LAHB) or left axis deviation from other causes

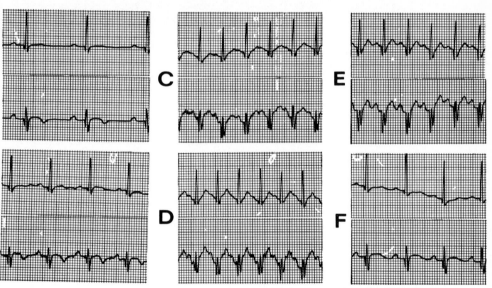

Fig. 12-22   This tracing is his exercise ECG which was ordered primarily for the assessment of his functional capacity. The strips A are his resting ECG, whereas the strips B to D were recorded during exercise. The strips E and F represent his post-exercise ECG. Note significant upsloping S-T segment elevation during and after exercise. He exercised up to the middle of stage 6, and his maximal heart rate was 168 beats/minute. His functional capacity was estimated to be class I. His exercise ECG test is still positive, however.

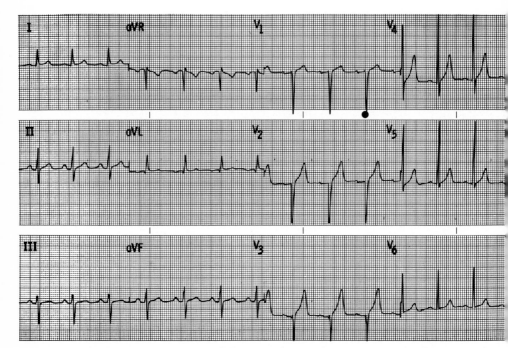

Fig. 12-23   Figures 12-23 and 24 were obtained from a 43-year-old man with a history of myocardial infarction 3 months previously. This figure shows sinus rhythm with a rate of 83 beats/minute and the evidence of old anterior myocardial infarction which is manifested by a loss of R waves in leads V_{2-3}.

is said to produce a false negative exercise ECG test.[59] However, abnormal S-T segment depression can be detected on the exercise ECG when multiple leads are utilized (Figures 12-36 and 37). Similarly, pre-existing bifascicular block (combination of RBBB and LAHB, or RBBB and left posterior hemiblock) does not seem to influence the interpretation of the exercise ECG test (Figures 12-38 and 39).

The extremely high incidence of false positive exercise ECG tests among individuals with Wolff-Parkinson-White (WPW) syndrome is well known (Figures 12-40 and 41). In my recent study dealing with 20 healthy individuals with known WPW syndrome, all subjects (16 out of 20) showing anomalous A-V conduction during exercise demonstrated a false positive exercise ECG test (Figures 12-40 and 41).[60] Thus, it is concluded that the exercise ECG test is invalid in individuals with known WPW syndrome. In addition, the high incidence of false positive exercise ECG tests in individuals with mitral valve prolapse syndrome is well recognized (Figure 12-42).

A common occurrence of exercise-induced S-T segment elevation in patients with previous myocardial infarction has been stressed previously (Figures 12-19 to 22). At times, however, exercise-induced S-T segment depression may be observed in patients with previous myocardial infarction

(Figures 12-17 and 18) and the exercise ECG test may be entirely negative in spite of old myocardial infarction in some cases (Figures 12-23 to 26).

In individuals with dextrocardia, the result of the exercise ECG test will be influenced by the coexisting cardiac anomaly. When there is a significant coronary heart disease, the diagnostic S-T segment depression is expected on the exercise ECG (Figures 12-43 and 44). The only problem, of course, is to use the right precordial leads (e.g., opposite side of CM$_5$) for individuals with dextrocardia.

(B) Cardiac Arrhythmias

Various cardiac arrhythmias may be provoked or suppressed by exercise in healthy individuals as well as in patients with coronary heart disease.

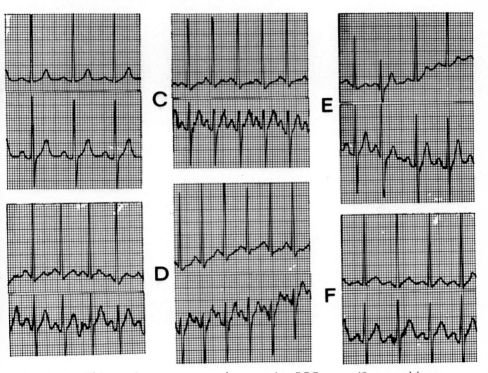

Fig. 12-24 This tracing represents the exercise ECG on a 43-year-old man with a previous history of anterior myocardial infarction. The exercise ECG was ordered to assess his functional capacity. The strips A represent a resting tracing. The strips B to D were taken during exercise whereas the remaining strips E and F represent post-exercise ECG. He was able to complete a 7-stage course without any difficulty and the maximal heart rate reached to 165 beats/minute. His functional capacity was excellent (functional class I) and the exercise ECG test is negative. Note a ventricular premature beat in strip E.

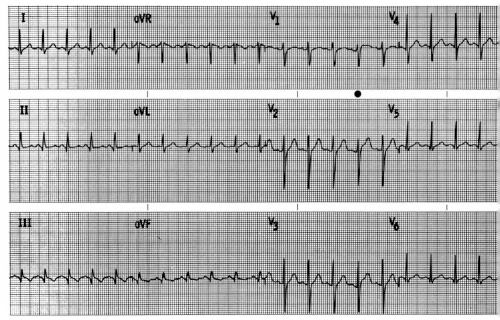

Fig. 12-25   Figures 12-25 and 26 were obtained from a 39-year-old man who had suffered from acute myocardial infarction 2 months previously. A 12-lead ECG shown in this figure reveals sinus tachycardia with a rate of 123 beats/minute and the evidence of old diaphragmatic myocardial infarction.

Nevertheless, certain ventricular arrhythmias such as frequent VPCs, multifocal VPCs, grouped VPCs and ventricular tachycardia provoked by minimal exercise (70% or less of maximal heart rate) are considered to be highly suggestive of coronary heart disease (see Table 12-6, Figure 12-45) even in the absence of diagnostic S-T segment alteration. Of course, many patients with proven coronary artery disease demonstrate the diagnostic S-T segment change associated with serious ventricular arrhythmias (Figures 12-16, 18, 44 and 46). Marked bradycardia often occurs in patients with advanced coronary artery disease during the immediate post-exercise period, and it is frequently associated with angina, hypotension and significant S-T segment depression (Figure 12-18).

Atrial or A-V junctional tachyarrhythmias during or after exercise are non-specific findings and they are clinically insignificant (Figure 12-47). Various ECG findings of equivocal or no value for the diagnosis of the exercise ECG test are summarized in Table 12-9. Detailed descriptions of exercise-induced cardiac arrhythmias are found elsewhere in this book (see Chapter 13).

(C) Inversion of U Waves

Inversion of U waves during or after exercise had received little attention until recently. Although it is rare, inverted U waves provoked by exercise in a patient with a normal resting ECG are highly suggestive of a positive exercise ECG test[3, 45] (see Table 12-6, Figure 12-48). It should be noted, however, that prominent U waves on the exercise ECG are indicative of hypokalemia and *not* myocardial ischemia.

(D) Intraventricular Blocks

Various intraventricular blocks including LBBB, RBBB, hemiblocks and bifascicular block may be observed during or after exercise, but their occurrence is merely a rate-dependent phenomenon. In other words, rate-

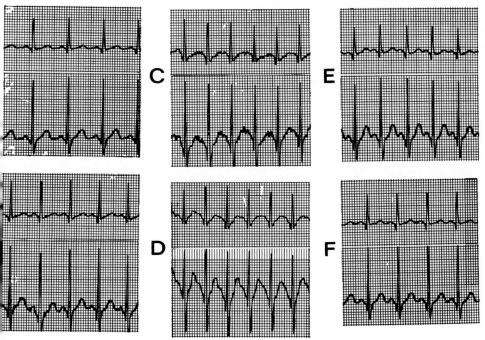

Fig. 12-26 This tracing was taken on a 39-year-old man with a history of diaphragmatic myocardial infarction 2 months previously. The exercise ECG was performed in order to assess his functional capacity. The strips A represent a resting ECG. The strips B to D were recorded during exercise, whereas the remaining strips E and F were obtained during the post-exercise period. He has completed a 7-stage course without any complaint, and his maximal heart rate reached to 176 beats/minute. The exercise ECG test is negative. His functional capacity is, therefore, functional class I.

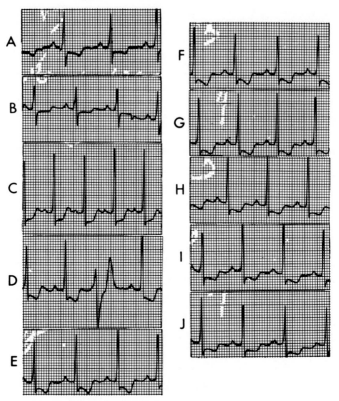

K.J., 50 M. - Angina and hypertension
Incomplete exercise ECG test because of chest pain

Fig. 12-27   This exercise ECG was taken on a 50-year-old man with angina pectoris and hypertension. The strips A and B were taken at rest on supine and standing position, respectively. The strip C was recorded during exercise, whereas the remaining strips D to J represent post-exercise ECG. The exercise test was terminated soon after the initiation of exercise because of severe chest pain associated with marked S-T segment depression (downsloping S-T segment depression preceded by horizontal S-T segment depression). Note also significant increment of the R wave amplitude during and after exercise. He was unable to exercise beyond stage 1 and his maximal heart rate was only 110 beats/minute. The exercise ECG test is positive (incomplete), and his functional capacity is class III. He required sublingual nitroglycerin for severe angina. Note a VPC in strip D.

dependent LBBB or RBBB may develop as the heart rate is accelerated by the exercise beyond the critical rate. Therefore, the development of intraventricular blocks during or after exercise alone is *not* diagnostic of coronary heart disease (Figures 12-28 and 29). On the other hand, the diagnostic S-T

segment depression may be observed during normal intraventricular conduction in patients with intermittent LBBB (Figures 12-49 and 50). Under
this circumstance, of course, the usual diagnostic criteria are applied (see
Table 12-7). Exercise-induced intraventricular blocks are discussed in Chapter 13 in detail.

(E) Increased R Wave Amplitude

As described previously, the amplitude of the QRS complex is often
reduced slightly in healthy individuals, especially during a near-maximal
exercise period or immediately after exercise as a physiologic phenomenon
(see Table 12-2). Recently, Christison et al.[40] studied the diagnostic value of
changes in R wave amplitude to compare with S-T segment alterations by
treadmill stress testing in 108 selected cases as a predictor of coronary artery
disease. They found that the S-T segment changes had a sensitivity of 49%
with a specificity of 74%, whereas the R wave amplitude changes had a
sensitivity of 68% with a specificity of 84%. In their study, an index formed
from the sum of the change in the R wave amplitude and the magnitude of
the S-T segment change, demonstrated a sensitivity of 74% with a specificity

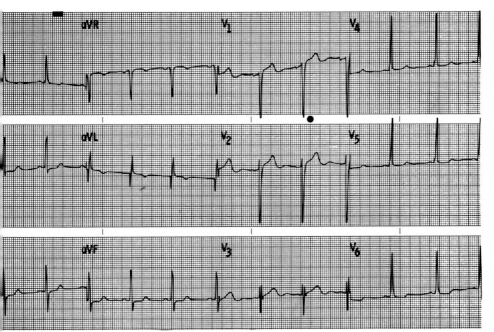

Fig. 12-28   Figures 12-28 and 29 were obtained from a 70-year-old woman
with hypertension and chest pain. Her resting ECG shown in this figure
reveals left ventricular hypertrophy.

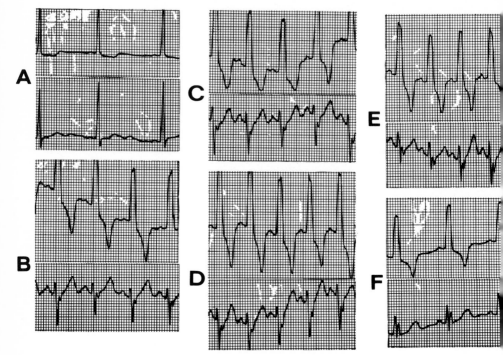

Fig. 12-29 This tracing shows her exercise ECG test. The strips A are her resting ECG, whereas the strips B to D were taken during exercise. The strips E and F represent post-exercise ECG. She developed left bundle branch block soon after the exercise was initiated as the heart rate increased. The exercise ECG test as a diagnostic tool is invalid in the presence of left bundle branch block. She reached the maximal heart rate of only 128 beats/minute (stage 3). Her functional capacity was estimated to be class II.

of 78%. It was interesting to note that 69% had no coronary artery disease, whereas 31% had significant lesions in those patients showing reduction of R wave amplitude. The clinically significant result was that 83% had coronary artery disease while 17% had no coronary heart disease in patients showing increment or no change in the R wave amplitude. Among 83% with coronary artery disease, 81% had 2- or 3-vessel disease (greater than 70% stenosis), whereas only 19% had a single-vessel disease. These authors concluded, from this study, that increment or no change of the R wave amplitude during treadmill exercise testing is a more reliable indicator of significant coronary artery disease than S-T segment changes.

Another study from the same laboratory,[41] using 159 patients (52 false positives and 107 false negatives) who were selected randomly by computer, demonstrated that the incidence of these false positive and negative tests was significantly reduced when the R wave amplitude changes were analyzed. The authors concluded that S-T segment depression with reduction of R wave amplitude is suggestive of a false positive test, whereas the increment of R wave amplitude without significant S-T segment depression is suggestive of a false negative exercise ECG test. However, the diagnostic value of the R wave amplitude change requires further investigation to increase the sensitivity and specificity of the exercise ECG test.

(F) Acute Myocardial Infarction

The precise incidence of acute myocardial infarction directly related to the exercise ECG test is difficult to assess, but it seems to be extremely rare. McHenry and Morris[45] reported 2 or 3 cases of unsuspected recent myocardial infarction of less than 48 hours in duration at the time of the pre-test examination among approximately 1,200 patients annually. In our laboratory, we have observed a similar annual incidence of unsuspected recent myocardial infarction before the exercise ECG test, but no patient developed acute myocardial infarction during or after exercise among 5,500 patients tested in the past 5 years.

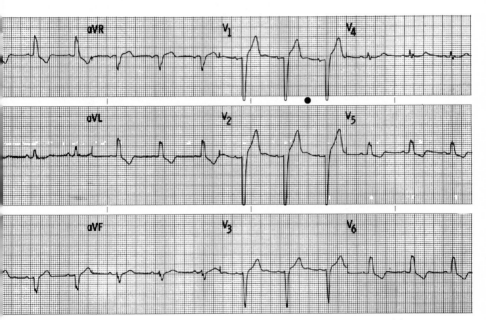

Fig. 12-30   Figures 12-30 and 31 were obtained from a 52-year-old woman with atypical chest discomfort of several months' duration. Her resting ECG shown in this figure reveals left bundle branch block.

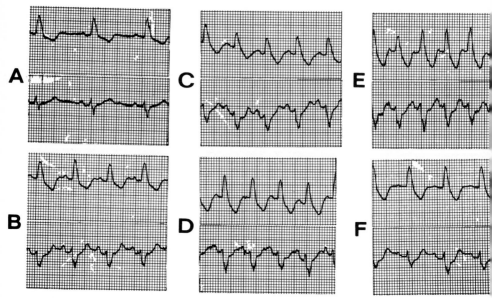

Fig. 12-31   This tracing is her exercise ECG. The strips A are her resting ECG while the strips B to E were taken during exercise. The strips F represent post-exercise ECG. Her maximal heart rate was 162 beats/minute (stage 6), and her functional capacity was estimated to be class I. Needless to say, her exercise ECG test is invalid because of pre-existing left bundle branch block as far as the diagnostic value is concerned.

Obviously, the exercise ECG test will be unequivocally positive when acute myocardial infarction is provoked by exercise testing.

(G) Miscellaneous Findings

Various electrocardiographic findings such as Q-X:Q-T ratio, Q-T interval change, alteration in the P wave or T wave morphology, etc., during or after exercise are non-specific or unreliable for the interpretation of the exercise ECG test (see Table 12-2).

2. Hemodynamic Changes

It has been well documented that the major determinants of increased myocardial oxygen requirements include increases in heart rate, intramyocardial tension and velocity of myocardial contraction. Physical exercise is proved to be a potent stimulus for all of these determinants. It has been shown that the simple product of heart rate and systolic blood pressure is a practical index for the clinical exercise laboratory.

As a physiologic phenomenon, acceleration of heart rate with elevation of systolic blood pressure is expected during and after exercise (see Table 12-2). When the expected increment in heart rate and/or blood pressure is not observed during exercise, abnormal hemodynamic alterations should be suspected. On the other hand, a more than expected rise in systolic blood pressure during exercise most likely represents labile hypertension.

(A) Hypotension

In healthy individuals, physical exercise causes an increment in systolic blood pressure associated with a slight reduction of diastolic blood pressure leading to a wide pulse pressure.[61, 62] Reduction of systolic blood pressure below a resting value at the onset of treadmill exercise-induced angina has been reported to be a reliable diagnostic sign for advanced multivessel coronary artery disease.[63] On the other hand, a reduction of systolic blood pressure below resting value has also been encountered during treadmill exercise testing in some patients with severe valvular, hypertensive or coronary heart disease.[64] In addition, a reduction of systolic blood pressure

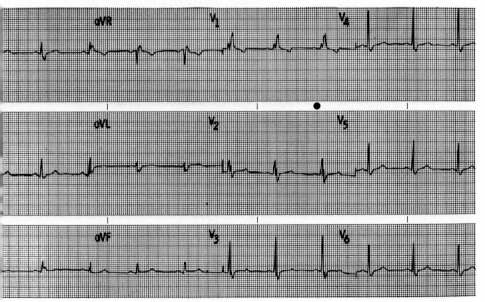

Fig. 12-32   Figures 12-32 and 33 were taken on a 50-year-old man with a history of angina for 6–8 months. A 12-lead ECG shown in this figure reveals sinus rhythm with a rate of 65 beats/minute and right bundle branch block which is manifested by RR' or M-shape QRS complex in leads V$_{1-2}$ with slurred S waves in leads I, aVL and V$_{4-6}$.

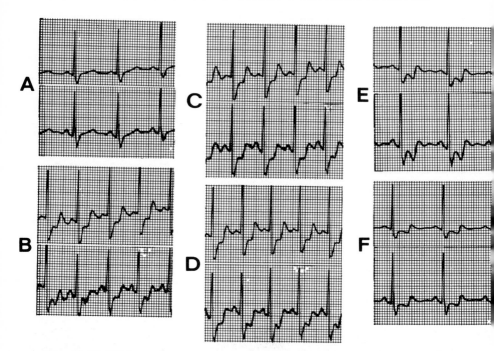

Fig. 12-33   This tracing represents the exercise ECG test taken on a 50-year-old man with angina. The strip A is a resting ECG. The strips B to D were taken during exercise, whereas the remaining strips E and F represent post-exercise ECG. The exercise ECG test was stopped in the middle of stage 4 because of significant chest pain associated with horizontal to downsloping S-T segment depression. The maximal heart rate reached to 130 beats/minute. The exercise ECG test is positive (incomplete). Note marked horizontal to downsloping S-T segment depression with biphasic to inverted T waves during and after exercise.

is reported to occur during exercise testing in the absence of significant coronary artery disease, especially in females.[65] In particular, very anxious subjects with excessive sympathetic tone at the beginning of the exercise test may show a temporary reduction of their heart rate and systolic blood pressure during the first 2–3 minutes of exercise.[45] Furthermore, it has been suggested that a reduction of systolic blood pressure may be a physiologic response in some healthy individuals during prolonged strenuous exercise.[66, 67]

Recently, Morris et al.[68] investigated the incidence of decreases in peak systolic blood pressure during treadmill exercise testing in 460 patients with definite or suspected coronary artery disease. Twenty-two patients with 75% or greater stenosis of one or more major coronary arteries showed a reduction of systolic blood pressure 10 mm. Hg or more during exercise. The reduction of blood pressure was reproducible in the 7 patients who underwent a second exercise ECG test; this blood pressure reduction was abolished in the 6 patients who exercised again following coronary bypass surgery. A reduction of systolic blood pressure of 10 mm. Hg or more was also observed during exercise testing in 3 patients with an obstructive cardiomyopathy. A reduction of systolic blood pressure was not encountered during 650 maximal exercise tests performed on 560 clinically healthy men.

These investigators concluded that a sustained exercise-induced reduction of peak systolic blood pressure of 10 mm. Hg or greater is a highly specific sign of multivessel coronary artery disease, provided that cardiomyopathy or significant valvular heart disease is excluded. The reduction of the systolic blood pressure is considered on the basis of acute left ventricular pump failure secondary to extensive myocardial ischemia.

Zohman and Kattus[8] further emphasized that progressive reduction of

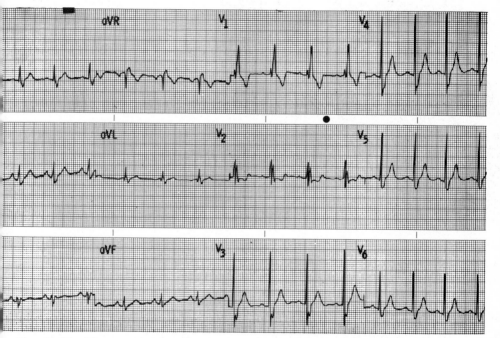

Fig. 12-34 Figures 12-34 and 35 were obtained from a 61-year-old male with chest discomfort from unknown cause. This figure shows a 12-lead ECG on this patient, and the diagnosis of right bundle branch block is obvious. Right bundle branch block is diagnosed on the basis of RR' or M-shape QRS complex in leads V_{1-2} with slurred S waves in leads I, aVL and V_{3-6}.

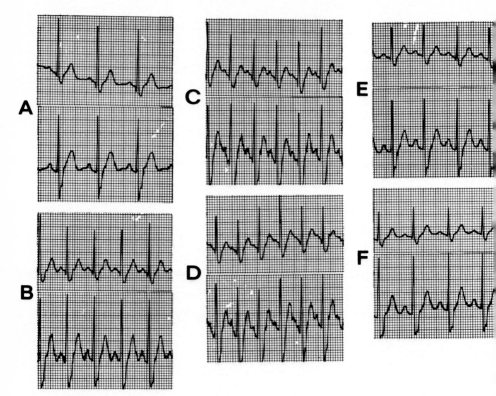

Fig. 12-35 This tracing represents the exercise ECG test on a 61-year-old man. He has performed a 7-stage course of the exercise ECG test without any difficulty. Chest discomfort was not produced by the exercise. His maximal heart rate reached to 175 beats/minute. The strips A represent a resting (control) ECG. The strips B to D were taken during exercise, whereas the remaining strips E and F are post-exercise ECG. The exercise ECG test is negative.

systolic blood pressure during increasing workloads is a strong indicator of myocardial ischemia even in the absence of chest pain or the diagnostic ECG abnormalities (see Tables 12-6 and 7). The blood pressure change during exercise, therefore, will be extremely valuable when there are various factors which may cause a false positive exercise ECG test (e.g., LBBB, WPW syndrome, left ventricular hypertrophy, pre-existing S-T, T wave abnormality, etc., see Table 12-4). It should be noted that various pharmacologic agents may significantly reduce cardiac output or augment the vasodilatation accompanying exercise. This fact should be kept in mind when evaluating the blood pressure change during exercise.

(B) Slowing of Heart Rate

In healthy individuals, a progressive acceleration of the heart rate is expected during a multistage exercise ECG test. The average increment of heart rate during submaximal or maximal exercise ECG test in healthy subjects is well established (see Chapter 9). Thus, a failure of the increment in heart rate during exercise may be an important abnormal response to exercise, and the finding may be a strongly suggestive sign of advanced coronary heart disease. On the other hand, insignificant acceleration of sinus rate (less than 120 beats/minute) during submaximal or maximal exercise may be indicative of sick sinus syndrome.[27] It should be emphasized, however, that physically active healthy individuals such as athletes may not exhibit the expected heart rate acceleration during exercise. In addition, beta-blockers such as propranolol (Inderal) will prevent acceleration of sinus rate.

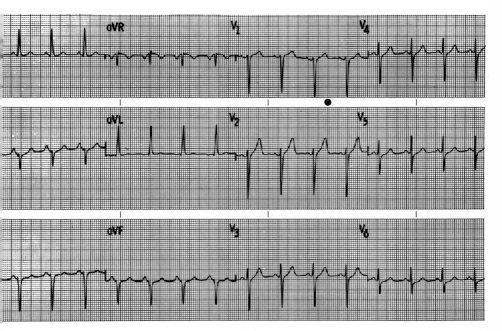

Fig. 12-36 Figures 12-36 and 37 were taken on a 50-year-old man who has been suffering from exertional chest pain for several months. A 12-lead ECG shown in this figure reveals sinus rhythm with a rate of 92 beats/minute, and left anterior hemiblock on the basis of marked left axis deviation of the QRS complexes (QRS axis: −45 degrees).

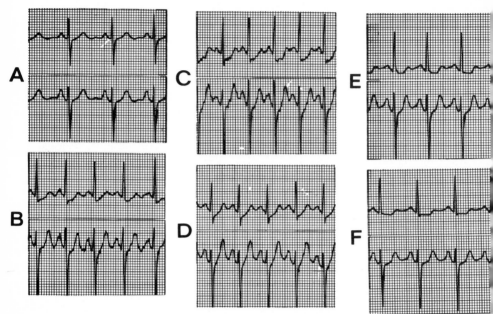

Fig. 12-37   This tracing shows the exercise ECG test on a 50-year-old man with chest pain. The exercise was stopped prematurely at the end of stage 5 because of significant chest pain. His maximal heart rate reached to 150 beats/minute. The strips A represent a resting (control) ECG. The strips B and C were taken during exercise, whereas the remaining strips D to F represent post-exercise ECG. The exercise ECG test is positive (incomplete). Note significant horizontal S-T segment depression in lead CM₅ during and after exercise. Only functional S-T segment depression is shown in lead II (bottom strips).

(C) Marked Hypertension

Unusual elevation of systolic blood pressure during exercise is also an abnormal response although it is *not* indicative of coronary heart disease. Most physicians believe that systolic pressure above 220 mm. Hg during exercise is an abnormal response. Labile hypertension is often suspected under these conditions. Exercise testing should be terminated when significant elevation (220 mm. Hg) of systolic pressure is recorded during exercise.

3. Symptoms and Signs

Various symptoms and signs may be observed during or after exercise, but the most common symptom is probably fatigue. Although some manifestations such as fatigue or dyspnea are nonspecific, others such as exercise-induced typical angina are highly diagnostic of coronary heart disease.

(A) Symptoms

Among various exercise-induced symptoms, typical chest pain provoked by exercise is the only reliable symptom of coronary artery disease. However, it should be noted that many patients with atypical or non-specific chest pain may also experience their "characteristic" pain during exercise. The most important aspect of evaluating chest pain is its reproducibility by exercise. In other words, typical angina pectoris can be reproduced with the same amount of exercise workloads or product of heart rate and blood pressure with repeated exercise testing. This reliable finding is highly suggestive of coronary artery disease even in the absence of the diagnostic S-T segment change.[8, 45, 69] This is particularly so if the angina is relieved by administration of nitroglycerin during continuous exercise testing.[8] Conversely, atypical (not true angina) or non-specific chest pain fails to show its reproducibility. In many cases, atypical chest pain can not be reproduced at workloads considerably higher than those the patient reaches during daily activities.

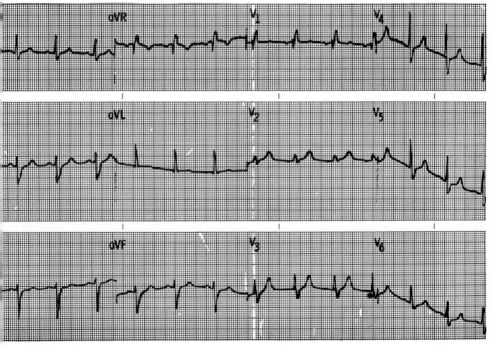

Fig. 12-38   Figures 12-38 and 39 were obtained from a 64-year-old man with occasional chest discomfort. A 12-lead ECG shown in this figure reveals sinus rhythm with a rate of 80 beats/minute and a bifascicular block. The bifascicular block consists of right bundle branch block and left anterior hemiblock (the QRS axis: −65 degrees).

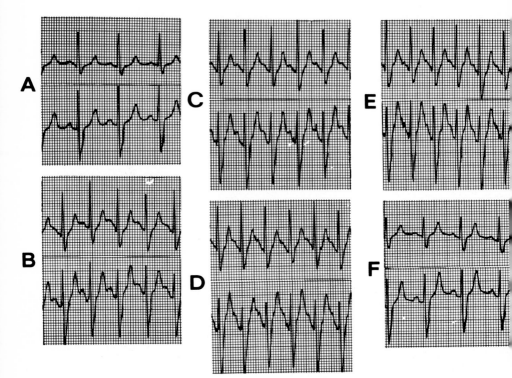

Fig. 12-39 This tracing demonstrates the exercise ECG test on a 64-year-old man. He has completed the exercise ECG test up to stage 6 without any problem, and the desired maximal heart rate (rate: 165 beats/minute) was reached. The strip A represents a resting ECG. The strips B to E were taken during exercise while the strips F demonstrate post-exercise ECG. The exercise ECG test is negative.

Recently, Cole and Ellestad[70] studied the significance of chest pain during treadmill exercise to correlate with coronary events (myocardial infarction, progression of angina and coronary death) in 1,402 patients with a positive maximal treadmill stress test. Coronary events were twice as frequent in patients with angina and S-T segment depression as in those without angina. In addition, the incidence of coronary events was more than twice as great when the angina was provoked by a light workload (4 METs) as when it was provoked by a heavier workload (8–9 METs). This study clearly demonstrated that the patients (men between the ages of 41 and 50) who developed angina during exercise had a 3-fold greater incidence of coronary events and a 4-fold greater incidence of myocardial infarction compared with their counterparts showing S-T segment depression alone. They concluded that exercise-induced angina identified 85% of true positive tests for coronary artery disease, whereas S-T segment depression alone identified only 64%.

Severe dyspnea, marked pallor or cyanosis and near-syncope or syncope are abnormal responses to exercise, but these manifestations are *not* diagnostic of coronary heart disease.

(B) Signs

The importance of recognizing various abnormal physical signs during or after exercise in patients with known or suspected coronary heart disease has not been fully appreciated. Among auscultatory findings, a clearly audible S_4 gallop provoked by exercise is considered an important diagnostic sign of myocardial ischemia even if the diagnostic S-T segment change is absent.[5, 9, 45] When the S-T segment abnormality or angina induced by

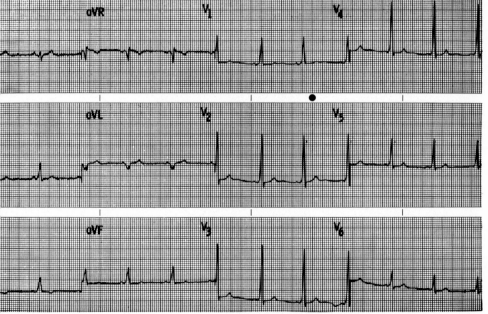

Fig. 12-40   Figures 12-40 and 41 were taken on a 48-year-old man as a part of the research program. A 12-lead ECG shown in this figure reveals sinus rhythm with a rate of 70 beats/minute, and the evidence of Wolff-Parkinson-White (WPW) syndrome, type A. Note a short P-R interval with broad QRS complex due to a delta wave (initial slurring of the QRS complex). The WPW syndrome, type A is diagnosed because the delta wave is directed anteriorly. Note that the QRS complexes are upright in all precordial leads.

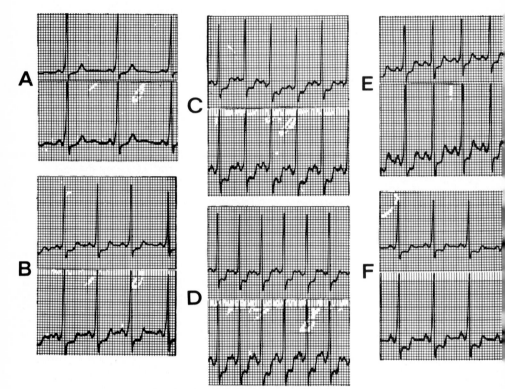

Fig. 12-41   This tracing shows the exercise ECG test on a 48-year-old man with the Wolff-Parkinson-White syndrome, type A. He has completed a 7-stage course exercise without any complaint, and his maximal heart rate reached to 170 beats/minute. The strips A represent a resting ECG. The strips B to D were taken during exercise, whereas the remaining strips E and F represent post-exercise ECG. According to the conventional diagnostic criteria, the exercise ECG test is unequivocally positive on this patient. However, it should be re-emphasized that a false positive exercise ECG test is the rule rather than the exception in patients with the WPW syndrome. The evidence of the WPW syndrome is shown throughout in the exercise electrocardiogram.

exercise is equivocal, a post-exercise S_4 gallop may be reliable confirmative evidence for the diagnosis of coronary heart disease. It should be noted, however, that patients with systemic hypertension or other forms of underlying heart disease may be exceptions to this rule regarding the S_4 gallop. A double impulse may be felt when an S_4 gallop is heard. In addition to S_4 gallop, a clearly audible S_3 gallop induced by exercise is also strongly suggestive of advanced coronary artery disease and myocardial dysfunction.[5, 9, 45] Another auscultatory sign is systolic murmurs induced by exercise and the finding is often due to papillary muscle dysfunction which is strongly suggestive of coronary artery disease. Other abnormal signs may include exercise-induced pulsus alternans, abnormal precordial bulges and palpable thrills which may be supportive evidence for the diagnosis of coronary artery disease in some cases.

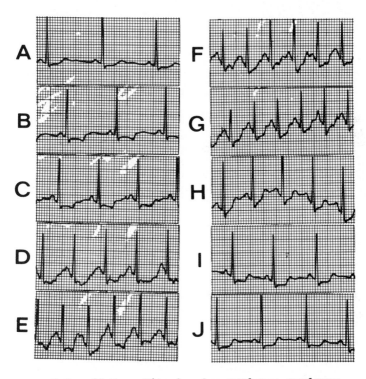

K.T., 45 F. - Mitral valve prolapse syndrome

Fig. 12-42 This exercise ECG was obtained from a 45-year-old woman with atypical chest pain. All rhythm strips represent lead CM5. The strips A and B were taken at rest, in supine and standing position, respectively. The strips C to G were recorded during exercise, whereas the remaining strips H to J represent post-exercise ECG. She had completed a 7-stage course exercise without any chest pain. Her maximal heart rate reached to 167 beats/minute. According to the standard criteria, her exercise ECG test is interpreted as a positive test. However, it is most likely a false positive test in view of her underlying cardiac disorder—mitral valve prolapse syndrome, confirmed by echocardiogram as well as cardiac catheterization. It is well documented that a false positive exercise ECG test is common in patients with mitral valve prolapse syndrome.

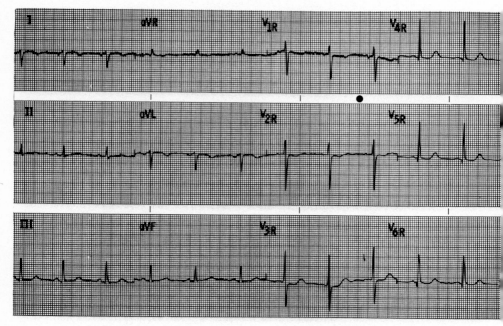

Fig. 12-43 Figures 12-43 and 44 were obtained from a 70-year-old woman with known dextrocardia. Her resting ECG (taken with right precordial leads) shown in this figure is within normal limits, except for dextrocardia.

Factors Modifying the Result of Exercise ECG Interpretations

There are many factors which influence the result of the exercise ECG test (see Table 12-1). Consequently, a false positive exercise ECG test may be produced by numerous factors (see Table 12-4), whereas various factors may cause false negative exercise ECG tests (see Table 12-5). Among these factors, the frequent occurrence of false positive exercise ECG tests in patients with digitalis therapy typifies the above-mentioned statements (Figures 12-51 and 52).

Various factors which influence the results of the exercise ECG test are discussed in Chapter 5; the effects of drugs and metabolic abnormalities on the exercise ECG test are described in Chapter 6.

Clinical Implications of the Result of the Exercise ECG Test[1-9, 15, 16, 45, 68, 70]

1. Symptomatic Patients

The multistage exercise ECG test is the most important and reliable non-invasive method in the diagnosis of coronary artery disease. The sensitivity of the exercise ECG test to diagnose triple-vessel coronary disease approaches near 100% (ranging between 86 and 100%) although the sensitivity

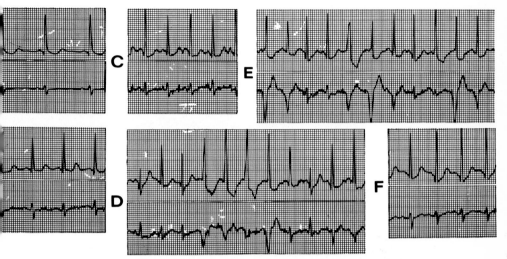

Fig. 12-44   This tracing shows her exercise ECG test. Each top strip represents right side lead CM₅ (opposite site of the usual CM₅). The strips A are her resting ECG, whereas the strips B to D were taken during exercise. The strips E and F represent post-exercise ECG. The exercise ECG test is positive (incomplete) on the basis of significant S-T segment depression and frequent multifocal and grouped VPCs. The exercise was prematurely terminated because of severe chest pain and fatigue associated with the above-mentioned ECG abnormalities. Her maximal heart rate was 140 beats/minute (stage 4).

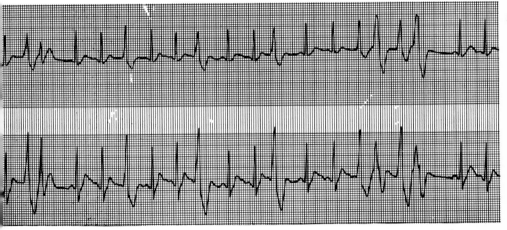

Fig. 12-45   This tracing is an exercise ECG on a 35-year-old man with palpitations. He developed frequent ventricular premature contractions with grouped beats by mild exercise (maximal heart rate: 130 beats/minute). This finding is an abnormal response to exercise, but it is *not* conclusive evidence of coronary artery disease.

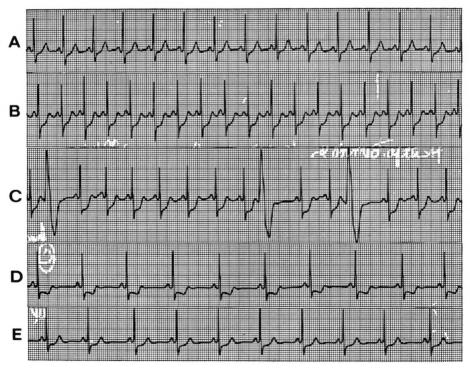

Fig. 12-46   This is an exercise ECG test on a 50-year-old man with angina. The strip A is a resting ECG, whereas the strip B was taken during exercise. The remaining strips C to E represent post-exercise ECG. The exercise ECG test is markedly positive (incomplete). The test was terminated prematurely because of severe chest pain associated with marked upsloping followed by horizontal and downsloping S-T segment depression.

for a single-vessel involvement is only 37–60%.[44-47] The sensitivity is further enhanced when other ischemic responses such as exercise-induced hypotension or typical angina pectoris are interpreted simultaneously. It has been shown that a reduction of systolic blood pressure of 10 mm. Hg or more below peak values during treadmill exercise testing is a reliable sign of multivessel coronary artery disease.[68] Typical true angina pectoris can be reproduced during repeated exercise testing with the same amount of exercise workloads in most cases. Atypical chest pain, on the other hand, is usually not reproducible by repeated exercise testing. Even in individuals with atypical chest pain, the diagnostic S-T segment change during or after exercise indicates an increasing probability of significant coronary artery disease, providing a false positive exercise ECG test is excluded.

The onset of significant S-T segment depression in relation to the amount of exercise workload is important to recognize. Namely, the diagnostic S-T segment depression induced by minimal exercise certainly indicates advanced multivessel disease in most cases, whereas the S-T segment depression that occurs only during near-maximal exercise most likely represents mild coronary artery disease.

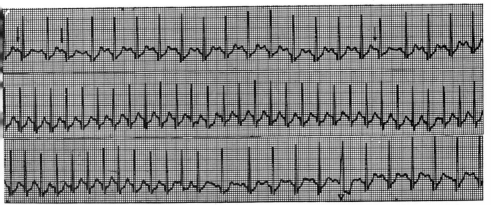

Fig. 12-47 This tracing is an exercise ECG on a 59-year-old woman with palpitations. The strips A to C represent post-exercise ECG. B and C are continuous. She developed paroxysmal atrial tachycardia (rate: 188 beats/minute) soon after the termination of exercise. This finding is a nonspecific response to exercise.

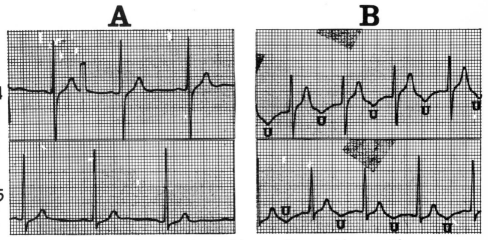

Fig. 12-48 This tracing was obtained from a 47-year-old man with angina. The 12-lead ECG at rest is within normal limits (only leads V₄₋₅ are shown—strip A). After exercise, he developed inverted U waves (marked U—strip B). The exercise ECG test is interpreted as probably positive.

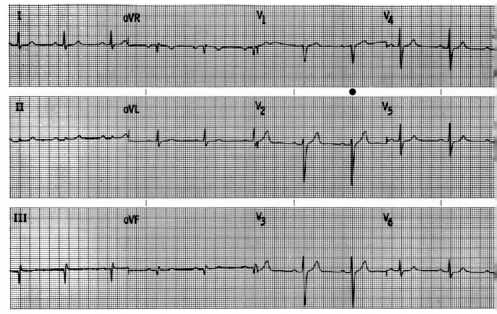

Fig. 12-49   Figures 12-49 and 50 were obtained from a 62-year-old man who had suffered from myocardial infarction 1 year previously. A 12-lead ECG shown in this figure shows sinus rhythm with a rate of 62 beats/minute and evidence of diaphragmatic myocardial infarction.

Various cardiac arrhythmias may be provoked by exercise in healthy individuals as well as in patients with coronary artery disease. In both healthy subjects and coronary patients, cardiac arrhythmias are usually abolished during rapid heart rate in peak exercise periods, but the arrhythmias often recur during the post-exercise period as the heart rate is reduced. Thus, the above-mentioned findings are meaningless clinically. Coronary artery disease is strongly suspected when serious ventricular arrhythmias such as multifocal VPCs, grouped (3 or more) VPCs or ventricular tachycardia are provoked by mild exercise (70% or less of the maximal heart rate). Under these circumstances, other myocardial ischemic responses, including the diagnostic S-T segment depression, typical angina pectoris or hypotension are usually present.

Clearly audible S_4 or S_3 gallop, and systolic murmur during the post-exercise period provide important supportive evidence for the diagnosis of coronary artery disease.

Exercise-induced S-T segment elevation is a relatively uncommon finding, and it is nearly always encountered in patients with previous myocardial infarction, particularly anterior wall involvement. Many patients with exercise-induced S-T segment elevation show ventricular aneurysm and areas of dyskinesis or akinesis of the ventriclar wall. Interestingly enough, the exercise ECG test is usually negative in patients with a variant angina (Prinzmetal's angina) in which S-T segment elevation is often observed during spontaneous angina.

It is well documented that the exercise ECG test provides useful infor-

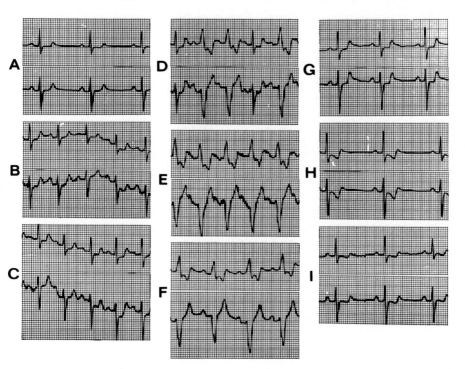

Fig. 12-50   The exercise ECG test shown in this tracing was performed on a 62-year-old man with a history of myocardial infarction 1 year ago because of recurrent chest pain on exertion. The strips A represent a resting ECG. The strips B to E were taken during exercise, whereas the remaining strips F to I represent post-exercise ECG. He was unable to continue the exercise after the end of stage 3 because of chest pain, and the test was stopped prematurely. His maximal heart rate reached only to 108 beats/minute. The exercise ECG test is positive (incomplete). It is interesting to note that intermittent left bundle branch block is observed in the strips D to F. However, the appearance of left bundle branch block alone is *not* diagnostic of a positive exercise ECG test. In this patient, however, the exercise ECG test is interpreted as positive on the basis of horizontal to downsloping S-T segment depression with biphasic to inverted T waves during normal intraventricular conduction. His functional capacity is estimated to be class II.

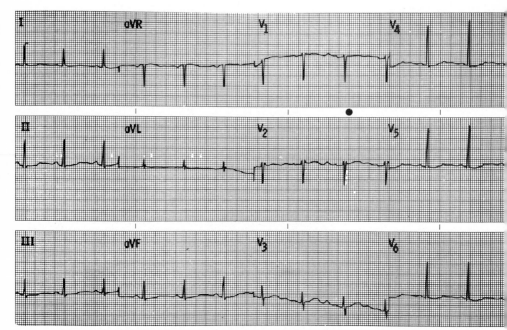

Fig. 12-51 Figures 12-51 and 52 were obtained from a 59-year-old woman during digitalis therapy. Her resting ECG shows non-specific S-T segment and T wave abnormality compatible with digitalis effect. In addition, left ventricular hypertrophy is suggested.

mation on the functional capacity in a given individual with coronary artery disease. In other words, functional classification is possible by evaluating the symptom-limited exercise workloads (see Table 12-10). Patients with functional class IV may be unable to exercise at all (1 MET), whereas functional class I patients may be able to perform exercise with 6–8 METs workloads. Functional class II and III patients can perform 4–6 METs and 2–3 METs exercise workloads, respectively. In patients with functional class II or more, coronary angiography should be considered in order to determine whether significant coronary artery stenosis is present. Aortocoronary by-pass surgery should be recommended on an individual basis according to the angiographic findings in conjunction with other ischemic responses. In functional class I patients, invasive diagnostic study is probably not war-ranted. Under these circumstances, the patients may be treated with vaso-dilators, prevention or elimination of any additional risk factors for coronary heart disease and a medically supervised and prescribed exercise program. The exercise test should be repeated at intervals of 6–12 months in order to assess whether the clinical status is stable, improving or deteriorating. An invasive diagnostic test with a possible surgical approach is in order when the clinical status is deteriorating.

2. Asymptomatic Individuals

There is a significant controversy regarding the clinical implications of positive exercise ECG tests in asymptomatic individuals. Nevertheless, an abnormal ECG response to exercise in asymptomatic subjects is shown to be predictive of an increased incidence of future coronary events. It has been shown that the risk of developing clinical manifestations of coronary artery disease in subsequent years was 14–20 times greater if the exercise test was positive than if it was negative.[71, 72] In addition, a change from a negative to positive exercise ECG test in the same individual is shown to be a more accurate prediction for the presence of asymptomatic coronary artery disease. Borer et al.[73] and Froelicher et al.[71] reported, in highly selected groups of asymptomatic subjects, that approximately 40% had significant coronary artery disease. Another study by Erikssen et al.[74] on a group of clinically healthy subjects (more representative of the general population), indicated that 64% of the subjects with a positive exercise ECG test had significant coronary artery stenosis. The vast majority showed 75% or more stenosis in one or more coronary arteries.

It is extremely important to remember that the predictive accuracy of an abnormal S-T segment response to near-maximal exercise in clinically healthy individuals is not as great as in symptomatic patients. In addition,

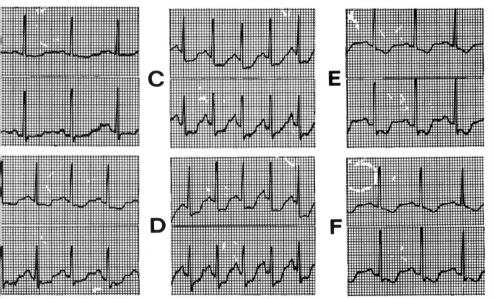

Fig. 12-52   This tracing is her exercise ECG. The strips A are the resting ECG, whereas the strips B to D were taken during exercise. The remaining strips E and F represent post-exercise ECG. This tracing is a typical example of a false positive exercise ECG test due to digitalis effect.

the natural history of patients with coronary artery disease manifested only by an abnormal S-T segment response to near-maximal exercise is not yet certain.

It is well documented that false positive exercise ECG tests can occur in both sexes, but the incidence of false positive tests is approximately 3 times greater in women than men. Cumming et al.[75] clearly demonstrated this fact on 357 asymptomatic women between the ages of 20 and 83. Ellestad and Halleday[76] reported a false positive exercise ECG test among women undergoing catheterization to be 54% according to the diagnostic S-T segment change alone. Another study by Sketch et al.[77] showed 67% false positive tests among 56 women by correlating exercise-induced S-T segment change and coronary arteriographic findings. In addition, a borderline or equivocal exercise ECG test result is extremely common among apparently healthy women between the ages of 30 and 60. The reason for the peculiar reactions of women to exercise testing is not clearly understood. This fact should be kept in mind when interpreting the exercise ECG test on all women, particularly in asymptomatic individuals.

In asymptomatic individuals who develop S-T segment change only, every effort should be made to eliminate possible causes for false positive exercise ECG tests (see Table 12-4). When no direct cause (e.g., digitalis, mitral valve prolapse syndrome) for a false positive test is found, an isolated S-T segment change should be considered as one of the "risk factors", and not as conclusive diagnostic evidence of coronary artery disease. Both physicians and patients should make every effort to reduce or eliminate other risk factors such as hyperlipidemia, obesity, hypertension, diabetes mellitus, smoking, etc. Every asymptomatic individual with a positive exercise ECG test should be well educated by a physician regarding early warning symptoms of coronary heart disease, particularly chest pain, which he should report to his physician immediately. Periodic exercise ECG testing (every 3–6 months) in order to detect new symptoms or earlier development of and more marked S-T segment depression may also be valuable. Invasive cardiac procedures with possible coronary bypass surgery should be considered when the patient's clinical picture and/or exercise ECG test results

Table 12-10. Relationship Between New York Heart Association Functional Classification and MET

1. Cardiac patient is able to perform exercise workloads:	
• *Functional Class I:*	6–10 METs
• *Functional Class II:*	4–6 METs
• *Functional Class III:*	2–3 METs
• *Functional Class IV:*	1 MET
2. Healthy subject is able to perform exercise workloads:	
• *Healthy sedentary individuals:*	Beyond 10–11 METs
• *Physically active individuals:*	Beyond 16 METs

become worse than previous examination. The same diagnostic and therapeutic principles should be applied when asymptomatic individuals with a previous negative test demonstrate a positive exercise ECG test on subsequent testing. It is difficult to establish fixed guidelines as to the frequency of the exercise ECG test in asymptomatic individuals. However, any individual with various coronary risk factors should have a periodic exercise ECG test (every 6–12 months) for early detection of coronary artery disease.

Summary

1. The exercise ECG test is the most reliable non-invasive diagnostic tool for coronary artery disease. The test result should be evaluated in conjunction with the information obtained from the history, physical examination, resting 12-lead electrocardiogram and other routine laboratory findings.

2. There are 3 major myocardial ischemic responses to exercise, including electrocardiographic, hemodynamic and symptomatic. These responses should be interpreted together.

3. Many factors influence the result of the exercise ECG test (see Table 12-1).

4. Physiologic responses versus abnormal responses to exercise are summarized in Tables 12-2 and 3. Various physiologic S-T segment changes such as functional S-T segment depression, S-T segment depression in vasoregulatory asthenia, etc. should not be confused with the diagnostic S-T segment depression (see Table 12-7).

5. There are numerous factors which may cause a false positive (see Table 12-4) and false negative exercise ECG test (see Table 12-5). In particular, digitalis, LBBB, WPW syndrome and left ventricular hypertophy most commonly produce a false positive exercise ECG test. Propranolol and other anti-anginal drugs frequently cause a false negative test.

6. Development of exercise-induced hypotension and typical angina pectoris is extremely valuable evidence for diagnosis of coronary artery disease. A unique feature of true angina pectoris is its reproducibility of chest pain by the same exercise workloads.

7. Exercise-induced S_3 or S_4 gallop and systolic murmurs are reliable supportive evidence for the diagnosis of coronary artery disease.

8. Various cardiac arrhythmias may be provoked or abolished by exercise in healthy individuals as well as in patients with coronary artery disease. However, the development of serious ventricular arrhythmias such as frequent VPCs, multifocal VPCs, grouped VPCs and ventricular tachycardia provoked by minimal exercise workloads (70% or less of the maximal heart rate) is nearly always indicative of advanced multivessel coronary artery disease.

9. Horizontal or downsloping S-T segment depression of 1 mm. or greater is the most reliable finding for a positive exercise ECG test (see Table 12-7).

Table 12-11. Report of Exercise ECG Test Result

1. Indicate whether the test is positive or negative, borderline or equivocal.
2. Describe abnormal responses to exercise in detail (type and magnitude of S-T segment change, etc.).
3. Specify the reason for termination of the test.
4. Specify symptoms (e.g., chest pain—typical or atyical) during or after exercise.
5. Indicate the maximal heart rate and the maximal stage reached.
6. Indicate abnormal blood pressure or heart rate response.
7. Describe cardiac arrhythmias provoked during or after exercise.
8. Describe the reason if the test is considered to be false negative or positive.
9. Indicate functional classification (New York Heart Association) if possible.
10. Indicate whether the test should be repeated and explain why.

10. S-T segment elevation is uncommon, and it is almost always encountered in patients with previous myocardial infarction associated with ventricular aneurysm, and/or areas of akinesis or dyskinesis of the ventricular wall.

11. The exercise ECG test is often negative in patients with variant angina.

12. The development of supraventricular tachyarrhythmias, LBBB, RBBB or hemiblocks has no diagnostic value in exercise ECG testing. Exercise-induced intraventricular blocks are usually rate-dependent.

13. Alteration of T wave configuration alone has no diagnostic value.

14. Functional classification of coronary patients can be determined on the basis of the exercise workloads (METs).

15. A false positive test is extremely common in women, more so than in men, and many female patients show borderline or equivocal exercise ECG test results.

16. In asymptomatic individuals, abnormal S-T segment change on the exercise ECG should be treated as one of the risk factors for coronary artery disease.

17. The proper way of reporting exercise ECG test results is summarized in Table 12-11.

REFERENCES

1. Naughton, J.: Stress electrocardiography in clinical electrocardiographic correlations, *in* Cardiovascular Clinics, edited by J. C. Rios, Vol. 8, pp. 127–139, Philadelphia, F. A. Davis, 1977.
2. Fortuin, N. J. and Weiss, J. L.: Exercise stress testing. Circulation, 56:699, 1977.
3. Faris, J. V., McHenry, P. L. and Morris, S. N.: Concepts and applications of treadmill exercise testing and the exercise electrocardiogram. Am. Heart J., 95:102, 1978.
4. Kattus, A. A.: Exercise electrocardiography: Recognition of the ischemic response, false-positive and false-negative patterns, *in* Exercise in Cardiovascular Health and Disease, Edited by E. A. Amsterdam, J. H. Wilmore and A. N. DeMaria, pp. 161–178, New York, Yorke Medical Books, 1977.

5. Ellestad, M. H.: Stress Testing. Principles and Practice, pp. 85–156, Philadelphia, F. A. Davis, 1976.
6. Blackburn H.: The exercise electrocardiogram in diagnosis. Cardiology, 62:190, 1977.
7. Detry, J-M.R., Kapita, B. M., Cosyns, J. et al.: Diagnostic value of history and maximal exercise electrocardiography in men and women suspected of coronary heart disease. Circulation, 56:756, 1977.
8. Zohman, L. R. and Kattus, A. A.: Exercise testing in the diagnosis of coronary heart disease: A perspective. Am. J. Cardiol., 40:243, 1977.
9. Linhart, J. W.: Stress testing in angina. Resident & Staff Physician, pp. 79–89, Feb. 1978.
10. Bruce, R. A. and Hornstein, T. R.: Exercise stress testing in evaluation of patients with ischemic heart disease. Prog. Cardiovasc. Dis., 11:371, 1969.
11. Lozner, E. C. and Morganroth, J.: New criteria to enhance the predictability of coronary artery disease by exercise testing in asymptomatic subjects. Circulation, 56:799, 1977.
12. McNeer, J. F., Margolis, J. R., Lee, K. L. et al.: The role of the exercise test in the evaluation of patients for ischemic heart disease. Circulation, 57:64, 1978.
13. Simoons, M. L. and Hugenholtz, P. G.: Estimation of the probability of exercise-induced ischemia by quantitative ECG analysis. Circulation, 56:552, 1977.
14. Ascoop, C. A., Distelbrink, C. A. and DeLang, P. A.: Clinical value of quantitative analysis of ST slope during exercise. Br. Heart J., 39:212, 1977.
15. Ellestad, M. H., Savitz, S., Berdall, D. and Teske, J.: The false positive stress test. Multivariate analysis of 215 subjects with hemodynamic, angiographic and clinical data. Am. J. Cardiol., 40:681, 1977.
16. McHenry, P. L.: The actual prevalence of false positive ST-segment responses to exercise in clinically normal subjects remains undefined. Circulation, 55:683, 1977.
17. Redwood, D., Borer, J. and Epstein, S. E.: Whither the ST segment during exercise? Circulation, 54:703, 1976.
18. Sheffield, L. T., Reeves, T. J., Blackburn, H. et al.: The exercise test in perspective. Circulation, 55:681, 1977.
19. McHenry, P. L. and Fisch, C.: Clinical applications of the treadmill exercise test. Mod. Concepts Cardiovasc. Dis., 46:21, 1977.
20. Master, A. M. and Jaffe, J. L.: The electrocardiographic changes after exercise in angina pectoris. J. Mt. Sinai Hospital, New York, 7:629, 1941.
21. Master, A. M.: The Master two step test. Am. Heart J., 75:809, 1968.
22. Master, A. M. and Rosenfeld, I.: Clinical application of the two step exercise test. J.A.M.A., 178:283, 1961.
23. McConahay, D. R., McCallister, B. D. and Smith, R. E.: Post-exercise electrocardiography: correlations with coronary arteriography and left ventricular hemodynamics. Am. J. Cardiol., 28:1, 1971.
24. Most, A. S., Kemp, H. G. and Gorlin, R.: Post exercise electrocardiography in patients with arteriographically documented coronary artery disease. Ann. Intern. Med., 71:1043, 1969.
25. Demaney, M. A., Tambe, A. and Zimmerman, H. A.: Correlation between coronary arteriography and the post-exercise electrocardiogram. Am. J. Cardiol., 19:526, 1967.
26. Cohen, L. S., Elliott, W. C., Klein, M. D. and Gorlin, R.: Coronary heart disease. Clinical, cinearteriographic and metabolic correlations. Am. J. Cardiol., 17:153, 1966.
27. Chung, E. K.: Sick sinus syndrome and brady-tachyarrhythmia syndrome, in Artificial Cardiac Pacing: Practical Approach, edited by E. K. Chung, Baltimore, Williams & Wilkins, 1979.
28. Yu, P. N., Bruce, R. A., Lovejoy, F. W., Jr. and Pearson, R.: Observations on changes of ventricular systole (QT interval) during exercise. J. Clin. Invest., 29:279, 1950.
29. Roman, L. and Bellet, S.: Significance of the QX/QT ratio and the QT ratio (QTr) in the exercise electrocardiogram. Circulation, 32:435, 1965.
30. Sjorstrand, T.: Experimental variations in T-wave of electrocardiogram. Acta Med. Scand., 138:191, 1950.
31. Sandberg, L.: Studies in electrocardiogram changes during exercise tests. Acta Med. Scand., 169:(Suppl. 365), 1969.
32. Friesinger, G. C., Biern, R. O., Likar, J. and Mason, R. E.: Exercise ECG and vasoregulatory abnormalities. Am. J. Cardiol., 30:733, 1972.

33. Holmgren, A., Jonsson, B., Linderholm, H. et al.: ECG changes in vasoregulatory asthenia and the affect of physical training. Acta Med. Scand., *165:*259, 1959.
34. Holmgren, A. and Ström, G.: Vasoregulatory asthenia in a female athlete and Da Costa's syndrome in a male athlete successfully treated by physical training. Acta Med. Scand., *164:*113, 1959.
35. Scherf, D.: Fifteen years of electrocardiographic exercise test in coronary stenosis. N. Y. State J. Med., *47:*2420, 1947.
36. Scherf, D. and Schoffer, A. I.: The electrocardiographic exercise test. Am. Heart J., *43:*44, 1952.
37. Lloyd-Thomas, J.: The effect of exercise on the electrocardiogram in healthy subjects. Br. Heart J., *23:*260, 1961.
38. Bellet, S., Deliyiannis, S. and Eliakim, M.: The electrocardiogram during exercise as recorded by radioelectrocardiography. Comparison with the post-exercise electrocardiogram (Master's two-step test). Am. J. Cardiol., *18:*385, 1961.
39. Yu, P. N. G. and Soffer, A.: Studies of electrocardiographic changes during exercise (modified double two-step test). Circulation, *6:*183, 1952.
40. Christison, G. W., Bonoris, P. E., Greenberg, P. S. et al.: Comparison of changes in R-wave amplitude and ST segments in treadmill stress testing as a predictor of CAD (Abstract), Am. J. Cardiol., *41:*376, 1978.
41. Bonoris, P. E., Greenberg, P. S., Christison, G. W. et al.: Ability of R-wave amplitude changes to reduce false negative and false positive responses by ST depression in treadmill stress testing (Abstract), Am. J. Cardiol., *41:*378, 1978.
42. Kahn, K. A. and Simonson, E.: Changes of mean spatial QRS and T vectors and of conventional electrocardiographic items in hard anaerobic work. Circ. Res., *9:*629, 1957.
43. Bellet, S., Eliakim, M., Deliyiannis, S. and Figallo, E. M.: Radioelectrocardiographic changes during strenuous exercise in normal subjects. Circulation, *225:*686, 1962.
44. Martin, C. and McConahay, D. R.: Maximal treadmill exercise electrocardiography. Correlations with coronary arteriography and cardiac hemodynamics. Circulation, *46:*956, 1972.
45. McHenry, P. L. and Morris, S. N.: Exercise electrocardiography. Current state of the art; in Advances in Electrocardiography, edited by J. W. Hurst and R. C. Schlant, New York, Grune & Stratton, 1976.
46. Goldschlager, N., Selzer, A. and Cohn, K.: Treadmill stress tests as indicators of presence and severity of coronary artery disease. Ann. Intern. Med., *85:*277, 1976.
47. Kaplan, M. A., Harris, C. N., Aronov, W. S. et al.: Inability of the submaximal treadmill stress test to predict the location of coronary disease. Circulation, *47:*250, 1973.
48. Stuart, R. J. and Ellestad, M. H.: Upsloping S-T segments in exercise stress testing. Six year follow-up study of 438 patients and correlation with 248 angiograms. Am. J. Cardiol., *37:*19, 1976.
49. Kurita, A., Chaitman, B. R. and Bourassa, M. G.: Significance of exercise-induced junctional S-T depression in evaluation of coronary artery disease. Am. J. Cardiol., *40:*492, 1977.
50. Detry, J. R.: Exercise Testing and Training in Coronary Heart Disease. Baltimore, Williams & Wilkins, 1973.
51. Chung, E. K.: Principles of Cardiac Arrhythmias, Second Edition, Baltimore, Williams & Wilkins, 1977.
52. Chahine, R. A., Raizner, A. E. and Ishimori, T.: The clinical significance of exercise-induced S-T segment elevation. Circulation, *54:*209, 1976.
53. Widlansky, S., McHenry, P. L. and Corya, B. C.: Coronary arteriographic, echocardiographic and electrocardiographic studies in a patient with variant angina due to coronary artery spasm. Am. Heart J., *90:*631, 1975.
54. Kemp, G. L.: Value of treadmill stress testing in variant angina pectoris. Am. J. Cardiol., *30:*781, 1972.
55. MacAlpin, R. N., Kattus, A. A. and Alvaro, A. B.: Angina pectoris at rest with preservation of exercise capacity. Circulation, *47:*946, 1973.
56. Kansal, S., Roitman, D. and Sheffield, L. T.: Stress testing with S-T segment depression at rest. An angiographic correlation. Circulation, *54:*636, 1976.
57. Whinnery, J. E., Froelicher, V. F. and Stewart, A. J.: The electrocardiographic response to maximal treadmill exercise of asymptomatic men with left bundle branch block. Am. Heart J., *94:*316, 1977.

58. Whinnery, J. E., Froelicher, V. F., Stewart, A. J. et al.: The electrocardiographic response to maximal treadmill exercise of asymptomatic men with right bundle branch block. Chest, *71*:335, 1977.
59. Peskoe, S., McHenry, P. L. and Richmond, H. W.: Masking of exercise-induced S-T segment depression by rate-dependent left axis deviation. Heart Lung, *6*:1031, 1977.
60. Zuckerman, G. and Chung, E. K.: Exercise response in Wolff-Parkinson-White syndrome (In prep.), 1978.
61. Fraser, R. S. and Chapman, C. B.: Studies on the effect of exercise on cardiovascular function, II. The blood pressure and pulse rate. Circulation, *9:*193, 1954.
62. Bruce, R. A., Gey, G. O., Jr., Cooper, M. N. et al.: Seattle Heart Watch: initial clinical, circulatory and electrocardiographic responses to maximal exercise. Am. J. Cardiol., *33*:459, 1974.
63. Thomson, P. D. and Keleman, M. H.: Hypotension accompanying the onset of exertional angina. Circulation, *52*:28, 1975.
64. Bruce, R. A., Cobb, L. A., Katsura, S. et al.: Exertional hypotension in cardiac patients. Circulation, *19*:543, 1959.
65. Baker, T., Levites, R. and Anderson, G. J.: The significance of hypotension during treadmill exercise testing (Abstract). Circulation, *54:* Suppl. II:II–11, 1976.
66. Saltin, B. and Sternberg, J.: Circulatory response to prolonged severe exercise. J. Appl. Physiol., *19:*833, 1964.
67. Smith, E. E., Guyton, A. C., Manning, R. D. et al.: Integrated mechanisms of cardiovascular response and control during exercise in the normal human. Prog. Cardiovasc. Dis., *18*:421, 1976.
68. Morris, S. N., Phillips, J. F., Jordan, J. W. and McHenry, P. L.: Incidence and significance of decreases in systolic blood pressure during graded treadmill exercise testing. Am. J. Cardiol., *41:*221, 1978.
69. Kelemen, M. H., Gillilan, R. E., Bouchard, R. J. et al.: Diagnosis of obstructive coronary disease by maximal exercise and atrial pacing. Circulation, *48*:1227, 1973.
70. Cole, J. P. and Ellestad, M. H.: Significance of chest pain during treadmill exercise: Correlation with coronary events. Am. J. Cardiol., *41:*227, 1978.
71. Froelicher, V. F., Thompson, A. J., Longo, M. R., Jr. et al.: Value of exercise testing for screening asymptomatic men for latent coronary artery disease. Prog. Cardiovasc. Dis., *18:*265, 1976.
72. Bruce, R. A. and McDonough, J. R.: Stress testing in screening for cardiovascular disease. Bull. N.Y. Acad. Med., *45:*1288, 1969.
73. Borer, J. S., Brensike, J. F., Redwood, D. R. et al.: Limitations of the electrocardiographic response to exercise in predicting coronary-artery disease. N. Engl. J. Med., *293:*368, 1975.
74. Erikssen, J., Enge, I., Forfang, K. and Storstein, O.: False positive diagnostic tests and coronary angiographic findings in 105 presumably healthy males. Circulation, *54:*371, 1976.
75. Cumming, G. R., Dufresne, C., Kich, L. and Samm, J.: Exercise electrocardiogram patterns in normal women. Br. Heart J., *35:*1055, 1973.
76. Ellestad, M. H. and Halleday, W. K.: Stress testing for the prognosis and management of ischemic heart disease. Angiology, *28:*149, 1977.
77. Sketch, M. H., Mohuddin, S. M., Lynch, J. D. et al.: Significant sex differences in the correlation of electrocardiographic exercise testing and coronary arteriograms. Am. J. Cardiol., *36:*196, 1976.

13

Exercise-Induced Cardiac Arrhythmias

Edward K. Chung, M.D., F.A.C.P., F.A.C.C.

General Considerations[1-19]

It is well documented that various cardiac arrhythmias may be observed in clinically healthy subjects as well as in individuals with diseased hearts. Although almost every known type of cardiac arrhythmia may be induced by exercise (see Table 13-1), the primary concern is ventricular arrhythmias which have been reported to be closely related to coronary heart disease and sudden death.

Numerous investigators have attempted to assess in depth the prognostic significance of ventricular arrhythmias to correlate with various aspects of exercise, but there is no clear conclusion. For example, the clinical significance of ventricular premature contractions (VPCs) at rest, induced during exercise, abolished by exercise, occurring during post-exercise period, multifocal VPCs and grouped VPCs varies markedly.

Various supraventricular arrhythmias induced by exercise are relatively uncommon compared with ventricular arrhythmias. Clinically, exercise-induced supraventricular arrhythmias are considered relatively benign in most cases.

A-V conduction time is often altered by exercise. The P-R interval may be shortened or prolonged by exercise, and at times, a transient Wenckebach A-V block may be induced by exercise. The clinical significance of these A-V conduction alterations is uncertain, although some investigators feel that exercise-induced first or second degree A-V block is definitely a pathologic condition in the heart.

Various intraventricular blocks seem to be related to the heart rate (rate-dependent) in most cases, and this finding is *not* sufficient for a positive exercise ECG test (see Chapter 12). When there is pre-existing left bundle branch block (LBBB), however, the exercise ECG test is unreliable because of the high incidence of false positive exercise ECG tests[16] (see Chapter 12). The pre-existing right bundle branch block (RBBB) does not significantly alter the result of the exercise ECG test.[17]

Table 13-1. Classification of Exercise-induced Cardiac Arrhythmias

Sinus arrhythmias:
  Sinus bradycardia
  Sinus tachycardia
  Sinus arrhythmia
  Sinus arrest
  Sino-atrial block
  Wandering atrial pacemaker in the sinus node
Atrial arrhythmias:
  Atrial premature contractions
  Atrial tachycardia
  Atrial flutter
  Atrial fibrillation
A-V Junctional arrhythmias:
  A-V junctional premature contractions
  A-V junctional tachycardia
  A-V junctional escape rhythm
  Wandering pacemaker between sinus and A-V node
Ventricular arrhythmias:
  Ventricular premature contractions
  Ventricular tachycardia
  Ventricular fibrillation and flutter
A-V Conduction disturbances:
  Varying A-V conduction time
  First degree A-V block
  Second degree A-V block
  Complete A-V block
Intraventricular blocks:
  Hemiblocks
  Right bundle branch block
  Left bundle branch block
  Bifascicular blocks
Brady-tachyarrhythmia syndrome
Wolff-Parkinson-White syndrome
Miscellaneous:
  Parasystole
  Aberrant ventricular conduction
  Fusion beats

Exercise may provoke or abolish anomalous A-V conduction in the Wolff-Parkinson-White (WPW) syndrome. However, more commonly, anomalous conduction is caused by exercise, and it often continues during the entire procedure of the exercise ECG test. The exercise ECG test is invalid in most cases with the WPW syndrome because of the extremely high incidence of false positive exercise ECG tests.[18]

The exercise ECG test has been utilized to evaluate the efficacy of antiarrhythmic drug therapy, but the result of the commonly used drugs (e.g., quinidine and procaine amide) has been disappointing.[14]

In addition, the exercise ECG test has been used as a provocative test to assess the function of the sinus node.[19] In general, the diagnosis of the sick sinus syndrome is strongly suspected when the sinus rate does not increase beyond 120 beats/minute by submaximal or maximal exercise ECG test.

In this chapter, current knowledge of the electrophysiologic response of the heart to exercise in conjunction with classification, the diagnosis and the clinical significance of various exercise-induced cardiac arrhythmias will be reviewed.

Proper Lead System[1, 5, 9, 20, 21]

It is essential to apply an appropriate skin preparation and proper electrodes in order to minimize or prevent excessive noise and artifacts for optimal recognition and classification of exercise-induced arrhythmias (see Table 13-1). Proper use of electrodes and skin preparation has been discussed in detail elsewhere (see Chapter 1).

As far as the lead systems are concerned, a single lead system is insufficient to identify various types of exercise-induced arrhythmias. Although a modified bipolar lead V_5 (e.g., CM_5) is the most important lead to detect S-T segment alteration, it is not ideal for identification of arrhythmias. It is, therefore, ideal to add at least another inferior lead (e.g., lead II or aVF, or Y lead of the orthogonal lead system). The reason for this is that the P wave is best registered in the inferior lead. In addition, the presence of VPCs, as the heart rate is accelerated during exercise, the coupling interval (the interval from the ectopic beat to the preceding sinus beat) commonly becomes almost equal to the R-R interval of the basic rhythm leading to frequent occurrences of ventricular fusion beats. Consequently, it is often difficult to distinguish between atrial premature contractions (APCs) with aberrant ventricular conduction and VPCs. Another reason is that VPCs may not be detected readily in a single lead system when the QRS complex of the ectopic beat happens to be similar to that of the basic rhythm during fast rate.

In our laboratory, a 2-channel ECG recording system including leads II and modified V_5 (CM_5) is utilized with satisfying results.

Electrophysiologic Effects of Exercise

It is well documented that exercise may alter the electrical events in the myocardium which may lead to production or inhibition of ectopic impulse formation. In addition, A-V conduction as well as the intraventricular conduction may be improved or depressed by the exercise. Depending upon the amount of exercise performed and depending upon the status of cardiac function in a given individual, the net result of the exercise varies significantly.

It is known that the exercise often induces various ectopic arrhythmias which are not present at rest. The exercise-induced arrhythmias are generated by enhanced sympathetic tone and/or increased myocardial oxygen demand. The increased sympathetic tone to the myocardium may stimulate the ectopic Purkinje pacemaker activity by accelerating the phase 4 depolarization which provokes its spontaneous discharge leading to increased automaticity.[22, 23]

Local tissue hypoxia is produced when the increased myocardial oxygen demand is not matched by oxygen supply. Myocardial hypoxia induces a temporal dispersion of depolarization and repolarization in addition to the alterations of the cardiac conduction velocity. As a result, myocardial ischemia can provide a suitable background for the initiation of ectopic arrhythmias via automaticity and reentry mechanism.[24]

Myocardial ischemia is commonly produced by exercise in patients with coronary heart disease. Myocardial oxygen consumption (MVO_2) is determined by various factors including the heart rate, myocardial contractility and intramyocardial tension.[25] The effect of exercise upon these factors augments MVO_2, and consequently myocardial ischemia is produced if oxygen demand exceeds supply. The imbalance between oxygen demand and supply can be observed not only during high-level exercise but also during the immediate post-exercise period. Peripheral arteriolar dilatation induced by exercise, and reduced cardiac output resulting from diminished venous return secondary due to sudden termination of muscular activity, may lead to a reduction of blood pressure as well as coronary perfusion while the cardiac rate is still fast.

On the other hand, exercise may abolish various cardiac arrhythmias which are present at rest. The reason for this phenomenon is most likely due to the over-drive suppression of ectopic impulse formation by marked sinus tachycardia induced by exercise—vagal withdrawal and increased sympathetic stimulation. In addition, it has been suggested that exercise-induced sinus tachycardia may inhibit automaticity of an ectopic focus because of the fact that rapid stimulation may result in reduced automaticity of Purkinje tissue.[26]

Value of Holter Monitor ECG Versus Exercise ECG Test in Detecting Arrhythmias

The Holter monitor ECG is proven to be the best diagnostic tool to detect transient and occult cardiac arrhythmias which may not be diagnosed on the resting electrocardiogram.[27] Although the Holter monitor ECG is capable of detecting mild exercise-induced (ordinary daily activity) arrhythmias as well as arrhythmias unrelated to physical exercise, arrhythmias provoked only by near-maximal or maximal exercise cannot be detected by this method. Thus, the submaximal or maximal exercise ECG test has a definite role in detecting certain arrhythmias under these circumstances. The primary concern is the identification of ventricular arrhythmias during and immediately after exercise.

Kosowsky et al.[28] evaluated the capability of detecting ventricular arrhythmias in 81 patients with and without coronary heart disease by using the Holter monitor ECG versus the exercise ECG test. In this study, among 66 patients with a normal resting ECG, ventricular arrhythmias were detected by 12-hour Holter monitor ECG in 27%, whereas the exercise ECG test provoked the arrhythmia in 39%. On the other hand, another study[29] from the same institution using the 24-hour Holter monitor ECG demonstrated ventricular premature contractions (VPCs) in 88% of patients with coronary heart disease, compared with the exercise ECG test which produced the arrhythmias in 56% of these patients. Similarly, Amsterdam et al.[30] reported that the 10- to 12-hour Holter monitor ECG detected VPCs in 82% of 22 patients with angiographically documented coronary heart disease, whereas exercise provoked the arrhythmia only in 59% of these patients.

Recently, Kennedy et al.[7] studied the quantitative and qualitative aspects of ventricular arrhythmias detected 24 hours before and 24 hours after the maximal exercise ECG test by the Holter monitor ECG in 67 patients with coronary heart disease and 23 normal subjects in order to determine if the maximal exercise treadmill test influences ventricular arrhythmias in the hours following exercise. It was interesting to note that the maximal treadmill exercise test did not significantly influence the development of ventricular arrhythmias in the hours after exercise, either in patients with coronary artery disease (New York Heart Association Class I–II) or in normal subjects.

In conclusion, from the above observations and my own experience, the Holter monitor ECG is definitely superior to the exercise ECG test in detecting almost all types of cardiac arrhythmias. However, the exercise ECG test is a supplementary diagnostic tool to detect arrhythmias which may only be provoked by submaximal or maximal exercise. Another important role of the exercise ECG test is in the evaluation of the efficacy of various anti-arrhythmic drugs (will be discussed later in this chapter).

Evaluation of Anti-arrhythmic Drug Therapy

The exercise ECG test has significant value in assessing the efficacy of various anti-arrhythmic drugs and digitalis.[4, 31] It is common knowledge that the ventricular rate (60–80 beats/minute) is ideally controlled in patients with chronic atrial fibrillation by digitalis in the resting state, but the ventricular rate is disproportionately accelerated as soon as the patient engages in any type of physical activity.[31, 32] This fact can be clearly delineated by the exercise ECG test. When the ventricular rate is markedly enhanced by the exercise in atrial fibrillation during long-term digitalization, digitalis dosage may be carefully increased or an additional drug such as propranolol (Inderal) may be prescribed, providing that DC cardioversion is not feasible. Similarly, anti-arrhythmic drug therapy is proven to be unsatisfactory when the patient with sinus rhythm at rest develops paroxysmal atrial fibrillation during exercise in various clinical circumstance, including rheumatic heart disease, hyperthyroidism and Wolff-Parkinson-White syndrome (Fig. 13-1 through 3).

Jelinek and Lown[4] studied the efficacy of 2 commonly used anti-arrhythmic drugs for ventricular arrhythmias—quinidine and procaine amide (Pronestyl)—utilizing the exercise ECG test. Procaine amide was effective in only 8 of 23 patients (12 patients with coronary artery disease; 7 with various other myocardial disease, and 4 healthy subjects). Four of these patients required 6.0 gm. to achieve this therapeutic effect. Toxic manifestations were observed in 10 of 16 patients requiring these larger doses. The success rate with quinidine was similar to that of procaine amide. The arrhythmia was controlled in only 7 of 21 patients (33%). Side effects were observed in 7 of 16 patients requiring 1.8 gm. daily.

The above study clearly indicates that ventricular arrhythmias are well controlled by quinidine or procaine amide at rest, but the arrhythmia is easily provoked by exercise even when a large dosage of these drugs is used

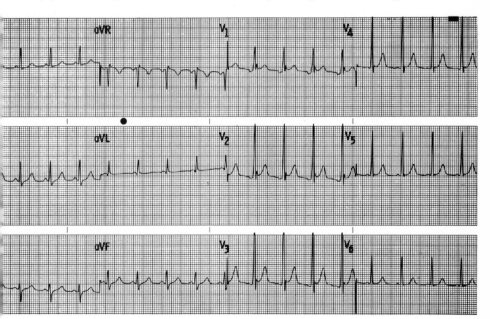

Fig. 13-1   Figures 13-1 to 3 were obtained from a 55-year-old man with the WPW syndrome associated with hyperthyroidism. Figure 13-1 taken before exercise shows sinus rhythm (rate: 96 beats/minute) and WPW syndrome, type A.

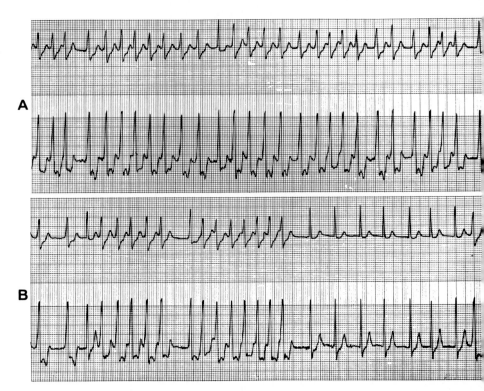

Fig. 13-2 The rhythm strips A and B were taken during mild exercise (treadmill) and they are not continuous. The upper strip represents modified bipolar lead V_5 (CM_5) whereas the bottom strip is lead II. All of the following figures showing 2 strips simultaneously consist of leads CM_5 and II, unless specified otherwise. The cardiac rhythm is atrial fibrillation with intermittent anomalous A-V conduction which closely resembles ventricular tachycardia. Note marked S-T segment depression during anomalous A-V conduction (false positive exercise ECG test). In this patient, atrial fibrillation was provoked by treadmill exercise.

(Figures 13-4 and 5). In our institution, Norpace (disopyramide phosphate, 150 mg. every 6 hours by mouth) was effective to control frequent VPCs with paroxysmal ventricular tachycardia in a patient with triple-vessel coronary artery disease. In this case, larger doses (near toxic doses) of quinidine (0.4 gm. every 4 hours) and/or procaine amide (750 mg. every 3 hours) were ineffective, but Norpace was capable of suppressing the ventricular arrhythmias even during the submaximal exercise ECG test. We, of course, need further investigation regarding the efficacy of Norpace for ventricular arrhythmias compared with other commonly used anti-arrhythmic agents.

Cardiac Arrhythmias and Termination of the Exercise ECG Test

There is no uniform agreement as to when to terminate the exercise prematurely in cases of ventricular arrhythmias provoked by the exercise ECG test. Although the presence of significant ventricular arrhythmias is considered a relative contraindication to the exercise ECG test by some investigators, this author's policy is that the exercise ECG test is *not* contraindicated when the patient's condition is stable without any acute problem other than relatively benign ventricular arrhythmia (Figures 13-6 and 7) alone on resting electrocardiogram.[31, 32] However, the exercise ECG test is contraindicated in patients with serious ventricular arrhythmias such as frequent multifocal VPCs, VPCs with the R-on-T phenomenon, grouped VPCs and paroxysmal ventricular tachycardia (see Chapter 8). For the same reason, the exercise ECG test should be terminated prematurely when the above-mentioned serious ventricular arrhythmias are produced by exercise with (Figure 13-8) or without S-T segment alteration (Figure 13-9). The exercise ECG test may be continued when the patient develops benign supraventricular arrhythmias such as APCs, atrial group beats or short runs

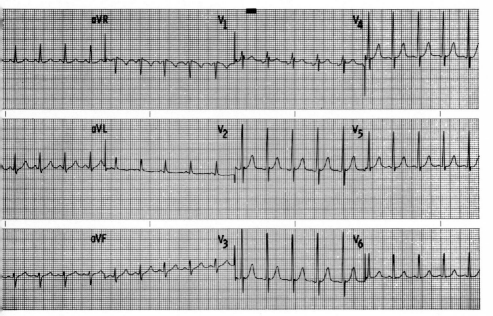

Fig. 13-3 This ECG was obtained following a termination of atrial fibrillation by administration of procaine amide (Pronestyl) 500 mg. every 4 hours by mouth. The rhythm is sinus tachycardia (rate: 125 beats/minute) with WPW syndrome, type A. It should be noted that the configuration of the QRS complexes is slightly different in this tracing compared with that shown in Figure 13-1. These findings may indicate dual anomalous pathways.

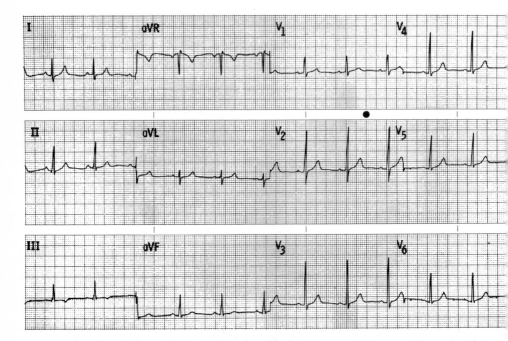

Fig. 13-4   Figures 13-4 and 5 were obtained from a 51-year-old man with a history of myocardial infarction 3 months previously. Figure 13-4 taken before exercise reveals sinus rhythm (rate: 74 beats/minute) and old posterior myocardial infarction.

of atrial tachycardia (Figure 13-10). The development of unifocal VPCs alone (Figure 13-11) during exercise without R-on-T phenomenon, S-T segment alteration, significant chest pain or hypotension is *not* an indication for premature termination of the test. The exercise ECG test should be stopped, however, when atrial fibrillation or flutter is provoked by the exercise (Figure 13-2).

Classification, Diagnosis and Clinical Significance of Exercise-Induced Arrhythmias

Almost every known cardiac arrhythmia may be induced by exercise, whereas some arrhythmias may be abolished by exercise. Some conduction disturbances, particularly bundle branch blocks or hemiblocks are observed during exercise, but this phenomenon is often rate-dependent. Classification of exercise-induced cardiac arrhythmias is summarized in Table 13-1.

Sinus Arrhythmias

Progressive acceleration of the sinus rate causing marked sinus tachycardia is expected during the multistage exercise ECG test. Depending upon the individual's age, the predicted submaximal and maximal sinus rate varies markedly—anywhere between 150 to 200 beats/minute (see Chapter 9). When the expected increment of the sinus rate is not observed during the exercise ECG test, however, dysfunction of the sinus node—the sick sinus syndrome may be suspected.[19] The sinus rate is seldom accelerated beyond 120 beats/minute by the usual exercise protocol (see Chapter 9) in the sick sinus syndrome.[19]

Sinus arrhythmia with areas of slight sinus bradycardia and wandering atrial pacemaker are relatively common during the immediate post-exercise period[33] (Figures 13-12 and 13). The presence of these arrhythmias alone has no clinical significance. On rare occasions, sinoatrial block and sinus arrest may be observed during the exercise ECG test, usually after the termination of exercise.[33] Again, the sick sinus syndrome is a possibility

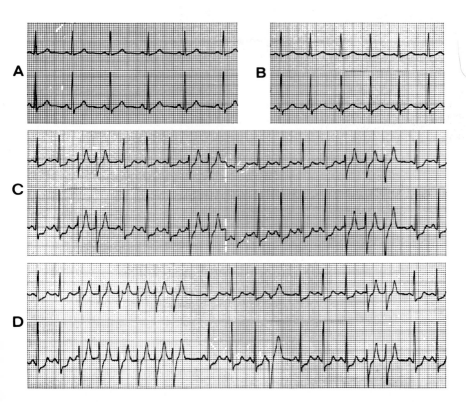

Fig. 13-5 These rhythm strips are his exercise ECG. The strips A and B were obtained at rest in supine and standing positions, respectively. The strips C and D were taken during exercise, but they are *not* continuous. The exercise was stopped prematurely because he developed ventricular tachycardia (rate: 150 beats/minute) associated with chest pain and S-T segment depression. The exercise ECG test is definitely positive.

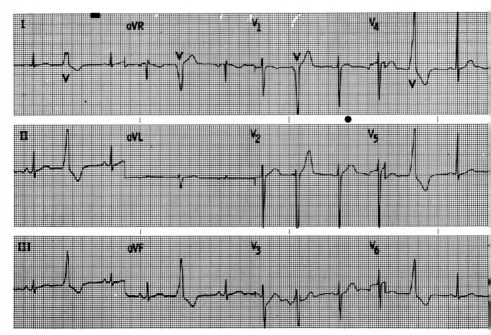

Fig. 13-6 Figures 13-6 and 7 were obtained from a 19-year-old man who complains of palpitations. A 12-lead ECG shown in Figure 13-6 reveals sinus rhythm with frequent ventricular premature contractions (VPCs) producing ventricular trigeminy (marked V). By analyzing the configuration of the VPCs, the VPCs are considered to be originating from the right ventricle. His ECG is within normal limits other than high left ventricular voltage.

when there are frequent episodes of marked sinus bradycardia, sinus arrest and sinoatrial block.[19]

Atrial Arrhythmias

Exercise-induced atrial premature contractions (APCs) and atrial group beats (Figure 13-10) are not uncommon in either normal or diseased hearts. Because of the rapid sinus rate during exercise, differentiation between APCs with aberrant ventricular conduction (Figure 13-14) and VPCs is often difficult. A concept of the full compensatory pause in VPCs and non-full compensatory pause in APCs cannot be applied readily during very rapid sinus tachycardia because the coupling interval in both situations approaches the R-R interval of the basic rhythm.[32] The frequent occurrence of ventricular fusion beats from VPCs makes it more difficult to distinguish from APCs with aberrant ventricular conduction (Figure 13-14) under these circumstances. Sustained atrial tachycardia induced by exercise is very rare, and it was observed only in 5 of 3,000 patients exercised.[33] It was interesting to note that no episode of supraventricular (reciprocating) tachycardia was encountered by this author during the submaximal treadmill exercise ECG test among 20 subjects with proven Wolff-Parkinson-White syndrome.[18]

Atrial fibrillation and flutter induced by exercise have been observed occasionally by different investigators,[3, 31–37] but in most cases, these arrhythmias are transient. Transient atrial fibrillation or flutter may be induced by exercise in patients with rheumatic heart disease, hyperthyroidism, Wolff-Parkinson-White syndrome (Figures 13-1 to 3), cardiomyopathy (Figure 13-15), and even in healthy individuals. The development of these atrial arrhythmias by exercise alone, therefore, is not indicative of a positive exercise ECG test (see Chapter 12). The important role of the exercise ECG

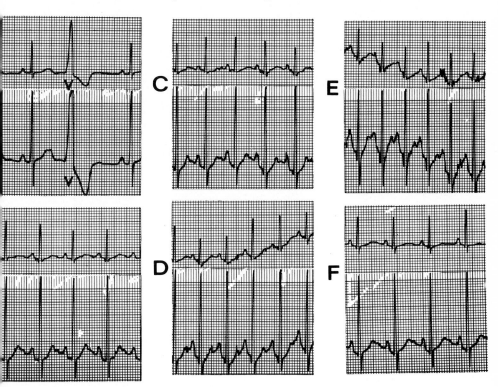

Fig. 13-7   This ECG is the exercise ECG test on this 19-year-old male. The exercise ECG test was ordered primarily to determine the nature of the VPCs in relation to exercise. The strips A represent a resting ECG. The strips B to E were taken during exercise, whereas the strips F represent the post-exercise ECG. He had completed a full 7-stage exercise program without any difficulty and his maximal heart rate reached 170 beats/minute. It is noteworthy that the VPCs (marked V) have been abolished completely by the exercise. In general, right VPCs as well as the VPCs abolished by exercise are often found in healthy individuals. The exercise ECG test is negative.

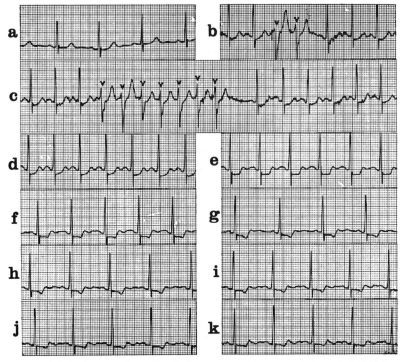

Fig. 13-8 These rhythm strips were recorded from a patient with known angina pectoris, and lead CM₅ was recorded throughout. The strip a was taken at rest whereas the strips b and c were obtained during exercise. The strips d to k represent post-exercise ECG. The exercise was terminated prematurely because ventricular tachycardia (marked V) was provoked by the exercise associated with marked S-T, T wave changes. The exercise ECG test is markedly positive.

test in assessing the status of digitalization in patients with chronic atrial fibrillation has been emphasized previously in this chapter.

A-V Junctional Arrhythmias

The exact incidence of exercise-induced A-V junctional premature contractions (JPCs) is uncertain because most investigators do not separate JPCs from APCs. In addition, in a practical sense, it is usually difficult to distinguish between these two arrhythmias, and its differentiation is often arbitrary.[32] For a similar reason, the incidence of exercise-induced A-V junctional tachycardia is unknown because the term "supraventricular tachycardia" is commonly used to designate paroxysmal atrial as well as A-V junctional tachycardia.[32]

Nevertheless, paroxysmal A-V junctional tachycardia is observed during exercise only on rare occasions in our laboratory. Recently, a 40-year-old, apparently healthy man developed paroxysmal A-V junctional tachycardia without any other abnormal findings during submaximal exercise in our exercise laboratory (Figures 13-16 to 18). The tachycardia was successfully terminated by carotid sinus stimulation (Figure 13-17). No underlying cause was demonstrated in this patient for the development of exercise-induced A-V junctional tachycardia. When there is aberrant ventricular conduction under these circumstances, ventricular tachycardia is closely simulated.

The clinical significance of JPCs and paroxysmal A-V junctional tachycardia induced by exercise is probably the same as that of APCs and atrial tachycardia. Thus, the presence of these A-V junctional arrhythmias alone is not indicative of a positive exercise ECG test.

A transient episode of A-V junctional escape rhythm with or without wandering atrial pacemaker is not uncommon during the early post-exercise

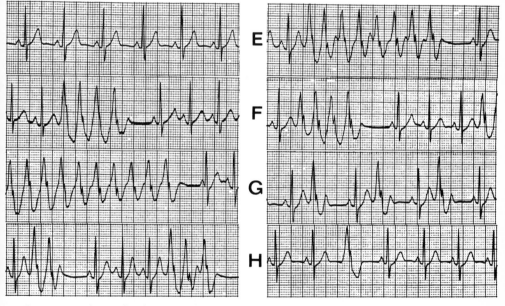

Fig. 13-9 These rhythm strips were obtained from a 41-year-old man with a history of palpitations. All rhythm strips represent lead CM_5. The 12-lead ECG was within normal limits. The strip A represents a resting ECG. The strips B to D were taken during exercise, whereas the remaining strips E to H were recorded after exercise. The exercise ECG test was terminated prematurely because of paroxysmal ventricular tachycardia. After the termination of exercise, his ventricular tachycardia subsided spontaneously. There is no S-T segment or T wave alteration. Cardiomyopathy was considered his underlying heart disease.

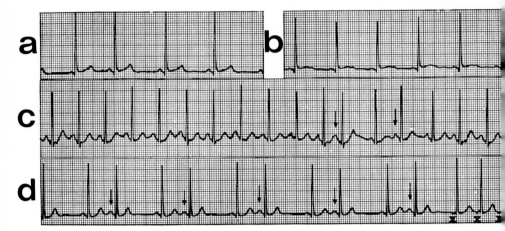

Fig. 13-10 Exercise-induced APCs (indicated by arrows) with supraventricular grouped beats (marked X). The strips a and b were taken at rest in supine and standing positions, respectively. The strips c and d represent post-exercise ECG.

period (Figures 13-12 and 13). However, the diagnosis of the sick sinus syndrome may be suspected when slow A-V junctional escape rhythm persists after exercise, especially when it is preceded by an inappropriate increment of the sinus rate by exercise.[19]

Ventricular Arrhythmias

It is well documented that ventricular arrhythmias, particularly ventricular premature contractions (VPCs), may be induced or abolished by exercise in normal subjects as well as in patients with organic heart disease, especially coronary heart disease.[1-12] However, there is a significant controversy among investigators[1-12] regarding the clinical significance of VPCs in considering various aspects, including:

(1) Site of the origin of VPCs (right versus left VPCs)
(2) VPCs at rest
(3) VPCs induced by exercise (onset of VPCs in relation to the amount of exercise)
(4) VPCs abolished by exercise
(5) Unifocal versus multifocal VPCs
(6) Grouped versus isolated VPCs
(7) Relation to the development of ventricular tachycardia or fibrillation
(8) Relation to the presence or absence of coronary heart disease (e.g., single-, double- versus triple-vessel disease, etc.)
(9) Relation to the risk of developing future coronary event and
(10) Relation to sudden death.

Isolated, unifocal VPCs are frequently encountered in healthy individuals at rest as well as during maximal or submaximal exercise ECG tests (Figure 13-11).[38][39] On the other hand, multifocal VPCs and grouped VPCs (3 or more) or ventricular tachycardia are obviously much more common in patients with coronary heart disease[1-3] (Figures 13-4, 5 and 8).

Diagnosis

As far as the diagnosis of ventricular arrhythmias is concerned, it is often difficult to differentiate between ventricular tachycardia and supraventricular tachycardia with aberrant ventricular conduction or pre-existing bundle branch block (Figures 13-17 and 18). Similarly, supraventricular tachyarrhythmias, particularly atrial fibrillation with anomalous A-V conduction in the Wolff-Parkinson-White syndrome closely simulates ventricular tachycardia or even ventricular fibrillation[32] (Figures 13-1 to 3). Another example is multifocal VPCs which may be diagnosed erroneously by recognizing frequent ventricular fusion beats in unifocal VPCs during rapid basic heart rate induced by exercise. In addition, atrial or A-V junctional premature contractions with aberrant ventricular conduction may mimic VPCs (Figure 13-14). Differential diagnosis of these arrhythmias is often difficult, but it is important to distinguish between them because of their markedly different

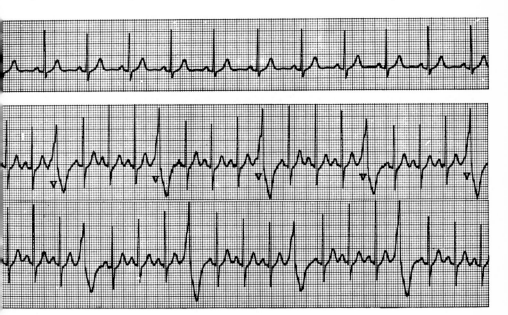

Fig. 13-11 Exercise-induced VPCs (marked V) causing ventricular quadrigeminy. Strip A is a resting ECG whereas the strips B and C represent post-exercise ECG. All strips represent lead CM_5.

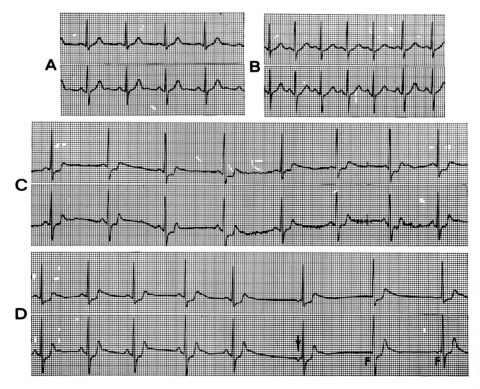

Fig. 13-12   Figures 13-12 and 13 were obtained from a 67-year-old man with chest pain. In Figure 13-12, the strips A represent resting ECG whereas the strips B were taken during exercise. The strips C and D represent post-exercise ECG. Note marked slowing of the sinus rate immediately after the termination of exercise (the strip C), and it is followed by intermittent A-V junctional escape beats (indicated by arrow) and atrial fusion beats (marked F). Thus, the pacemaker is wandering between sinus and A-V node. The exercise ECG test is positive (marked S-T segment depression in the strips C and D).

clinical significance. Different types of cardiac arrhythmias are fully discussed elsewhere by this author.[32]

Ventricular Arrhythmias Induced by Exercise

It has been pointed out that the presence of organic heart disease is most likely responsible for the production of VPCs during mild exercise.[35] This view is in accordance with my own experience that the initiation of VPCs induced by less than 70% of maximal exercise is nearly always indicative of underlying heart disease, most commonly coronary heart disease (Figure 13-19). In most cases with mild exercise-induced VPCs there is also significant S-T segment alteration in patients with coronary heart disease (Figure 13-19). In addition, the VPCs are often multifocal in origin. It has been repeatedly stressed that exercise-induced ventricular tachycardia is nearly always indicative of underlying organic heart disease.[35] The diagnosis of coronary heart disease is almost certain when there is coexisting S-T segment alteration (Figures 13-4, 5 and 8). On the other hand, exercise-induced ventricular tachycardia may be encountered in patients with other clinical entities, particularly mitral valve prolapse syndrome or cardiomyopathy (Figure 13-9). The absence of significant S-T segment alteration in exercise-induced ventricular tachycardia makes the diagnosis of coronary artery disease less likely.

Recently, I observed the development of frequent VPCs, grouped VPCs, and a short run of ventricular tachycardia associated with ventricular

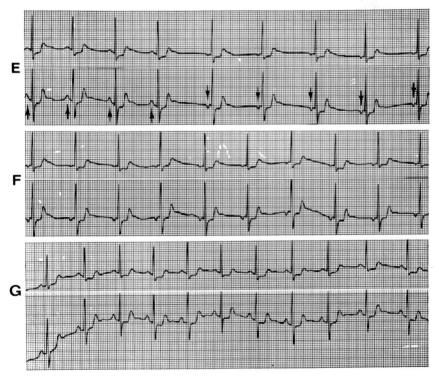

Fig. 13-13 Figure 13-13 was obtained a few minutes later and the rhythm strips E, F and G were taken with 1 minute intervals. Wandering pacemaker between sinus (indicated by upward arrows) and A-V node (indicated by downward arrows) persists in the strips E, but A-V junctional escape rhythm is established momentarily in the strips F until stable sinus rhythm is restored in the strips G.

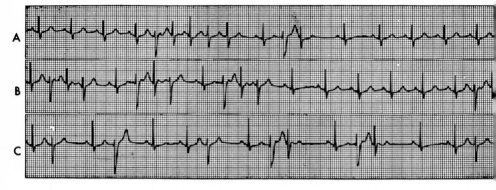

Fig. 13-14 These rhythm strips were taken on a 58-year-old man with palpitations. The rhythm strips A to C represent lead CM5 and they are continuous. He developed frequent atrial premature contractions with aberrant ventricular conduction, atrial group beats and short runs of atrial tachycardia during and after exercise. The strips A to C represent post-exercise ECG. These atrial arrhythmias have subsided with rest without any medication.

parasystole in a 54-year-old man with previous diaphragmatic myocardial infarction (Figures 13-20 to 22). There was a significant S-T segment depression associated with chest pain, and the ventricular parasystole persisted for 12 minutes after the termination of exercise although ordinary VPCs and short runs of ventricular tachycardia had subsided soon after the end of the exercise (Figure 13-22). The clinical significance of exercise-induced ventricular parasystole is uncertain, but its occurrence is rare.

Correlation with Angiographic Findings

As far as the correlation between exercise-induced ventricular arrhythmias and angiographic findings is concerned, Zaret and Conti[40] demonstrated that coronary artery disease was found in 72% of a group of patients with exercise-induced ventricular irritability. In this study, multiple-vessel disease was much more common in patients with exercise-induced arrhythmias than in a group of patients without ventricular arrhythmia. Another study by Goldschlager et al.[41] found that significant coronary artery stenosis was demonstrated in 89% of patients with exercise-induced VPCs. They further demonstrated a significantly higher prevalence of double- and triple-vessel coronary artery disease and abnormal left ventricular motion in this group than in patients with coronary artery disease without ventricular arrhythmias. Exercise-induced arrhythmias were observed more frequently during the post-exercise period in their study, and in many patients with significant coronary artery disease, VPCs were abolished during exercise. On the other hand, a study by Helfant et al.[42] showed that VPCs were provoked or increased in frequency with exercise in 22 of 38 patients with coronary artery disease. In this investigative work, the vast majority of these patients had evidence of multiple-vessel involvement with ventricular dyssynergy. An important conclusion of this study was that 20 of the 22 patients with exercise-induced ventricular arrhythmias also demonstrated marked S-T segment depression (2 mm. or more). Their result coincides with my own experience (Figures 13-5, 8 and 19).[43]

A recent study by McHenry et al.[1] in 360 patients undergoing coronary arteriography for known or suspected coronary artery disease, demonstrated that exercise-induced ventricular arrhythmias were observed in 25% of the normal patients (37 of 149) and 38% of the patients with significant (greater than 50% stenosis) coronary artery disease (80 of 211). Among 117 patients with exercise-induced ventricular arrhythmias, 32% were normal subjects whereas 68% showed coronary artery disease. In this study, the incidence of exercise-induced frequent unifocal VPCs (10 or more/minute) was statistically insignificant between normal subjects and coronary patients. Similarly, ventricular arrhythmias abolished by excercise during progressive workloads

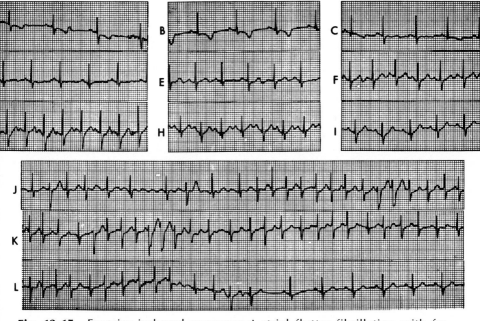

Fig. 13-15   Exercise-induced paroxysmal atrial flutter-fibrillation with frequent aberrant ventricular conduction (strips J to L). Strips A and B were taken at rest, in supine and standing positions, respectively. The strips C to G were recorded during exercise whereas the strips H to L represent post-exercise ECG. Lead CM₅ was recorded.

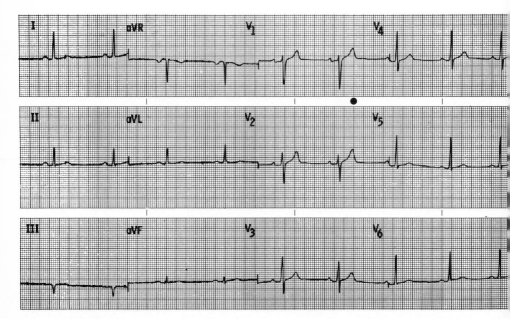

Fig. 13-16 Figures 13-16 to 18 were obtained from a 37-year-old obese man who has been suffering from palpitations for the past several years. The exercise ECG test was performed in order to assess the relationship between the occurrence of ectopic tachycardia and physical exercise. There was no known heart disease, hyperthyroidism or WPW syndrome. Figure 13-16 taken at rest shows mild sinus bradycardia (rate: 52 beats/minute) and within normal limits, otherwise.

with increased heart rates were equally common in normal individuals as well as coronary patients. The incidence of 2 grouped VPCs and VPCs from 2 foci was, likewise, almost the same between normal subjects and coronary patients in this study. Their result is similar to my experience in our exercise laboratory.[43] The most striking conclusion of the investigative work by McHenry et al.[1] is that 3 or more grouped VPCs (may be termed "ventricular tachycardia") were observed only in patients with coronary artery disease, and multifocal VPCs originating from 3 or more foci were much more common in patients with coronary artery disease than in normal subjects. Another study from the same laboratory[9] documented in 482 subjects with and without coronary artery disease that patients with 3-vessel coronary artery disease and abnormal left ventricular wall motion had a significantly higher incidence of exercise-induced ventricular arrhythmias.

Clinical Significance of the Origin of Ventricular Arrhythmias

As far as the clinical significance of the site of the ventricular ectopic focus is concerned, there is some evidence that right VPCs are more common in healthy subjects, whereas left VPCs are much more frequent in patients with diseased hearts. The diagnosis of the right VPCs is made on the basis of upright QRS complexes in the left precordial leads and primarily downward (negative) QRS complexes in the right precordial leads (left bundle branch block pattern).[32] On the other hand, left VPCs are diagnosed by recognizing right bundle branch block pattern of the ectopic beat.[32]

Bodenheimer et al.[11] studied 39 patients with right and left VPCs who were undergoing coronary arteriography for evaluation of chest pain. Among 19 patients with VPCs, 15 had coronary artery disease (12 with 2- or 3-vessel obstruction and 3 with single-vessel disease), whereas 4 had normal arteriographic study. On ventriculography, asynergy was found in 12 patients with left VPCs. Similar angiographic findings were demonstrated among 17 patients with right VPCs in that 11 had coronary artery disease (8 with triple-vessel disease and 3 with isolated obstruction of the left anterior descending coronary artery), whereas 6 had normal findings. Asynergy was also observed among 8 of the 11 coronary patients with right VPCs. All 3 patients demonstrating both right and left VPCs had coronary artery disease. Their conclusion[11] is that in patients with chest pain there is no relationship between the site of origin of VPCs and the prevalence or severity of coronary artery disease.

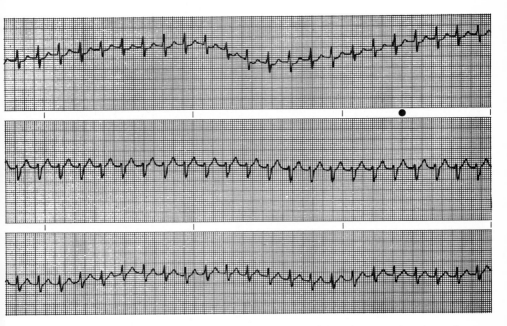

Fig. 13-17 This ECG tracing was taken immediately after termination of exercise. The cardiac rhythm is supraventricular (most likely A-V junctional) tachycardia (rate: 148 beats/minute) with aberrant ventricular conduction.

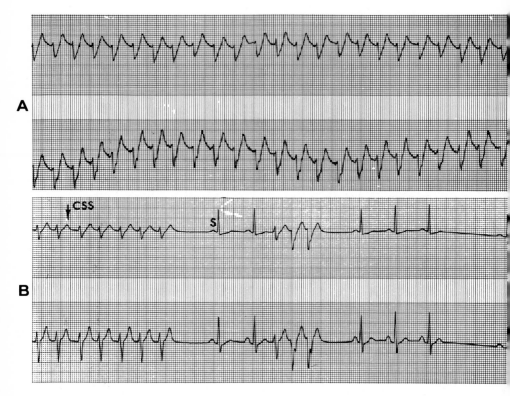

Fig. 13-18 Supraventricular (most likely A-V junctional) tachycardia with aberrant ventricular conduction (rate: 148 beats/minute) was provoked by mild exercise (treadmill) and the strips A and B represent post-exercise ECG. The tachycardia was successfully terminated by carotid sinus stimulation (marked CSS) and sinus rhythm (marked S) was restored. No further episode of the supraventricular tachycardia was observed in this patient following prescription of propranolol (Inderal) 10 mg. 4 times daily. Inderal is proven to be the best agent for exercise-induced tachyarrhythmias. No direct cause of the patient's tachycardia was determined.

Pietras et al.[14] reported recently the clinical significance of chronic recurrent left versus right ventricular tachycardia in correlation with hemodynamic and angiographic findings. The 15 patients with left ventricular tachycardia were older (mean age 43 years) and predominantly male (male-female ratio 10:5), and all (100%) had evidence of organic heart disease. On the other hand, the 12 patients with right ventricular tachycardia were younger (mean age 32 years) and mostly female (male-female ratio 4:8), and only 3 had evidence of organic heart disease. Patients with left ventricular tachycardia showed lower cardiac output and a much higher incidence of abnormal left ventricular and coronary angiograms than patients with right ventricular tachycardia. This study clearly indicates that left ventricular tachycardia is much more serious and clinically significant than right ventricular tachycardia.

In my experience,[31, 32, 43] right VPCs are extremely common in healthy individuals and the arrhythmia is often abolished by exercise (Figures 13-6 and 7). On the other hand, left VPCs and septal VPCs (Figures 13-20 and 21) are much more common in older individuals with diseased hearts (not

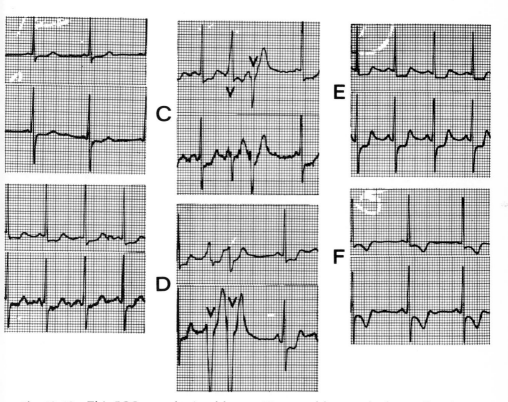

Fig. 13-19 This ECG was obtained from a 68-year-old man who has suffered from angina on exertion for several years. He was unable to continue the exercise beyond stage 3 because of significant chest pain associated with frequent multifocal ventricular premature contractions (marked V) and ventricular group beats. His maximal heart rate reached only 120 beats/minute. The strips A represent a resting ECG. The strips B and C were taken during exercise, whereas the remaining strips D to F represent post-exercise ECG. The exercise ECG test is positive (incomplete). Note significant S-T segment depression associated with biphasic to inverted T waves. Ventricular arrhythmias provoked by minimal exercise (less than 70% of the predicted maximal heart rate) are definitely an abnormal response to exercise and the underlying problem is usually coronary artery disease.

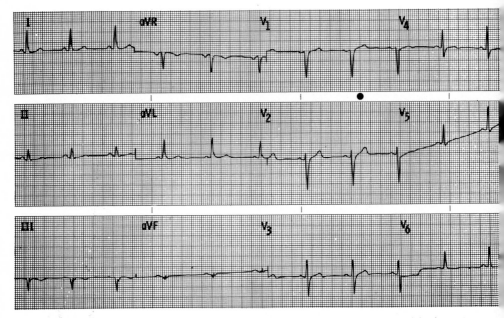

Fig. 13-20 Figures 13-20 to 22 were obtained from a 54-year-old physician with a previous history of myocardial infarction complaining of atypical chest pain and dyspnea on exertion for 2–3 weeks. His 12-lead ECG taken at rest shows sinus rhythm (rate: 65 beats/minute) and evidence of old diaphragmatic myocardial infarction.

necessarily coronary artery disease) and digitalis intoxication. Septal VPCs are diagnosed on the basis of upright QRS complexes in both left and right precordial leads. Exercise-induced unifocal VPCs (even 10 or more/minute) without S-T segment alteration (Figure 13-11) are *not* indicative of organic heart disease. Similarly, the development of ventricular tachycardia by exercise alone without S-T segment alteration (Figure 13-9) is not necessarily indicative of coronary artery disease.[43]

Reproducibility of Exercise-induced Ventricular Arrhythmias

Recently, the prevalence and reproducibility of exercise-induced ventricular arrhythmias during maximal exercise testing in 543 male Indiana state policemen at an average interval of 2.9 years has been studied by Faris et al.[10] In this study, the group (81 subjects) with known or suspected cardiovascular disease demonstrated a trend toward greater reproducibility with repeated exercise testing. The marked variability of exercise-induced ventricular arrhythmias during repeated maximal exercise ECG tests was observed in a clinically normal group (462 subjects).

Exercise-induced Ventricular Fibrillation

Ventricular fibrillation is a very rare complication of the exercise ECG test. In my own experience,[43] no incidence of ventricular fibrillation was observed during 5,500 exercise ECG tests. Similarly, Fox experienced no episode of ventricular fibrillation in approximately 30,000 exercise ECG tests.[44] However, Fletcher and Cantwell[8] reported recently that 5 patients with coronary artery disease who developed ventricular fibrillation in a medically supervised exercise program were successfully resuscitated. Four patients had successful myocardial revascularization, and 3 have returned to an exercise prescription of reduced intensity. As can be expected, ventricular fibrillation is primarily observed in patients with multivessel coro-

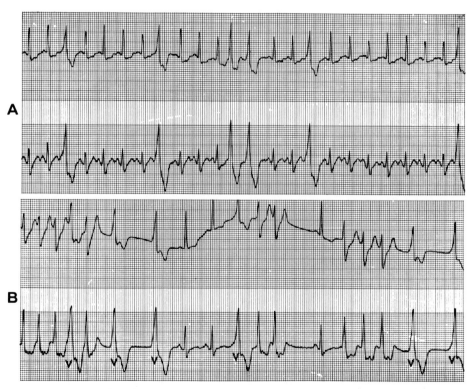

Fig. 13-21   He developed frequent multifocal VPCs with grouped beats and short runs of ventricular tachycardia at the last portion of the exercise protocol. In addition, parasystolic ventricular tachycardia (marked V, rate: 72 beats/minute) can be diagnosed. Note significant S-T segment depression with biphasic to inverted T wave. The strips A were taken during the end stage of exercise, whereas the strips B represent post-exercise ECG. The exercise ECG test is positive on this patient.

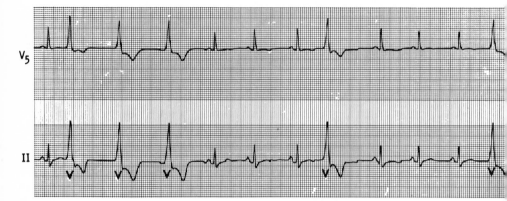

Fig. 13-22   These rhythm strips were recorded 6 minutes after the termination of exercise. Ordinary VPCs were subsided but ventricular parasystolic tachycardia (marked V) is still present.

nary disease, but the arrhythmia may occur unpredictably during the exercise program over a period of 2–48 months.

Predictive Implications for Future Coronary Events

Udall and Ellestad[6] studied the incidence of future coronary events (myocardial infarction, angina and cardiac death) on 6,500 patients who had undergone exercise ECG tests. In this study, 1,327 patients developed VPCs induced by exercise, and 83% of all patients had known or suspected cardiovascular disease. The annual incidence of new coronary events during the 5 year follow-up period among 1,067 subjects without VPCs or S-T segment alteration was reported to be 1.7%; 6.4% in 758 patients with VPCs alone; 9.5% among 609 patients with S-T segment alteration alone; and 11.4% in 569 patients with VPCs associated with S-T segment alteration. Their conclusion was that exercise-induced VPCs with or without S-T segment alteration represent a definite risk factor for future coronary events.

Conclusion

Although a controversy still remains, the relationship between ventricular arrhythmias and exercise may be summarized as follows from available data:[1-12, 14, 30-44]

(1) Exercise-induced ventricular arrhythmias are much more common in patients with coronary artery disease than in healthy subjects.
(2) Coronary patients who develop ventricular arrhythmias from exercise have a greater frequency of multivessel disease and left ventricular dysfunction.
(3) Ventricular arrhythmias induced by minimal or mild exercise with less than

70% of the predicted maximal heart rate strongly suggest the presence of coronary artery disease.

(4) VPCs are often abolished by exercise as the sinus rate is markedly accelerated. This finding does not prove or exclude the possibility of coronary artery disease.

(5) On the other hand, VPCs not suppressed by exercise do not indicate the presence or absence of coronary artery disease, although the finding favors the possibility of a diseased heart.

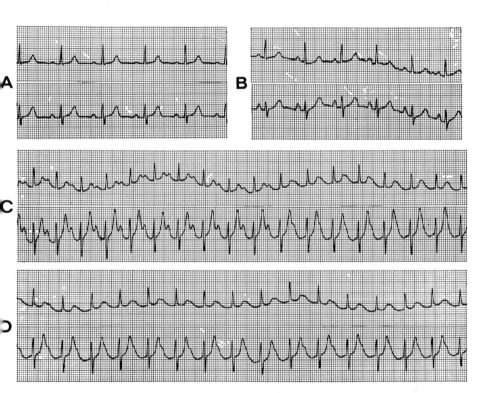

Fig. 13-23   An exercise ECG test was performed on a 33-year-old woman for the evaluation of atypical chest discomfort. Her 12-lead ECG at rest was within normal limits. The strips A and B were taken at rest in supine and standing position, respectively. The strips C were recorded immediately after the termination of exercise, whereas the strips D were taken 2 minutes later. It is noteworthy that the P-R intervals progressively lengthen (strips C), and marked first degree A-V block (P-R interval: 0.32 second) persists thereafter (later portion of strips C and entire strips D). She never developed Wenckebach A-V block, and her P-R intervals gradually returned to normal within 6 minutes. There was no S-T segment or T wave alteration during or after exercise. Thus, her exercise ECG test is negative. She failed to demonstrate any evidence of organic heart disease.

(6) Ventricular arrhythmias are very common during the post-exercise period in healthy subjects as well as in patients with coronary artery disease.

(7) Exercise-induced VPCs or ventricular tachycardia without S-T segment alteration do not necessarily indicate coronary artery disease. Mitral valve prolapse syndrome or cardiomyopathy may be responsible for the production of ventricular arrhythmias by exercise.

(8) Frequent (10 or more beats/minute) unifocal VPCs induced by exercise alone are not an indication of coronary artery disease.

(9) Grouped (2 consecutive) VPCs and multifocal (from 2 foci) VPCs may be found during exercise in healthy subjects as well as in coronary patients, but

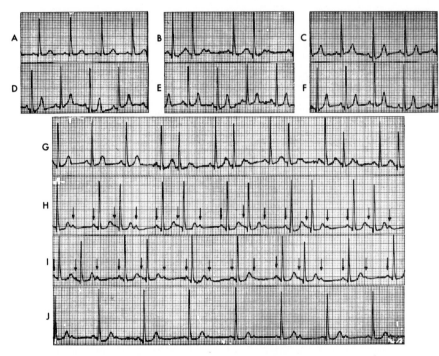

Fig. 13-24 Figures 13-24 to 26 were obtained from a 59-year-old Russian-born woman physician. She was referred to me from her family physician for the evaluation of her cardiac rhythm problem. She has been experiencing shortness of breath and marked weakness whenever she feels a slow heart rate and her symptoms seem to be pronounced during physical exercise (e.g., walking fast, climbing stairs, etc.). These rhythm strips are her exercise (treadmill) ECG. The strip A is a resting ECG, whereas the strips B to F were taken during exercise. The remaining strips G to J represent post-exercise ECG. She developed 3:2 Mobitz type II A-V block and intermittent 2:1 A-V block induced by mild exercise. Arrows indicate sinus P waves. The site of A-V block is most likely in the His bundle itself (intra-His block) in view of normal (narrow) QRS complexes of the conducted beats. Note occasional aberrant ventricular conduction (strip G). She denied chest pain.

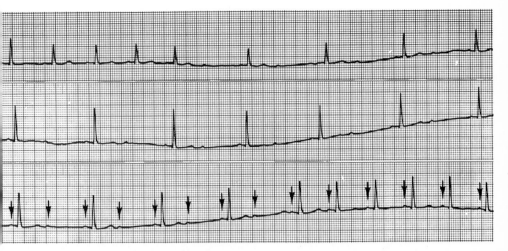

Fig. 13-25 The strips A to C represent her ambulatory (Holter monitor) ECG, and they are not continuous. Arrows indicate sinus P waves. Mobitz type II A-V block with intermittent 2:1 A-V block was documented during her ordinary daily activities. In more than 50% of the Holter monitor ECG, A-V block was recorded.

they are more common in diseased hearts. Multifocal VPCs from 3 or more foci, and 3 or more grouped VPCs are strongly indicative of coronary artery disease.

(10) The clinical significance of the origin of VPCs varies markedly depending upon the population studied. Either right or left VPCs may be induced by exercise in coronary patients. However, VPCs encountered in healthy subjects frequently originate in the right ventricle. In my experience, septal VPCs and left VPCs are similar in clinical significance—common in older individuals with diseased heart. Nevertheless, a possibility of coronary heart disease is not proven nor excluded from the viewpoint of the origin of VPCs.

(11) The reproducibility of exercise-induced ventricular arrhythmias is much more common in coronary patients than in healthy subjects.

(12) In general, exercise-induced ventricular arrhythmias seem to predict a definite risk of developing new coronary events, including sudden death, particularly in patients with known coronary artery disease.

(13) The clinical significance of exercise-induced ventricular parasystole is uncertain.

A-V Conduction Disturbances

It is not uncommon to observe alteration of the P-R interval during and/or immediately after exercise (Figure 13-23) in healthy individuals as well as in the patients with diseased heart.[43] Actual shortening of the P-R interval up to 0.10 or 0.11 second during exercise as the sinus rate increases

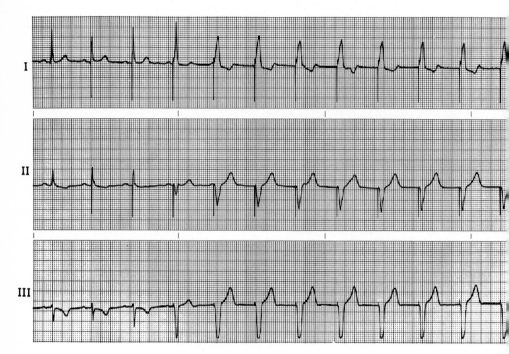

Fig. 13-26 This ECG tracing was recorded following permanent pacemaker (demand ventricular) implantation. It shows demand ventricular pacemaker rhythm (rate: 72 beats/minute) with occasional sinus beats (1st beat) and ventricular fusion beats (2nd, 3rd and 4th beats).

is extremely common, probably because of increased sympathetic tone. The shortening of the P-R interval during exercise seems to be seen more frequently among young, healthy individuals. The changing P-R interval or actual shortening of the P-R interval is clinically insignificant.

First Degree A-V Block

First degree A-V block is occasionally observed in the exercise laboratory during the late portion of the exercise or immediate post-exercise period (Figure 13-23). This finding is probably related to increased vagal tone, and it has no clinical significance in most cases. On the other hand, Sandberg[45] reported that 2 patients developed first degree A-V block induced by exercise and both patients had a history of myocarditis. One of them had some evidence of myocarditis while exercising. The other patient also developed Wenckebach A-V block immediately after exercise.

It can be said, regarding the development of first degree A-V block by exercise, that the finding may be observed in apparently healthy individuals although any factors which may produce the prolongation of the A-V conduction time (e.g., digitalis, propranolol, myocarditis, etc.) certainly will predispose to the lengthening of the P-R interval. Exercise-induced first degree A-V block per se is *not* indicative of coronary heart disease.

Second Degree A-V Block

Although the occurrence of Wenckebach (Mobitz type I) A-V block induced by exercise has been reported,[45] it is extremely rare indeed. Among 5,500 exercise ECG (treadmill) tests in our laboratory[43] and 30,000 exercise tests by Fox's experience,[44] no case demonstrating typical Wenckebach A-V block during or after exercise was encountered. On the other hand, Meytes et al.[13] reported 3 healthy youths who developed Wenckebach A-V block during vigorous exercise among 126 athletes. The development of Wenckebach A-V block by exercise is probably due to increased vagal tone as in exercise-induced first degree A-V block. Therefore, exercise-induced Wenck-

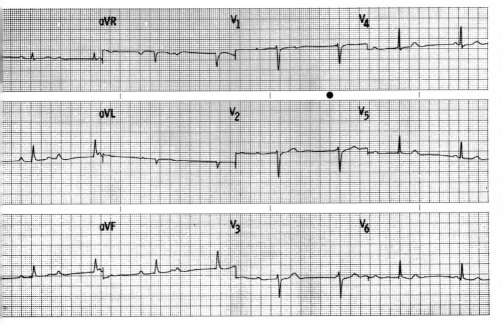

Fig. 13-27 Figures 13-27 and 28 were taken on a 35-year-old woman with known congenital complete A-V block. Exercise ECG test was performed in order to assess her functional capacity. There was no evidence of any other cardiac problem. Her resting 12-lead ECG shows sinus rhythm (atrial rate: 76 beats/minute) with A-V junctional escape rhythm (ventricular rate: 50 beats/minute) due to complete A-V block, and within normal limits, otherwise.

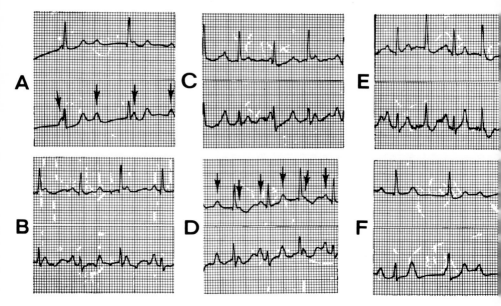

Fig. 13-28 This tracing is her exercise ECG. The strips A are resting ECG whereas the strips B to E were recorded during exercise. The strips F represent post-exercise ECG. Arrows indicate sinus P waves. The maximal atrial rate reached 190 beats/minute, but the maximal ventricular rate was only 138 beats/minute. Complete A-V block persisted throughout the exercise test. Her exercise capacity was excellent.

ebach A-V block may be physiologic in many cases, and the finding is probably insignificant.

Recently, Mobitz type II A-V block induced by exercise was observed in a 59-year-old woman (Figure 13-24). She becomes symptomatic (e.g., shortness of breath, weakness, etc.) as soon as she develops Mobitz type II A-V block with intermittent 2:1 A-V block causing a slow ventricular rate, even during ordinary daily activities (such as climbing stairs, walking fast, running, etc.) or during the treadmill exercise ECG test. Mobitz type II A-V block was also demonstrated by a 24-hour Holter monitor ECG during physical exercise on this patient (Figure 13-25). One point somewhat against the diagnosis of Mobitz type II A-V block in this patient was the narrow (normal) QRS complexes of the conducted beats. Thus, the site of the block is considered to be most likely in the His bundle itself—intra-His block.[32] This woman had experienced intermittent Mobitz type II A-V block for at least 3–4 years, and the A-V block had progressively increased over the past year. A permanent demand ventricular pacemaker was implanted with an excellent result (Figure 13-26).

The clinical significance of exercise-induced Mobitz type II A-V block is uncertain, but the finding may be a rate-related phenomenon. This finding is probably analogous to the development of bundle branch block during exercise as the sinus rate is accelerated—rate-dependent bundle branch block (will be discussed later in this chapter). Namely, Mobitz type II A-V block is produced as the sinus rate increases beyond the critical rate due to any means (e.g., exercise, atropine injection, etc.). Thus, the development of Mobitz type II A-V block is unlikely to be caused by a purely exercise-related phenomenon. It should be noted that Mobitz type II A-V block represents infra-nodal block which is irreversible.[32]

Complete A-V Block

Complete A-V block at rest is a relative contraindication to the exercise ECG test, particularly when the A-V block is acquired form (see Chapter 8). However, the exercise ECG test can be given to patients with congenital complete A-V block unless there is a coexisting significant congenital cardiac anomaly.

Ikkos and Hanson[15] studied the exercise response in 11 patients with congenital complete A-V block ranging from 7–23 years of age using an electrically braked bicycle ergometer for two 6-minute periods. Among the 11 subjects, the atrial rate was increased as expected (160–185 beats/minute) in all except one patient who had 143 beats/minute, but the maximal

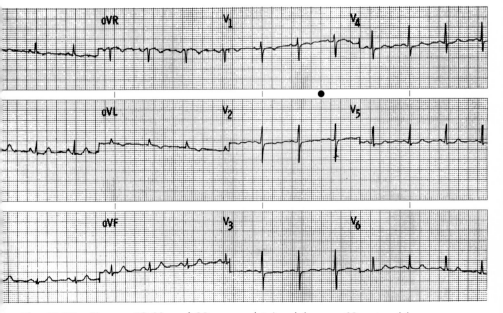

Fig. 13-29 Figures 13-29 and 30 were obtained from a 68-year-old woman with angina. Her resting 12-lead ECG shows sinus rhythm (rate: 76 beats/minute) with low voltage and slight non-specific T wave abnormality—within normal limits, otherwise.

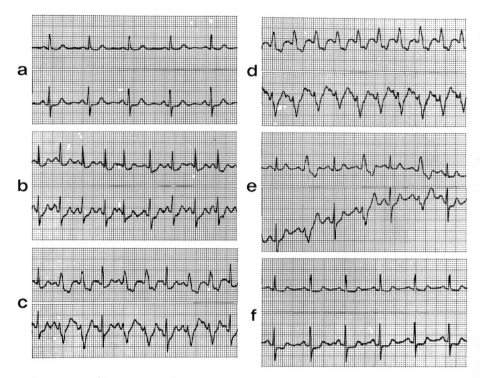

Fig. 13-30   This tracing is her exercise ECG. The strips a are resting ECG. The strips b to d were taken during exercise while the strips e and f represent post-exercise ECG. She developed intermittent LBBB as the sinus rate was accelerated, but normal conduction returned later on resting (strip f). There is an APC in strips b. The exercise ECG test is positive in view of S-T segment depression during normal conduction.

ventricular rate by exercise was only below 102 beats/minute in 8 subjects. The maximal ventricular rate induced by exercise was 130 beats/minute in one subject. Six patients developed VPCs during exercise and 4 had ventricular bigeminy.

I recently encountered a 35-year-old, apparently healthy woman with congenital complete A-V block. Her resting ECG demonstrated sinus rhythm (atrial rate: 75 beats/minute) with A-V junctional escape rhythm (ventricular rate: 50 beats/minute) due to complete A-V block and within normal limits, otherwise (Figure 13-27). Her exercise tolerance was excellent, and the maximal ventricular rate rose to 138 beats/minute during exercise (Figure 13-28). The maximal sinus rate was 190 beats/minute (Figure 13-28).

The physical working capacity in patients with uncomplicated congenital complete A-V block is normal or it may be slightly reduced.[15, 43] The degree of increment of sinus rate by exercise in congenital complete A-V block is normal, but the ventricular rate does not increase significantly in many cases. The acceleration of the ventricular rate during exercise is unrelated to the resting ventricular rate, atrial rate or cardiac size.[15]

Intraventricular Blocks

Various forms of intraventricular blocks may be observed during exercise ECG tests, but their occurrence is primarily a rate-related phenomenon— rate-dependent. In other words, right or left bundle branch block occurs during exercise as the sinus rate is increased beyond the critical rate of a given individual because of the pre-existing concealed bundle branch block (Figures 13-29 and 30). Thus, rate-dependent bundle branch block is *not* purely an exercise-related phenomenon, because bundle branch block may be produced by accelerating the heart rate via many other means (e.g., atropine injection, rapid atrial pacing, etc.). In addition to left or right bundle branch block, exercise may induce left anterior or posterior hemiblock and a bifascicular block (a combination of right bundle branch block and left anterior or posterior hemiblock).[46] These rate-dependent intraventricular blocks alone during and/or after exercise are *not* indicative of a positive exercise ECG test (see Chapter 12).

The interpretation of the exercise ECG test becomes extremely difficult when dealing with pre-existing left bundle branch block (LBBB) because of a very high incidence of false positive exercise ECG tests[16] (see Chapter 12). On the other hand, the pre-existing right bundle branch block (RBBB) does not influence significantly the interpretation of the exercise ECG test.[17] Clinically, many patients with exercise-induced LBBB in the general hospital population show positive exercise ECG tests because of the coexisting coronary heart disease.[43] In contrast, LBBB may be found in apparently healthy individuals, especially when dealing with a large population of young, healthy people such as Air Force personnel.[16] Therefore, the clinical significance of either rate-dependent or fixed LBBB largely depends upon a given population studied. In my experience, the incidence of coronary heart disease in patients with rate-dependent or fixed RBBB is much lower than those with LBBB.[43, 46] RBBB is, of course, relatively common in apparently healthy individuals.[17]

It can be said that it is impossible to predict the result of the exercise ECG test when dealing with any type of intraventricular block. In addition, intraventricular blocks observed during the exercise ECG test are *not* indicative of a positive test.

Brady-Tachyarrhythmia Syndrome

The term "brady-tachyarrhythmia syndrome" is used when the cardiac rhythm consists of a component of tachyarrhythmia and a component of bradyarrhythmia due to various mechanisms.[32] Brady-tachyarrhythmia syndrome is often a manifestation of advanced sick sinus syndrome.[19] Brady-tachyarrhythmia syndrome is only occasionally observed in older individuals with diseased hearts in the exercise laboratory.

Wolff-Parkinson-White Syndrome

Exercise may provoke or abolish anomalous A-V conduction in individuals with known Wolff-Parkinson-White (WPW) syndrome.[32] However, it is more common to bring out anomalous A-V conduction by exercise as the sinus rate is accelerated (Figure 13-31).

Recently, the exercise response in the WPW syndrome was investigated, in our exercise laboratory, in 20 subjects with known WPW syndrome

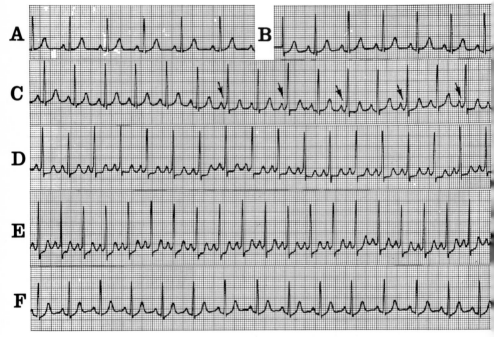

Fig. 13-31   This tracing is an exercise ECG on a 47-year-old woman. Her resting 12-lead ECG was within normal limits. The strips A and B were taken at rest in supine and standing position, respectively. The strips C to E were recorded during exercise, whereas the strip F represents post-exercise ECG. The exercise was stopped at the end of stage 4, prematurely, and her maximal heart rate reached to only 135 beats/minute. Intermittent WPW syndrome is obvious (indicated by arrows) in the strip C. In the strips D and E, a false positive exercise ECG test is diagnosed because of the WPW syndrome. As soon as the heart rate is reduced by rest, a normal conduction has returned, and the S-T segment depression is no longer present in the strip F.

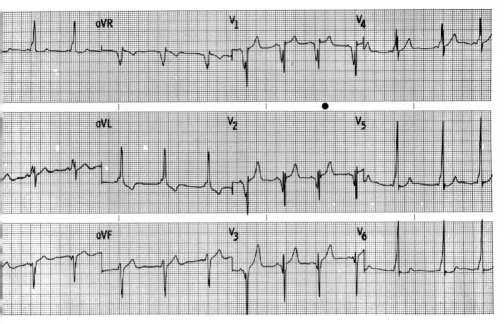

Fig. 13-32 Figures 13-32 and 33 were obtained from a 14-year-old boy in a research program for the assessment of the exercise response in WPW syndrome. His resting 12-lead ECG shows sinus arrhythmia (rate: 60–78 beats/minute) and WPW syndrome, type B.

without any organic heart disease.[18] Anomalous A-V conduction was observed in all but 4 subjects, and significant S-T depression was induced by exercise in all (16) subjects with anomalous A-V conduction which meets the criteria of the conventional positive exercise ECG test (see Chapter 12). In other words, the incidence of false positive exercise ECG tests was 100% among individuals showing anomalous A-V conduction during and/or after exercise (Figures 13-32 and 33). It is concluded from our study that the exercise ECG test is invalid in patients with WPW syndrome when anomalous A-V conduction is present during the test.[18] Another interesting observation was that no patient with WPW syndrome developed ectopic tachyarrhythmia during and/or after exercise in this study, although physical exercise has been considered a predisposing factor to initiate the tachyarrhythmia in the WPW syndrome. On the other hand, a 55-year-old man with known WPW syndrome associated with hyperthyroidism developed paroxysmal atrial fibrillation with anomalous A-V conduction by mild exercise in our exercise laboratory (Figures 13-1 to 3). His arrhythmia was successfully terminated by administration of procaine amide (Pronestyl, 500 mg. every 4 hours by mouth). This patient was relatively asymptomatic during paroxysmal atrial fibrillation except for palpitations.

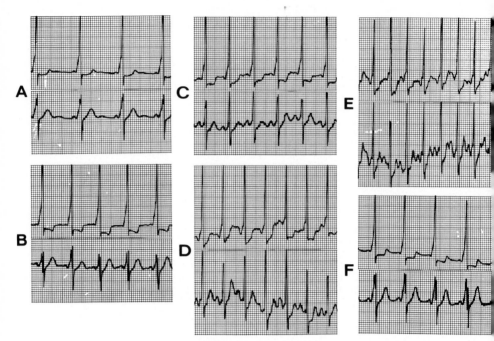

Fig. 13-33 This tracing is his exercise ECG. The strips A are a resting ECG. The strips B to E were recorded during exercise, whereas the strips F represent post-exercise ECG. Note marked S-T segment depression—false positive exercise ECG test.

Miscellaneous

Various other electrophysiologic events may be observed during and/or after exercise. Aberrant ventricular conduction is very common in APCs or A-V junctional premature beats because of a short coupling interval and rapid basic sinus rate (Figure 13-14). In addition, aberrant ventricular conduction is frequently observed in various supraventricular tachyarrhythmias because of rapid rate (Figures 13-15, 17 and 18). A common occurrence of ventricular fusion beats from frequent VPCs associated with rapid sinus tachycardia induced by exercise has been stressed previously.

A rare occurrence of exercise-induced parasystole has been described, and, in most cases, the parasystole is ventricular in origin (Figures 13-21 and 22). Occasionally, slow ventricular parasystolic tachycardia (rate: 60–100 beats/minute) induced by exercise may be observed. Exercise-induced parasystole does not seem to have any clinical significance.

Summary

(1) There is a significant controversy regarding the clinical significance of exercise-induced arrhythmias.

(2) Exercise may provoke almost every known type of cardiac arrhythmia (see Table 13-1), and it may abolish the pre-existing arrhythmias.

(3) Exercise-induced arrhythmias alone are not indications of organic heart disease.

(4) Cardiac arrhythmias abolished by exercise do not necessarily mean a benign nature.

(5) Ventricular arrhythmias are the primary concern in the exercise laboratory, and VPCs are the most common exercise-induced arrhythmia.

(6) Exercise-induced supraventricular arrhythmias are relatively uncommon and their occurrence is clinically insignificant in most cases.

(7) In general, exercise-induced ventricular arrhythmias are much more common in patients with coronary artery disease than in healthy subjects.

(8) Coronary artery disease is strongly suspected when ventricular arrhythmias are provoked by minimal exercise with less than 70% of the predicted maximal heart rate.

(9) In healthy subjects as well as the patients with coronary heart disease, VPCs are often abolished by exercise when the sinus rate is markedly accelerated, and the VPCs frequently reappear during recovery (post-exercise) period.

(10) Exercise-induced VPCs or ventricular tachycardia alone without S-T segment change are not sufficient to diagnose coronary heart disease. Individuals with mitral valve prolapse syndrome and cardiomyopathy frequently develop ventricular arrhythmias during exercise.

(11) Coronary heart disease is strongly suspected when exercise provokes multifocal VPCs from 3 or more foci, or 3 or more grouped VPCs.

(12) Left VPCs as well as right VPCs may be induced by exercise in patients with coronary artery disease, but VPCs in healthy individuals are commonly originating from the right ventricle. Thus, left VPCs and septal VPCs are more common in older subjects with diseased hearts and digitalis toxicity.

(13) Reproducibility of exercise-induced ventricular arrhythmias is a common occurrence in coronary patients.

(14) Alteration of the A-V conduction by exercise is insignificant clinically.

(15) Exercise may induce first degree or Wenckebach A-V block especially during the post-exercise period, even in healthy individuals.

(16) The occurrence of exercise-induced bundle branch block or hemiblock is a rate-dependent phenomenon, and this finding alone is not indicative of coronary heart disease.

(17) In congenital complete A-V block, the exercise tolerance is excellent in most cases unless there is a coexisting congenital cardiac anomaly.

(18) Exercise is not a predisposing factor for the initiation of ectopic tachyarrhythmias in individuals with the WPW syndrome.

(19) Parasystole is rarely produced by exercise and it is clinically insignificant.

REFERENCES

1. McHenry, P. L., Morris, S. N. and Kavalier, M.: Exercise-induced arrhythmias —Recognition, classification, and clinical significance, *in* Complex Electrocardiography— 2, edited by C. Fisch, Cardiovas. Clin., *6:*246–254, Philadelphia, F. A. Davis, 1974.
2. DeMaria, A. N., Vera, Z., Amsterdam, E. A. and Mason, D. T.: Disturbances of cardiac rhythm and conduction induced by exercise: diagnostic, prognostic and therapeutic implications, *in* Exercise In Cardiovascular Health And Disease, edited by E. A. Amsterdam, J. H. Wilmore and A. N. DeMaria, pp. 209–217, New York, Yorke Medical Books, 1977.
3. Ellestad, M. H.: Stress Testing: Principles and Practice, pp. 125–156, Philadelphia, F. A. Davis, 1975.
4. Jelinek, M. V. and Lown, B.: Exercise stress testing for exposure of cardiac arrhythmia. Prog. Cardiovasc. Dis., *16:*497, 1974.
5. DeBacker, G., Jacobs, D., Prineas, R. et al.: Ventricular premature beats: Reliability in various measurement methods at rest and during exercise. Cardiology, *63:*53, 1978.
6. Udall, J. A. and Ellestad, M. H.: Predictive implications of ventricular premature contractions associated with treadmill stress testing. Circulation, *56:*985, 1977.
7. Kennedy, H. L., Caralis, D. G., Khan, M. A. et al.: Ventricular arrhythmia 24 hours before and after maximal treadmill testing. Am. Heart J., *94:*718, 1977.
8. Fletcher, G. F. and Cantwell, J. D.: Ventricular fibrillation in a medically supervised cardiac exercise program. Clinical, angiographic, and surgical correlations. J.A.M.A., *238:*2627, 1977.
9. McHenry, P. L., Morris, S. N., Kavalier, M. and Jordan, J. W.: Comparative study of exercise-induced ventricular arrhythmias in normal subjects and patients with documented coronary artery disease. Am. J. Cardiol., *37:*609, 1976.
10. Faris, J. V., McHenry, P. L., Jordan, J. W. and Morris, S. N.: Prevalence and reproducibility of exercise-induced ventricular arrhythmias during maximal exercise testing in normal men. Am. J. Cardiol., *37:*617, 1976.
11. Bodenheimer, M. M., Banka, V. S. and Helfant, R. H.: Relation between the site of origin of ventricular premature complexes and the presence and severity of coronary artery disease. Am. J. Cardiol., *40:*865, 1977.
12. Sheps, D. S., Ernst, J. C., Briese, F. R. et al.: Decreased frequency of exercise-induced ventricular ectopic activity in the second of two consecutive treadmill tests. Circulation, *55:*892, 1977.
13. Meytes, I., Kaplinsky, E., Yahini, J. H. et al.: Wenckebach A-V block: A frequent feature following heavy physical training. Am. Heart J., *90:*426, 1975.
14. Pietras, R. J., Mautner, R., Denes, P. et al.: Chronic recurrent right and left ventricular tachycardia: Comparison of clinical, hemodynamic and angiographic findings. Am. J. Cardiol., *40:*32, 1977.
15. Ikkos, D. and Hanson, J.: Response to exercise in congenital complete atrioventricular block. Circulation, *22:*583, 1960.
16. Whinnery, J. E., Froelicher, V. F., Stewart, A. et al.: The electrocardiographic response to maximal treadmill exercise of asymptomatic men with left bundle branch block. Am. Heart J., *94:*316, 1977.
17. Whinnery, J. E., Froelicher, V. F., Stewart, A. et al.: The ECG response to maximal treadmill testing in asymptomatic men with right bundle branch block. Chest, *71:*335, 1977.
18. Zuckerman, G. and Chung, E. K.: The exercise response in the Wolff-Parkinson-White syndrome (In preparation), 1978.
19. Chung, E. K.: Sick sinus syndrome and brady-tachyarrhythmia syndrome, *in* Artificial Cardiac Pacing: Practical Approach, edited by Edward K. Chung, Baltimore, Williams & Wilkins, 1979.
20. Blackburn, H.: The exercise electrocardiogram. Technological, procedural and conceptual developments, *in* Measurement in Exercise Electrocardiography, edited by H. Blackburn, pp. 220–258, Springfield, Ill., Charles C Thomas, 1969.
21. Hornsten, T. R. and Bruce, R. A.: Computed ST forces of Frank and bipolar exercise electrocardiograms. Am. Heart J., *78:*346, 1969.

22. Vassalle, M., Levine, M. J. and Stuckey, J. H.: Sympathetic control of ventricular automaticity: the effects of stellate ganglion stimulation. Circ. Res., *23*:249, 1968.
23. Vassalle, M., Stuckey, J. H. and Levine, M. J.: Sympathetic control of ventricular automaticity: role of the adrenal medulla. Am. J. Physiol., *217*:930, 1969.
24. Rosen, M. R. and Hoffman, B. F.: Mechanisms of action of anti-arrhythmic drugs. Circ. Res., *32*:1, 1973.
25. Sonnenblick, E. H. and Skelton, C. L.: Oxygen consumption of the heart: physiologic principles and clinical implications. Mod. Concepts Cardiovasc. Dis., *40*:9, 1971.
26. Alanis, J. and Benitez, D.: The decrease in the automatism of the Purkinje pacemaker fibers provoked by high frequencies of stimulation. Jpn. J. Physiol., *17*:556, 1967.
27. Chung, E. K.: Holter monitor electrocardiography, *in* Artificial Cardiac Pacing: Practical Approach, edited by Edward K. Chung, Baltimore, Williams & Wilkins, 1979.
28. Kosowsky, B. D., Lown, B., Whiting, R. et al.: The occurrence of ventricular arrhythmias with exercise as compared to monitoring. Circulation, *44*:826, 1971.
29. Ryan, M., Lown, B. and Horn, H.: Comparison of ventricular ectopic activity during 24-hour monitoring and exercise testing in patients with coronary heart disease. New Engl. J. Med., *292*:224, 1975.
30. Amsterdam, E. A., DeMaria, A. N., Vismara, L. A. et al.: Lethal arrhythmias in the pathogenesis of pre-hospital sudden death, *in* Concepts on the Mechanisms and Treatment of Arrhythmias, edited by G. Gensini, pp. 29–37, Mt. Kisco, N. Y., Futura Publishing Company, 1974.
31. Chung, E. K.: Clinical Electrocardiography, Part 9, Exercise Electrocardiography. New York, Medcom, 1978.
32. Chung, E. K.: Principles of Cardiac Arrhythmias, Second Edition. Baltimore, Williams & Wilkins, 1977.
33. Gooch, A. S.: Exercise testing for detecting changes in cardiac rhythm and conduction. Am. J. Cardiol., *30*:741, 1972.
34. Gooch, A. S. and McConnell, D.: Analysis of transient arrhythmias and conduction disturbances occurring during submaximal treadmill exercise testing. Prog. Cardiovasc. Dis., *13*:293, 1970.
35. Sandberg, L.: The significance of ventricular premature beats or runs of ventricular tachycardia developing during exercise tests. Acta Med. Scand., *169*:1, 1961.
36. Vedin, J. A., Wilhelmsson, C. E., Wilhelmsson, L. et al.: Relations of resting and exercise-induced ectopic beats to other ischemic manifestations and to coronary risk factors. Men born in 1913. Am. J. Cardiol., *30*:25, 1972.
37. Bryson, A. L., Parisi, A. F., Schecter, E. et al.: Life threatening arrhythmias induced by exercise: cessation after coronary bypass surgery. Am. J. Cardiol. *32*:995, 1973.
38. McHenry, P. L., Fisch, C., Jordan, J. W. and Corya, B. R.: Cardiac arrhythmias observed during maximal treadmill exercise testing in clinically normal men. Am. J. Cardiol., *29*:331, 1972.
39. Blackburn, H., Taylor, H. L., Hamrell, B. et al.: Premature ventricular complexes induced by stress testing. Their frequency and response to physical conditioning. Am. J. Cardiol., *31*:441, 1973.
40. Zaret, B. L. and Conti, C. R., Jr.: Exercise-induced ventricular irritability: hemodynamic and angiographic correlation (Abstr) Am. J. Cardiol., *29*:298, 1972.
41. Goldschlager, N., Cake, D. and Cohn, K.: Exercise-induced ventricular arrhythmias in patients with coronary artery disease. Their relation to angiographic findings. Am. J. Cardiol., *31*:434, 1973.
42. Helfant, R., Pine, R., Kabde, V. and Banka, V.: Exercise-related ventricular premature complexes in coronary heart disease. Ann. Intern. Med., *80*:589, 1974.
43. Chung, E. K.: Exercise ECG (treadmill) tests in 5,500 subjects (Unpublished data).
44. Fox, S.: Personal communication, 1978.
45. Sandberg, L.: Studies in electrocardiogram changes during exercise tests. Acta Med. Scand. *169* (Suppl. 365): 1969.
46. Chung, E. K.: Electrocardiography: Practical Applications with Vectorial Principles. Hagerstown, Md., Harper & Row, 1974.

14

Myocardial Perfusion Imaging with Thallium-201: Correlation with Exercise Electrocardiography and Coronary Angiography

Elias Botvinick, M.D., F.A.C.P.,
David Shames, M.D. and
William W. Parmley, M.D., F.A.C.P., F.A.C.C.

General Considerations

During the past 5 years, there have been rapid and impressive gains made in the evaluation of cardiac disease by nuclear medicine techniques. These advancements have been based on earlier established principles and have been made possible by the development of new radiopharmaceuticals, new instrumentation and imaginative new methods. Scintigraphic techniques are non-invasive and require only the intravenous injection of a radionuclide. In many cases, these studies enable us to gain information otherwise available only via expensive, painful and potentially dangerous invasive methods. In other situations, these non-invasive nuclear medicine studies enable us to evaluate cardiac structure and function in a more physiologic way than could be done, even during invasive catheterization. In yet other instances, scintigraphic studies allow evaluation of clinically valuable parameters measurable by no other technique, invasive or non-invasive. Nowhere have these techniques been more widely applied than for the evaluation of the patient with known or suspected ischemic heart disease.

Myocardial perfusion scintigraphy utilizes an intracellular cation to identify regions of reversible ischemia and irreversible infarction and indirectly delineate the coronary anatomy. The study may be applied in a dynamic fashion to the patient undergoing exercise. Stress-induced image abnormalities correspond to regional myocardial ischemia and correlate well with the presence of significant anatomic coronary stenosis in the appropriate coronary vessel on coronary angiography. The imaging technique has been found to be more sensitive and more specific for the diagnosis of significant coronary lesions than the simultaneously performed stress electrocardiogram (ECG). Imaging maintains its specificity and has been found capable of clarifying the ambiguous ECG findings in patients submitted to stress testing in the presence of conduction abnormalities, ventricular hypertrophy, drug effect and a multitude of other factors which make ECG interpretation tenuous. Myocardial perfusion scintigraphy seems especially valuable for the clinical evaluation of patients with atypical pain, and promises to serve as an objective indicator of the results of coronary bypass graft surgery. The method provides physiologic evidence of the significance of coronary lesions as opposed to the gross visual and often inexact anatomic methods available from invasive catheterization. Although seemingly nonspecific in nature, perfusion scintigraphy appears able to delineate myocardial ischemia caused by coronary disease from ischemia associated with other etiologies often of more benign prognosis. In association with rest perfusion imaging, stress perfusion scintigraphy can differentiate ischemia from infarcted myocardium, and facilitate therapy directed at the preservation of reversibly ischemic regions.

Historical Background

Intracellular cations have been used to image the myocardium since Love and coworkers first demonstrated myocardial deposition of radioactive potassium and its analogues over 20 years ago.[1] Clinical application of these observations was begun 5 years later when Carr and coworkers first utilized the method for imaging regions of myocardial infarction.[2,3] Using rubidium-86 and cesium-131, these observers demonstrated significant diminution of myocardial radioactivity in infarcted zones after intravenous administration of the radionuclide in experimentally infarcted animal preparations. Since that time, the presence of defects, radiopenic areas or "cold spots" have been noted in infarcted myocardial regions of both experimental animals and patients after the intravenous injection of a variety of intracellular cations, including potassium-42,[4] potassium-43,[5] cesium-129,[6] cesium-131,[2,3] and cesium-134 m.[7]

These agents were subsequently utilized for the visualization and localization of reversible ischemia during pathophysiologic conditions such as exercise stress. The slow extraction of cesium by the myocardium made it poorly suited for evaluation of alterations in perfusion during dynamic situations.[8] However, the myocardial extraction of potassium and rubidium was rapid and appeared to parallel relative myocardial perfusion after intravenous administration.[1,8,9] These agents have all been proven useful for the dynamic evaluation of stress-induced perfusion abnormalities and the indirect identification of significant coronary lesions. The extremely rapid physical half-life (4.2 hr) and method of production of rubidium-81 make daily acquisition of that radionuclide and close proximity to a cyclotron a necessity. Due to their high energies of emission, imaging of both potassium-43 and rubidium-81 can only be conducted using a rectilinear scanner with poor image resolution, or a specially constructed and cumbersome lead shield fitted over a pinhole collimator.[10] Rubidium-81 is often at a further disadvantage owing to the presence of rubidium-82 m radioactivity in the radiopharmaceutical which again emits high energy radiation with subsequent image degradation.

In an attempt to gain three-dimensional perspective on perfusion image abnormalities, nitrogen-13, a positron emitter, has been employed to obtain myocardial images with a scintillation camera[11] or a variety of new multicrystal positron cameras.[12] The ammonium ion has been found to behave similarly to potassium, and initial experimental studies utilizing this material for myocardial perfusion imaging have been encouraging.[11, 12] However, again nitrogen-13 is cyclotron-produced and has an extremely short half-life(10 min), making it available for study only in institutions with a cyclotron on the premises. Attempts to label the myocardium with a variety of radioactive metabolites has been made, and labeling fatty acids with radioactive technetium or other agents may provide another valuable approach.

The clinical development of myocardial perfusion scintigraphy utilizing intracellular cations has been prevented until recently by the factors related to nuclide production (rubidium-81 and nitrogen-13), physical behavior (cesium), short physical half-life (rubidium-81 and nitrogen13), and high energies of emission (potassium-43 and rubidium-81). Additionally, the need for cyclotron production often made such agents prohibitively expensive, as in the case of potassium-43.

Recent evaluation has demonstrated the superiority of thallium-201 (Tl-201) for myocaridal perfusion imaging. This agent, another intracellular cation, is also rapidly extracted by the myocardium and possesses a physical half-life of approximately 3 days, allowing a 1 week shelf life, permitting prolonged storage and facilitating emergency, as well as elective, patient evaluation.[13, 14] Although not optimal, the low energy emission of Tl-201 permits scintigraphy of relatively high quality using widely available conventional scintillation cameras and collimators without necessitating special shielding or other equipment. Tl-201 has been used for both the static evaluation of infarction and the dynamic evaluation of ischemia, and identification of significant coronary lesions.

Although not the ideal agent, Tl-201 provides a more optimal combination of physical characteristics, half-life, and emission energy, and has simplified myocardial perfusion scintigraphy and made quality evaluation widely available, permitting widespread investigation and clinical application. Mass production of the radionuclide in a commercial sphere promises also to reduce its cost. The remainder of this chapter will deal with the rationale, methodology and clinical experience with myocardial perfusion scintigraphy, particularly employing Tl-201. Emphasis will be placed on the relationship of these studies to the findings during simultaneous stress electrocardiography and the anatomic assessment of the vasculature at coronary angiography. Additionally, stress perfusion scintigraphy with Tl-201 will be related to rest scintigraphy and to other methods which might be utilized to diagnose the presence of coronary artery disease and determine the viability of the involved myocardium.

Rationale

Coronary artery disease is the leading cause of death in the United States. It accounts for a yearly mortality of 500,000 to 1,000,000 people and alters the lifestyle or totally incapacitates countless others. Owing to the size of this population and our increasing ability to influence the clinical course of many with this disease, there is growing emphasis on methods to accurately diagnose, localize and quantitate the severity and extent of coronary involvement. Direct visual evidence of coronary stenosis is available from selective coronary angiography where the coronary vascular bed is completely opacified following its injection with contrast media. This technique carries with it a small but finite risk, requires hospitalization, produces pain and anxiety and represents a significant expense. Additionally, this invasive method assesses the severity of stenosis in a rough, inprecise manner and requires assumptions regarding the pathophysiologic effect of the stenosis on myocardial blood supply and its relationship to symptoms. With this technique, there is no effort to objectively evaluate the determinants of myocardial ischemia, myocardial blood supply in relation to oxygen demands. Additionally, recent reports indicate the great variability of evaluating the significance of a coronary narrowing, simply on the basis of its anatomic appearance.[15]

A variety of parameters have been evaluated in an attempt to diagnose significant coronary lesions in a more physiologic, non-invasive manner. Certainly, the clinical history, at times aided by the physical examination, remains an important diagnostic tool. However, the history and physical are often misleading and fail to give adequate quantitative information, most frequently in those patients who present the greatest diagnostic dilemma. Graded exercise testing with electrocardiographic and hemodynamic monitoring potentially evaluates the determinants of myocardial ischemia and gives indirect evidence of the presence of a significant coronary lesion without necessitating visual evaluation of the coronary anatomy. However, stress electrocardiography has been shown to have problems of insensitivity and non-specificity.[16, 17] Many conditions, including conduction abnormalities, ventricular hypertrophy, drugs, electrolyte abnormalities and hyperventilation, have been shown to make interpretation of the stress electrocardiogram hazardous.[18-21] Even the female sex has been invoked as a potential cause for the false positive stress test.[22] Relative myocardial perfusion scintigraphy using Tl-201 is a graphic non-invasive method to diagnose pathologically significant coronary lesions by virtue of their pathophysiologic effects, without the burdensome need for direct anatomic assessment.

Myocardial perfusion scintigraphy utilizes a radioactive intracellular cation, currently Tl-201, to produce images of the myocardium, either at rest or in relation to exercise stress. After its intravenous administration, 70–80% of the radionuclide passing through the coronary circulation is extracted by the myocardium on its first pass.[13] The radionuclide is distributed to viable myocardial cells according to their relative perfusion.[14] Other determinants of thallium-201 distribution include the presence of a myocardial scar and, possibly, altered myocardial cell membrane function of any cause.[23] When the radionuclide is administered intravenously at rest, any of these factors may lead to a relative diminution in radionuclide content in one region of the myocardium compared to its neighbor. In patients without symptoms at the time of study, such abnormalities generally represent areas of infarction, but may conceivably be related as well to reversible, resting ischemia as might exist in a patient with crescendo angina. Image abnormalities related to transient, reversible conditions such as the myocardial ischemia related to angina pectoris, should normalize at a time following resolution of the underlying cause and resultant symptomatology. Similarly, abnormal heterogeneous patterns of myocardial blood flow may develop in association with exercise stress and give rise to abnormalities in the perfusion scintigram, which would not be visible in an image obtained at rest, indicating transient, stress-induced ischemia distal to a significantly stenotic coronary vessel.

The theoretical basis for Tl-201 stress myocardial perfusion scintigraphy is demonstrated in Figure 14-1 and depends on the fact that coronary blood flow at rest may be well maintained at normal levels in spite of high grade and nearly subtotal stenosis.[24] Such flow maintenance relies on the ability of the coronary vascular bed to decrease flow resistance in the stenotic vessel by compensatory dilatation in the affected coronary vascular bed distal to the stenosis. Utilizing such adaptation, normal flow may be maintained through a coronary vessel with significant stenosis at rest. With stress, flow through normal coronary vessels may increase 4- to 5-fold due to the diminution in distal flow resistance. However, due to the full distal dilatation, the significantly stenotic coronary vessel cannot further compensate and cannot fully supply the demands of stress. Although flow through the stenotic vessel may increase somewhat in response to stress, the incre-

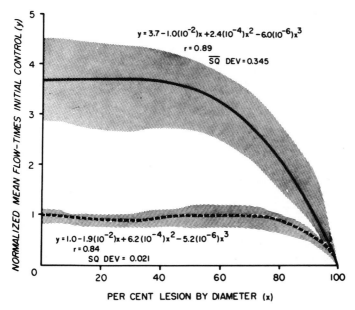

Fig. 14-1 Coronary flow. Shown graphically is the response to coronary flow distal to graded and sequential stenoses created in the left circumflex coronary artery of the dog(s) at rest (dotted line) and with stress (uninterrupted line). Measured flow was expressed in terms of multiples of the initial control resting flow (ordinate). At rest, flow was well maintained up to subtotal occlusion. With stress, here produced by the intracoronary administration of contrast medium, coronary flow uniformly increases, but fails to attain expected levels distal to significantly stenotic vessels, here appearing in the range of 60–80%. (From Gould, K. L. and coworkers: Physiologic Basis for Assessing Critical Coronary Stenosis. Am. J. Cardiol., *83*:87, 1974.)

ment of flow is significantly less than that which can occur through normal vessels. Whereas a significantly stenotic coronary vessel may maintain normal flow at rest and may increase flow in response to stress demands, it cannot match the flow response of normal or minimally stenotic vessels. "Significantly" stenotic coronary arteries may be defined in a pathophysiologic sense as those vessels demonstrating such a diminished "flow reserve" in response to stress. Such a definition contrasts with the anatomic definition of "significant" coronary stenosis which is defined in the coronary angiogram in anatomic terms as a vessel showing $\geq 75\%$ luminal narrowing.

Since flow through stenotic vessels may be well maintained at rest, most patients with significant coronary lesions are asymptomatic at rest. However, symptoms develop when flow demands cannot be met owing to a diminished "flow reserve." At rest, both normal and significantly stenotic vessels may accommodate similar and, in fact, normal flow. Myocardial regions perfused by both normal and stenotic vessels will show equal levels of radioactivity after T1–201 administration. However, with exercise, the normal pattern of homogeneous coronary perfusion is disrupted as the normal vessel provides flow far in excess of that through the stenotic vessel. At stress, the myocardial region supplied by the normal vessel is better perfused than that supplied by the significantly stenotic vessel. Stress produces a difference in perfusion between the region of the myocardium supplied by the normal vessel and that supplied by the stenotic vessel. Similarly, after T1–201 administration, myocardial regions supplied by stenotic vessels demonstrate a relative diminution in radioactivity compared to regions perfused by normal vessels. It is this heterogeneity of perfusion and radioactivity that allows identification of regions of stress-induced ischemia and indirectly enables us to identify significant coronary lesions. It is this relative decrement in perfusion and the resultant radiopenic image defect or "cold spot" that myocardial perfusion scintigraphy has as its basis.

Methods

When attempting to identify regions of stress-induced myocardial ischemia, the concepts outlined above are employed. Since maximal abnormalities of flow and radionuclide distribution are produced by stress, scintigraphy is initially performed in association with exercise, as is demonstrated in Figure 14-2. Most commonly, treadmill or bicycle exercise is employed. The patient is generally examined in the fasting state in order to minimize blood flow and resultant thallium distribution to the gastrointestinal tract. An intravenous line is begun to allow radionuclide administration at peak stress, and exercise is conducted in a routine manner utilizing any of a number of graded stress protocols. The ability of stress scintigraphy to identify significant ischemic regions will vary with the vigor of exercise in a manner similar to that defined for the stress electrocardiogram.[25] Symptomatic, electrocardiographic and hemodynamic monitoring of patients during exercise must be conducted as when performing stress testing without associated scintigraphy. As the patient nears the exercise end point, 2 millicuries of T1-201 are injected through the intravenous line and exercise is continued for an additional 30–60 seconds to allow optimal myocardial distribution. Continuous monitoring of the patient's electrocardiogram and blood pressure is conducted during the recovery period, as routinely performed in association with stress testing. Immediately after recovery, the patient is placed under a high resolution scintillation camera and cardiac imaging is performed in multiple projections using parallel collimation of medium to high sensitivity.

Image Interpretation

The normal T1-201 scintigram reveals radioactivity in all elements of the viable myocardium in proportion to perfusion. The greatest muscle mass will have the greatest relative perfusion and demonstrate the most intense radioactivity. For this reason, the left ventricular myocardial wall is best seen in the normal study. Figure 14-3 demonstrates the normal image in multiple projections, correlated with the appropriate cardiac muscular and vascular anatomy. The right ventricle is occasionally evident, but appears most commonly and most prominently in cases of right ventricular hypertrophy as demonstrated in Figure 14-4. The region of the ventricular base contains the membranous septum and valve planes and normally shows diminished radioactivity. For this reason, the myocardium in the normal T1-201 scintigram appears in a horseshoe configuration in the anterior and left lateral projections. The left anterior oblique projection looks directly up the long axis of the left ventricle and the scintigram frequently shows the myocardium in a horseshoe or doughnut configuration. The clear or radiopenic area in the center of myocardial radioactivity on each T1-201 scintigram corresponds to the blood filled ventricular cavity.

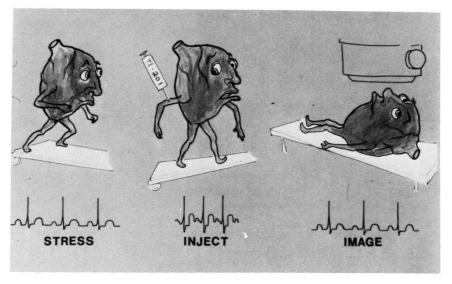

STRESS   **INJECT**   **IMAGE**

Fig. 14-2 Method of study. Thallium is injected through an established intravenous line at peak stress. After 30 seconds to 1 minute of continued exercise and a recovery period, the patient undergoes imaging in multiple projections. Alternatively, imaging may be conducted while monitoring the ECG in the recovery period.

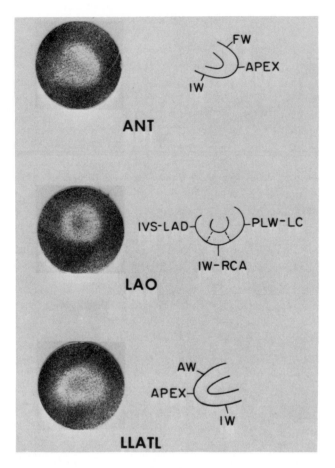

Fig. 14-3 Normal TI-201 myocardial perfusion scintigram. Shown are the normal TI-201 scintigrams in the anterior (ANT), left anterior oblique (LAO) and left lateral (LLATL) projections performed after peak treadmill stress in a patient with normal coronary arteries. Myocardial uptake in the left ventricle is intense and homogeneous. The right ventricle occasionally appears as a region of faint activity anterior to the left ventricle. The diagram to the right of each scintigram indicates ventricular as well as coronary anatomy. Abbreviations: AW—anterior wall; FW—free wall; IVS—interventricular septum; IW—left ventricular inferior wall; LAD— distribution of the left anterior descending coronary artery; LC—common region of distribution of the left circumflex coronary artery; PLW—left ventricular posterior lateral wall; RCA—common distribution of the right coronary artery. (From Botvinick, E. H. and coworkers: Thallium-201 myocardial perfusion scintigraphy for the clinical clarification of normal, abnormal and equivocal stress tests. Am. J. Cardiol., *41*:43, 1978.)

Since ventricular anatomy is well delineated on scintigram and since the relationship between coronary anatomy and ventricular anatomy is well established, perfusion abnormalities on the scintigram can be related to significant lesions in the coronary tree. These relationships are best evaluated in the left anterior oblique projection where the coronary anatomy exhibits the least degree of overlap and is therefore best defined (Figure 14-3). Generally, perfusion abnormalities in the interventricular septum correlate with significant stenosis of the left anterior descending coronary artery, whereas posterior lateral wall abnormalities generally imply circumflex lesions and inferior wall abnormalities are most frequently related to right coronary stenosis. Apical lesions may be the result of distal disease in any of the three major vessels, and can only be localized in the presence of other accompanying scintigraphic abnormalities.

Table 14-1 provides a general pattern of image interpretation. Since stress precipitates abnormalities or worsens those seen at rest, a rest image is not performed if the stress image is normal. If associated with vigorous exercise,

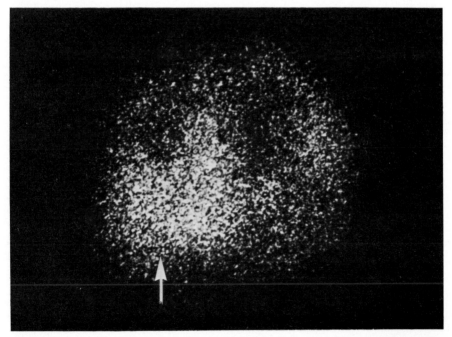

Fig. 14-4 Right ventricular hypertrophy. Shown is the myocardial perfusion scintigram performed with TI-201 in the left anterior oblique projection in a patient with cor pulmonale and known right ventricular hypertrophy. The typical owl's eye or omega configuration is seen due to the intense concentration of radioactivity in the right ventricular myocardium (arrow).

Table 14-1. Image Interpretation

Condition		Image Interpretation
Rest	Normal	No previous MI
Exercise	Normal	No reversible ischemia
Rest	Normal	No previous MI
Exercise	Abnormal	Reversible ischemia
Rest	Abnormal	Previous MI
Exercise	More abnormal	Reversible ischemia
Rest	Abnormal	Previous MI
Exercise	Unchanged from rest	No reversible ischemia

such normal stress scintigrams make the presence of significant coronary artery disease, reversible ischemia or permanent infarction, unlikely. However, if the stress image is abnormal, a rest scintigram must be performed to differentiate stress-induced ischemic abnormalities from permanent infarction. Persistent abnormalities in the rest scintigram are indicative of regional infarction. Rest scintigrams may be performed after a second radionuclide administration generally 1 week after the initial exercise study. More recently, some studies have indicated accurate assessment of the reversibility of stress-related image abnormalities with repeat imaging performed only hours after the initial exercise dose.[26] Such delayed imaging utilizes a single radionuclide dose for stress and subsequent rest scintigraphy and could potentially decrease the expense while increasing the convenience of the study, thereby allowing interpretation of the significance of stress image abnormalities during the course of a single work day. Defects persisting in the rest image are indicative of infarction, whereas those areas abnormal only in association with stress define a region of transient ischemia. Commonly, in patients with prior infarction, we see both rest image abnormalities and related areas of stress-induced ischemia. Similar to the assessment of the stress electrocardiogram, normal stress scintigrams performed in relation to suboptimal exercise stress (less than 85% of maximal predicted heart rate for age) can be seen in the presence of significant coronary disease.

The Clinical Utility of Stress Scintigraphy: Correlation with Stress Electrocardiography and Selective Coronary Angiography

General Relationships

There have been several well documented studies which attest to the clinical values of stress perfusion scintigraphy, and the accurate assessment of significant coronary lesions by this method. In early studies using rubidium-81 and potassium-43, we and others have documented the improved sensitivity and specificity of the method over stress electrocardiography for the diagnosis of coronary artery disease.[10, 14, 27–32] These same studies documented the sensitivity of historic evidence of typical anginal pain as a diagnostic indicator of significant coronary disease.[10] Such sensitivity was first proposed by Ross and Friesinger,[33] who showed the value of the careful history in a diagnosis of coronary disease. However, perfusion scintigraphy proved a useful diagnostic test even in patients with "typical" anginal pain and was extremely reliable among patients with atypical pain, a group difficult to evaluate by other methods. The presence of stress-induced perfusion abnormalities correlated extremely well with the presence of significant coronary stenosis as defined visually and anatomically on selective coronary angiography.

Image Sensitivity

Sensitivity of the imaging technique for the diagnosis of significant coronary lesions is defined as the percentage of patients with coronary disease who have an abnormal image. Image sensitivity varies from study to study, but generally is in the range of 75–90% using a variety of radionuclides, most recently Tl-201. Several studies have documented the improved diagnostic sensitivity of the scintigraphic technique when compared to maximal bicycle or treadmill stress electrocardiography where ischemic ECG changes are defined as horizontal or downsloping S-T segment depression 1 mm. beyond baseline, 0.08 second from the J-point at peak stress or during recovery employing one or multiple leads. Figure 14-5 demonstrates new stress-induced image and ECG abnormalities in a patient with angiographically documented coronary disease. However, Figure 14-6 demonstrates new stress-induced image abnormalities in the presence of a negative stress electrocardiogram in a patient proven to have significant coronary lesions in the vessel perfusing the region of image abnormality. Such false negative stress electrocardiograms are found most commonly in single-vessel disease, but rarely in triple-vessel disease.[10, 32]

The presence of a perfusion defect on scintigraphy correlates well with the presence of a stenotic lesion in the appropriate coronary artery. However, the absence of a perfusion defect in a given myocardial region does not exclude a coronary lesion in the vessel perfusing that segment. In a recent study evaluating the clinical utility of Tl-201 perfusion scintigraphy,[32] the image identified lesions in 41 of 89 (46%) significantly affected vessels. Stress scintigraphy using both rubidium-81 and Tl-201 has shown similar sensitivity for the demonstration of 1-, 2- and 3-vessel coronary involvement,[10, 32] and appears to demonstrate its greatest advantage over stress electrocardiography in the identification of patients with 1- and 2-vessel disease. An

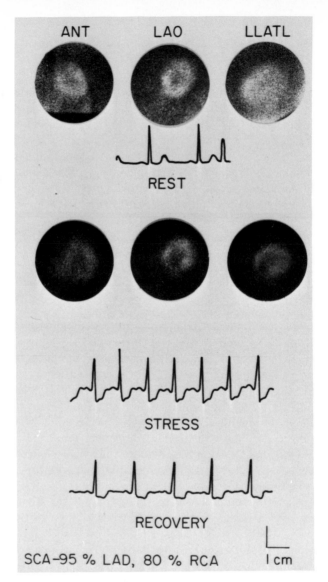

Fig. 14-5 True positive stress ECG. Shown are rest (above) and stress (below) ECGs and Tl-201 scintigrams in the anterior (ANT), left anterior oblique (LAO) and left lateral (LLATL) projections of a patient with selective coronary angiograms (SCA) demonstrating significant left anterior descending (LAD) and right coronary artery (RCA) lesions. The rest lesion is normal, whereas the stress image shows significant abnormalities involving the left ventricular apex and inferior wall, and distal aspect of the interventricular septum. Although both stress electrocardiogram and scintigram diagnosed the presence of significant coronary lesions, only the scintigram gave accurate localizing information. Note that the electrocardiogram, probably positive during stress, was definitely positive during recovery. (From Botvinick, E. H. and coworkers: Thallium-201 myocardial perfusion scintigraphy for the clinical clarification of normal, abnormal and equivocal stress tests. Am. J. Cardiol., *41*:43, 1978.)

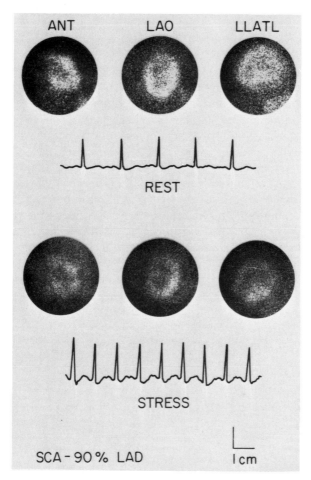

Fig. 14-6 False positive stress ECG. Shown are the rest (above) and stress (below) ECGs and Tl-201 perfusion scintigrams in the anterior (ANT), left anterior oblique (LAO) and left lateral (LLATL) projections in a patient with selective coronary angiography (SCA) demonstrating significant left anterior descending coronary artery (LAD) disease. The rest scintigram reveals homogeneous radioactivity. With stress, the interventricular septum and anterior left ventricular wall, the region supplied by the stenotic vessel, are barely visible. The electrocardiogram shows no ischemic change. (From Botvinick, E. H. and coworkers: Thallium-201 myocardial perfusion scintigraphy for the clinical clarification of normal, abnormal and equivocal stress tests. Am. J. Cardiol., *41:*43, 1978.)

additional manifestation of the improved sensitivity of stress scintigraphy for coronary diagnosis is its ability in occasional cases to identify significant coronary lesions even when obtained in association with a negative and suboptimal treadmill test in a patient who has undergone less than 85% of maximal predicted heart rate for age. Thus, while scintigraphy is an extremely sensitive technique for the identification of coronary disease in a given patient, it may not identify all sites of coronary involvement (see Figures 14-10 and 13). Table 14-2 combines the similar findings using rubidium-81 and T1-201[10, 32] to demonstrate the over-all sensitivity of stress electrocardiography and scintigraphy in relation to the number of vessels involved.

Perfusion scintigraphy utilizes regions of relative diminution of myocardial radioactivity to identify areas of stress-induced ischemia. Absolute measurements of blood flow are not made. Due to the relative nature of the technique, there were initial fears that the scintigraphic method may fail to identify the presence of severe triple-vessel disease due to generalized and uniform flow abnormalities brought on by a widespread diminution of coronary flow reserve. This fear never materialized, as numerous studies attest to the extremely high sensitivity of scintigraphic diagnosis of coronary artery disease in the setting of triple-vessel disease.[10, 14, 29–32] In most cases of triple-vessel disease, the scintigram merely identifies a region of ischemia related to one of the diseased vessels, likely the most severely involved vessel, responsible for ischemic symptoms or signs at the level of stress conducted. Occasionally, the image may demonstrate a pattern diagnostic of two-vessel disease (see Figure 14–10) and, on occasion, relative perfusion

Table 14-2. Sensitivity of Stress Electrocardiography and Scintigraphy in Relation to the Number of Coronary Vessels with Significant Stenosis*

Coronary Vessels Involved (no.)	Number of Patients	Abnormal Stress Test**		Equivocal Stress Test*** (no.)	Abnormal Scintigram	
		(no.)	(%)		(no.)	(%)
1	17	7	41	4	14	82
2	37	25	70	4	34	92
3	21	13	62	6	18	86

* This is a composite of tables appearing in Botvinick, E. H. and coworkers: Myocardial Stress Perfusion Scintigraphy with Rubidium-81 vs. Stress Electrocardiography. Am. J. Cardiol., 39:364, 1977 and Botvinick, E. H. and coworkers: Thallium-201 Myocardial Perfusion Scintigraphy for the Clinical Clarification of Normal, Abnormal and Equivocal Stress Tests. Am. J. Cardiol., 41: 43, 1978. The relative myocardial perfusion scintigram seems generally sensitive to the presence of single-, double- and triple-vessel involvement. Scintigraphy has its greatest advantage over stress electrocardiography in detecting single- and double-vessel disease and clarifying the equivocal stress test.
** Greater than or equal to 1 mm. of horizontal or downsloping S-T segment depression beyond an isoelectric baseline.
*** Electrocardiogram revealing significant baseline S-T segment depression greater than or equal to 1 mm.

abnormalities may be identified in the regions of all three involved coronary vessels (see Figure 14-12). In this manner, localization of ischemic myocardium and its associated stenotic vessel, which is simply and accurately performed scintigraphically, takes on more than academic importance. The prognosis of patients with main left coronary artery obstruction or triple-vessel involvement and most likely those with proximal left anterior descending coronary occlusion is far worse than those with coronary disease in general.[34] Identification of the extent and distribution of coronary involvement provides important clinical information which may have a profound bearing on the mode and timing of therapy. Such localization of coronary lesions cannot be well performed using evidence from the stress electrocardiogram alone.[35] In addition, scintigraphic localizing information may be of extreme value for the objective assessment of the patient after coronary bypass graft surgery[36] (see below).

Image Specificity

Image specificity for coronary diagnosis is defined as the percentage of patients without coronary disease who have a normal image. In those patients presenting with chest pain syndromes, but demonstrating normal coronary arteriograms, stress scintigraphy similarly demonstrated high diagnostic specificity for coronary artery disease in most studies ranging around 90%.[10,14,28–32] Since the initial study of Zaret and coworkers,[27] several studies have documented the ability of stress scintigraphy to identify the false positive stress test with the demonstration of improved image specificity over stress electrocardiography performed in association with one or multiple lead monitoring systems. Figure 14-7 demonstrates the negative stress scintigram and associated negative stress electrocardiogram in a patient with documented normal coronary arteriograms. Such correlation of normal scintigraphic, electrocardiographic and invasive arteriographic findings is the general rule in patients with normal coronary arteries. However, Figure 14-8 demonstrates the normal stress scintigram performed in association with a positive stress electrocardiogram in a patient who was documented to have normal coronary arteries. Such stress electrocardiograms may be said to be false positive for the diagnosis of significant large vessel coronary lesions. Regardless of the etiology of such stress-related ECG abnormalities, such changes occurring in the absence of significant coronary disease have a benign prognosis, not significantly different from normal. However, the true positive stress ECG bears the prognosis of the related coronary disease.[37] Such differentiation of the true positive from the false positive stress ECG is extremely difficult without scintigraphy, but obviously critical for the evaluation of prognosis and the delivery of therapy.

Whereas the stress electrocardiogram may be useful for the identification of myocardial ischemia unrelated to coronary disease, the stress scintigram

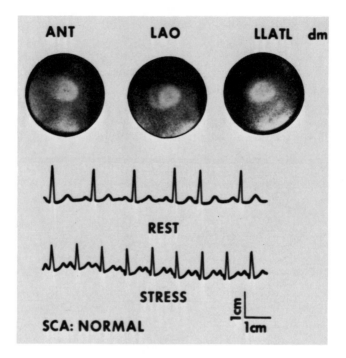

Fig. 14-7   Normal stress ECG and image. Shown are the normal stress TI-201 perfusion scintigrams in the anterior (ANT), left anterior oblique (LAO) and left lateral (LLATL) projections (above) and the rest and stress electrocardiograms (below) in patient DM with normal selective coronary angiograms (SCA). The stress electrocardiogram was similarly negative for ischemia.

does not appear to be too sensitive to myocardial ischemia on a noncoronary basis. Patients with aortic stenosis and left ventricular hypertrophy frequently develop ischemic pain and symptomatology as do those with mitral valve prolapse. In both cases, more certainly in the former, symptomatology may be related to myocardial ischemia of a generalized nature in the absence of significant coronary disease. Studies have determined that even in these settings relative myocardial perfusion scintigraphy can distinguish between those patients with ischemic pain on a coronary basis from those with similar symptoms but unrelated to large-vessel coronary disease.[38] Perfusion image abnormalities appear specific for segmental, localized malperfusion and, in this sense, appear more specific for coronary artery disease and extremely useful as a diagnostic and prognostic indicator in the presence of other possible ischemic syndromes. Simultaneous evaluation of perfusion imaging and myocardial metabolism in patients with known coronary anatomy have also documented this scintigraphic relationship with coronary disease. Image abnormalities may be induced via atrial pacing stress in regions perfused by significantly stenotic vessels.[39] Such pacing stress may serve a useful clinical purpose for the evaluation of pain syndromes in patients who are unwilling or unable to perform other forms of exercise stress. Pacing stress can also be used to provoke myocardial ischemia and evaluate the resultant metabolic abnormalities in association with scintigraphy. Pacing-induced scintigraphic abnormalities were only seen in relation to metabolic abnormalities precipitated in patients with significant coronary lesions. Metabolic abnormalities induced with extreme tachycardia or other conditions unrelated to significant coronary disease were generally seen in patients with normal stress scintigrams.

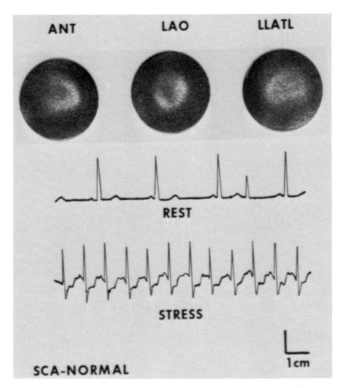

Fig. 14-8 False positive stress ECG. Shown are the stress Tl-201 perfusion scintigrams in the anterior (ANT), left anterior oblique (LAO) and left lateral (LLATL) projections (above) and the rest and stress electrocardiograms (below) in a patient with normal coronary arteries. Radionuclide distribution was also normal. However, the stress electrocardiogram showed distinct and significant horizontal S-T segment depression. Scintigraphy proved to be the valid clinical indicator. (From Botvinick, E. H. and coworkers: Thallium-201 myocardial perfusion scintigraphy for the clinical clarification of normal, abnormal and equivocal stress tests. Am. J. Cardiol., *41*:43, 1978.)

Although scintigraphic abnormalities appear specific for myocardial ischemia, and particularly that caused by coronary artery disease, such specificity is, of course, not absolute. Such image abnormalities have been documented in patients with granulomatous disease of the myocardium, cardiomyopathy or myocardial fibrosis of any cause. Extreme myocardial thinning and decreased radioactivity is demonstrated in the T1-201 scintigram shown in Figure 14-9 performed in a patient with idiopathic cardiomyopathy who demonstrated regional fibrosis in the absence of significant coronary disease on post-mortem examination.

Comparing scintigraphic, electrocardiographic and angiographic findings in 46 patients, T1-201 myocardial perfusion scintigraphy appeared to be more sensitive and specific than stress electrocardiography for the diagnosis of coronary disease. When the full population was examined, stress scintigraphy proved statistically more accurate than stress electrocardiography. The results of this study are shown in Table 14-3.

The Equivocal Stress ECG

The stress electrocardiogram has been shown to be inaccurate in the setting of resting baseline electrocardiographic abnormalities. The presence of right bundle branch block and resting S-T segment depression of a variety of causes has been shown to drastically diminish the sensitivity of stress electrocardiography for coronary disease diagnosis. On the other hand, the interpretation of stress-induced electrocardiographic changes is tenuous and generally lacks specificity in the presence of resting S-T segment depression due to left bundle branch block, left ventricular hypertrophy, digitalis preparations, electrolyte abnormalities, hyperventilation and a variety of other conditions.[18-22] Such resting baseline abnormalities occur frequently in the population evaluated for coronary disease and in some studies amount to as many as one-third to one-half of those evaluated.[25] It is in these patients that the diagnosis of coronary disease is often most difficult and at the same time most critical. We studied 22 patients with resting baseline electrocardiographic abnormalities by T1-201 stress scintigraphy, stress electrocardiography and coronary arteriography. There were 3 patients with right bundle branch block, 2 with left bundle branch block, 6 with left ventricular hypertrophy, 5 using digitalis preparations, 3 with hyperventilation changes, and 3 with baseline abnormalities of unknown cause. Among these 22 patients, 14 with stress-induced scintigraphic abnormalities had significant coronary lesions. The other 8 patients had normal stress perfusion scintigrams, 6 without evidence of coronary disease, but 2 with significant coronary lesions. Figure 14-10 illustrates the equivocal stress electrocardiogram in a patient taking digoxin. The scintigraphic study is grossly abnormal with new stress abnormalities involving the left ventricular inferior wall, distal aspect of the posterior lateral wall, interventricular septum and apex.

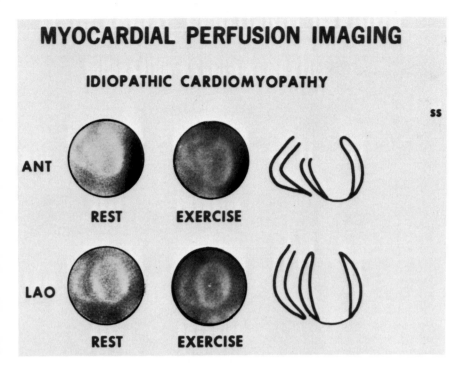

MYOCARDIAL PERFUSION IMAGING

IDIOPATHIC CARDIOMYOPATHY

SS

ANT

REST   EXERCISE

LAO

REST   EXERCISE

Fig. 14-9 Idiopathic cardiomyopathy. Shown are the Tl-201 test and exercise scintigrams in the anterior (ANT) and left anterior oblique (LAO) projections in patient SS with known non-coronary cardiomyopathy. Apparent are the large ventricular size bilaterally and areas of thinning and decreased radioactivity in the region of the cardiac apex. The region of apparent abnormality changes little with exercise and is demonstrated by a thin line in the accompanying schematic drawing. Similarly, an area of the distal right ventricular wall appears poorly labeled. Post-mortem examination revealed widespread myocardial scarring, particularly prominent in the apical region, without evidence of associated coronary disease.

In the presence of resting, drug-related S-T segment depression, the scintigram clearly documented the presence of significant right coronary, left anterior descending and, most likely, left circumflex coronary disease. This patient's coronary arteriogram revealed triple-vessel disease. Figure 14-11 illustrates the resting and stress electrocardiograms and scintigrams in a patient with severe left ventricular hypertrophy. Again, conduction abnormalities associated with left ventricular hypertrophy made ECG interpretation hazardous. The stress scintigram was entirely normal in this patient with normal coronary arteries. Figure 14-12 demonstrates new stress perfusion image abnormalities in a patient with left bundle branch block. Whereas the ECG was negative or, at best, equivocal, the stress scintigram

Table 14-3.* Analysis of T1-201 Results

Sensitivity Matrix

$$\text{Sensitivity} = \frac{TP}{TP + FN}$$

RMPS	SECG	
	TP	FN
TP	17	6
FN	1	3

Sensitivity: SECG–0.67
RMPS–0.85 $0.10 > p > 0.05$

Specificity Matrix

$$\text{Specificity} = \frac{TN}{TN + FP}$$

	SECG	
	TN	FP
TN	10	7
FP	2	0

Specificity: SECG–0.63
RMPS–0.89 $0.20 > p > 0.10$

Accuracy Matrix

$$\text{Accuracy} = \frac{TP + TN}{TP + TN + FP + FN}$$

	SECG	
	TP + TN	FP + FN
TP + TN	27	13
FP + FN	3	3

Accuracy: SECG–0.65
RMPS–0.87 $0.05 > p > 0.02$

* The results of stress electrocardiography (SECG) and the relative myocardial perfusion scintigram (RMPS) are compared and analyzed statistically. A true positive test (TP) refers to abnormal electrocardiographic or scintigraphic studies performed in patients with documented significant coronary lesions. A true negative test (TN) refers to a normal electrocardiographic or scintigraphic study in patients with documented normal or insignificantly narrowed coronary arteries. A false positive test (FP) refers to an abnormal electrocardiographic or scintigraphic study in patients with documented normal or insignificantly narrowed coronary arteries. A false negative test (FN) refers to a normal electrocardiographic or scintigraphic study in patients with documented significant coronary lesions. In evaluating our results, only the 46 patients with definitely positive or definitely negative stress electrocardiograms could be compared to the results of scintigraphy. Among this number, those 27 patients with abnormal coronary angiograms are considered under the sensitivity matrix, whereas those 19 patients with "normal" coronary angiograms are considered under the specificity matrix. The accuracy matrix attempts to simultaneously evaluate sensitivity and specificity and is a compilation of the preceding two matrices. Scintigraphy was more accurate than stress electrocardiography for the diagnosis of significant coronary lesions (from Botvinick, E. H. and coworkers: Thallium-201 Myocardial Perfusion Scintigraphy for the Clinical Clarification of Normal, Abnormal and Equivocal Stress Tests. Am. J. Cardiol., *41:* 43, 1978).

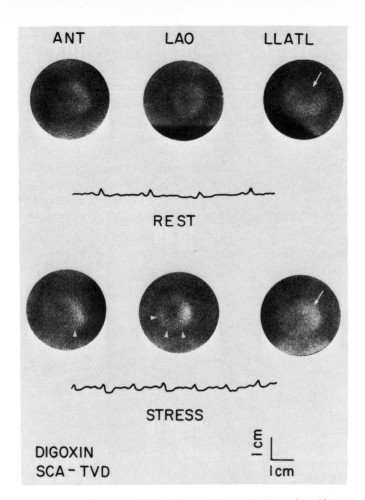

Fig. 14-10 Equivocal stress ECG with positive scintigraphy. Shown are the rest (above) and stress (below) ECGs and scintigrams in the anterior (ANT), left anterior oblique (LAO) and left lateral (LLATL) projections in a patient proven on coronary angiography (SCA) to have severe triple-vessel disease (TVD). The electrocardiogram showed resting S-T segment depression, which became somewhat deeper at stress. The patient was taking digoxin. Such drug-related S-T segment depression made the electrocardiogram interpretation difficult. However, the image showed clear stress-induced perfusion abnormalities involving the left ventricular inferior wall, distal aspect of the posterior lateral wall, interventricular septum and apex (arrow points), attesting to the severity and extent of coronary disease later documented angiographically. The redistribution of radioactivity is also prominent on the LLATL projection where the region of the ventricular base and lateral wall, relatively unlabeled at rest, become the most intense regions with stress (arrows), indicating "best" perfusion of the basal or proximal aspects of the ventricle and widespread distal abnormalities. The perfusion scintigram clarified the equivocal stress electrocardiogram. (From Botvinick, E. H. and coworkers: Thallium-201 myocardial perfusion scintigraphy for the clinical clarification of normal, abnormal and equivocal stress tests. Am. J. Cardiol., 41:43, 1978.)

documented severe, widespread coronary artery disease. The patient's coronary arteriogram documented triple-vessel disease which was, in fact, predicted scintigraphically. This study documents the ability of stress scintigraphy to simultaneously identify significant coronary lesions in all three major vessels in patients with triple-vessel disease. Another patient, illustrated in Figure 14-13, had an abnormally depressed resting baseline ECG S-T segment in the setting of atypical chest pain. The stress electrocardiogram showed significant S-T segment depression, but definite interpretation was made difficult due to the resting ECG abnormality. The stress scinti-

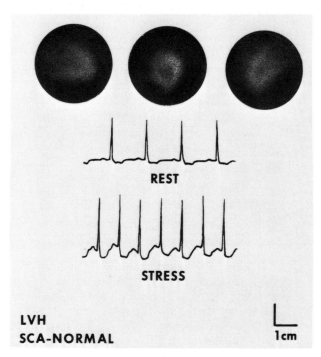

Fig. 14-11 Equivocal Stress ECG with normal scintigraphy. Shown are the rest (above) and stress (below) electrocardiograms and the stress scintigrams in the anterior (left), left anterior oblique (center) and left lateral (right) projections in a patient with troublesome chest pain and a history of hypertension. The full rest electrocardiogram revealed severe left ventricular hypertrophy (LVH). The monitored lead showed S-T segment depression which deepened with stress and was difficult to interpret in view of the resting depression. The perfusion image was normal, parallel to the coronary angiogram (SCA) and clarified the stress electrocardiogram. (From Botvinick, E. H. and coworkers: Thallium-201 myocardial perfusion scintigraphy for the clinical clarification of normal, abnormal and equivocal stress tests: Am. J. Cardiol., *41:*43, 1978.)

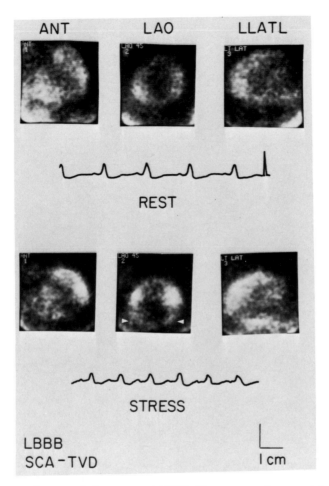

Fig. 14-12 Triple-vessel disease and LBBB. Shown are the rest (above) and stress (below) ECGs and scintigrams in the anterior (ANT), left anterior oblique (LAO) and left lateral (LLATL) projections in a patient with atypical chest pain. The rest ECG demonstrated left bundle branch block (LBBB) and could not be evaluated reliably for stress-induced ischemic changes. Nevertheless, the image reveals stress-induced perfusion abnormalities in the region of the interventricular septum, inferior and postero-lateral walls in the LAO projection (indicated by arrow). Selective coronary angiography (SCA) revealed triple-vessel disease (TVD).

gram clearly shows new perfusion abnormalities in the region of the left ventricular posterior lateral wall, septum and apex, indicating significant lesions in the left anterior descending, and left circumflex coronary arteries. The region supplied by the right coronary artery shows the best relative perfusion. Nevertheless, coronary arteriography again revealed severe triple-

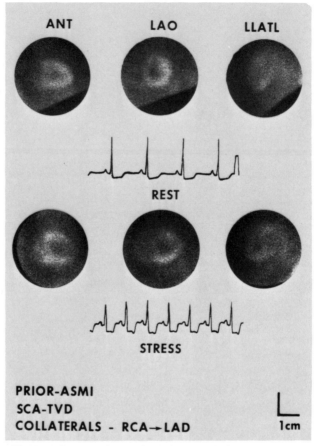

Fig. 14-13 Tl-201 scintigraphy and triple-vessel disease. Shown are the rest (above) and stress (below) ECGs and scintigrams in the anterior (ANT), left anterior oblique (LAO) and left lateral (LLATL) projections in a patient with atypical chest pain. The rest scintigram showed subtle diminution in relative septal activity, suggestive of a prior anteroseptal myocardial infarction (ASMI) in this region. Radionuclide distribution changed drastically with stress, exposing gross abnormalities of the left ventricular posterior lateral walls, septum and apex. The study is consistent with severe coronary disease and stress-induced malperfusion involving at least two vessels, the left anterior descending and the left circumflex coronary arteries. The region of right coronary perfusion appears "best" perfused. Since this is a relative study, it is not necessarily true that the region of "best" perfusion is the region of normal perfusion. Here, the right coronary artery has severe localized stenosis in the presence of severe triple-vessel disease (TVD). The frame from the patient's selective coronary angiogram is shown in Figure 14-14. The stress electrocardiogram in this case was difficult to interpret in the presence of resting S-T segment abnormalities in this patient taking digoxin. Abbreviations: see Figure 14-3. (From Botvinick, E. H. and coworkers: Thallium-201 myocardial perfusion scintigraphy for the clinical clarification of normal, abnormal and equivocal stress tests. Am. J. Cardiol., *41*:43, 1978.)

vessel disease. A frame from the patient's selective coronary arteriogram, shown in Figure 14-14, reveals evidence of significant right coronary disease. However, a prominent collateral circulation originated from the obstructed right coronary artery and supplied the region of perfusion of the obstructed left coronary artery. In this case, evidence that the right coronary artery was the source of collateral vasculature to other myocardial regions provides at least circumstantial evidence that the inferior left ventricular wall supplied by the patient's right coronary artery was indeed best, although not

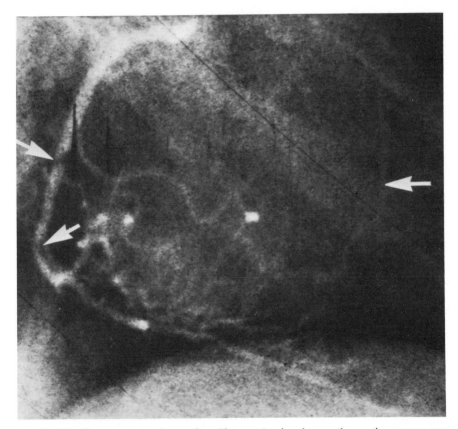

Fig. 14-14 Coronary angiography. Shown is the frame from the coronary angiogram performed after right coronary injection of the patient illustrated in Figure 14-13. The right coronary artery is well seen and clearly involved by at least two significant focal lesions (left arrows). However, this vessel gives rise to an extensive collateral circulation here shown filling the distal left anterior descending coronary artery (right arrow). Although diseased, from the circumstantial evidence presented by the collateral flow distribution, the right coronary artery appeared "best" perfused in this patient with triple-vessel disease.

normally, perfused. Such scintigraphic and anatomic correlations document the fact that in scintigrams with some evidence of malperfusion, those regions showing highest radioactivity may be best perfused but need not be normally perfused. Over-all, stress scintigraphy maintained its high sensitivity and specificity even in the face of resting baseline electrocardiographic abnormalities and equivocal stress electrocardiograms. Among the 16 patients with significant coronary lesions, 14 demonstrated stress-induced scintigraphic abnormalities, whereas only 9 showed evidence of further stress-induced S-T segment depression of an ischemic nature. However, among 6 patients with equivocal stress tests and normal coronary arteries, stress scintigrams were uniformly negative, whereas 5 of these 6 patients had impressive stress-induced S-T segment changes. Even applying S-T segment criteria to this group of patients with significant resting baseline electrocardiographic abnormalities, the scintigraphic accuracy of 89% was significantly better (p<0.05) than the 46% accuracy of the stress ECG in the presence of resting S-T segment depression.[32]

Stress Scintigraphy Following Bypass Graft Surgery

Another area of importance where the stress scintigram can be applied with great clinical utility is in the evaluation of the patient following coronary bypass graft surgery. Using potassium-43, Zaret and coworkers demonstrated that the method was of great potential value in the post-bypass setting.[40] We evaluated symptomatology, stress electrocardiography and Tl-201 stress scintigraphy in 24 patients following coronary bypass graft surgery. Symptomatic, electrocardiographic and scintigraphic findings were compared to those of coronary arteriography where significant post-operative lesions were represented by significant stenosis in the graft, distal vessel or an ungrafted native vessel. Post-operative chest pain lacked sensitivity (62%) and was totally non-specific (22%) for the identification of graft or native vessel coronary lesions. Stress electrocardiography was similarly insensitive (55%), but moderately specific (84%). Tl-201 scintigraphy was most sensitive (73%) and was 100% specific for coronary lesions. The scintigram was significantly more specific than the presence of post-operative pain and gave excellent localizing information, adding accuracy to the results of stress testing. The over-all accuracy of stress scintigraphy for the diagnosis of persistent coronary lesions following bypass graft surgery was 85%, similar to that found in the evaluation of native vasculature.[36] Although the relief of chest pain has been shown to correlate with graft patency following bypass graft surgery, additional factors, including the placebo effect of surgery, peri-operative infarction and possibly surgical denervation complicate the interpretation of symptomatic relief. Stress scintigraphy should provide an important objective parameter for evaluating and monitoring the results of such surgery. Figure 14-15 shows the scinti-

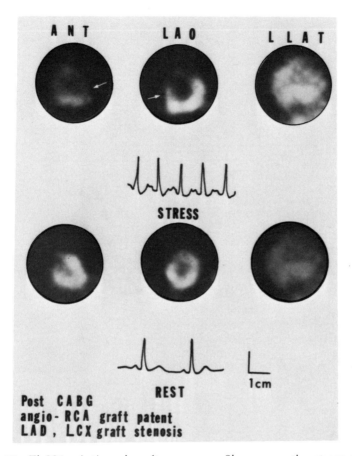

Fig. 14-15 TI-201 scintigraphy after surgery. Shown are the stress (above) and rest (below) ECGs and TI-201 scintigrams in the anterior (ANT), left anterior oblique (LAO), and left lateral (LLATL) projections of a patient with documented stenosis of coronary bypass grafts to the left anterior descending (LAD) and left circumflex (LCX) coronary arteries. Stress-induced image abnormalities are clearly seen in the anterior, apical and septal walls (arrows) paralleling the anatomic findings of graft stenosis. This stress ECG was negative for ischemia.

graphic evidence of poor perfusion in a patient with double graft stenosis following surgery. Figure 14-16 demonstrates scintigraphic evidence of reperfusion in a patient with an excellent clinical result.

Other Implications

In all of the studies referred to above, the standard for disease diagnosis was the anatomic assessment of coronary angiography. Whereas scinti-

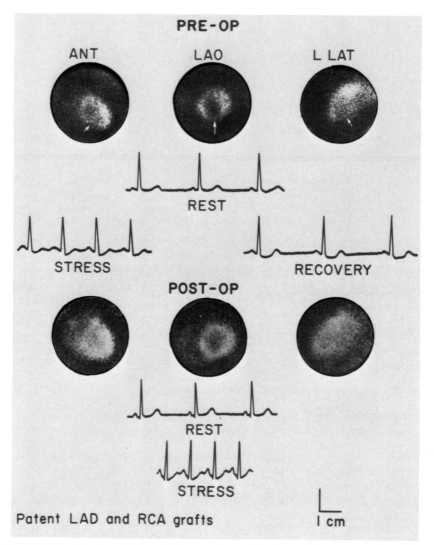

Fig. 14-16 Scintigraphic evidence of reperfusion. Shown are the Tl-201 stress scintigrams performed before (above) and after (below) coronary bypass graft surgery. In the preoperative study, the patient developed an inferior wall perfusion abnormality seen best in the left anterior oblique (LAO) projection (arrow) and ischemic electrocardiographic response at a low level of exercise stress. After surgery and the placement of a right coronary artery (RCA) graft, the patient became symptom-free and demonstrated normal scintigraphic and electrocardiographic findings at much increased exercise stress. Scintigraphy documents reperfusion in this patient. Abbreviations: ANT—anterior projections; LAD—left anterior descending coronary artery; LLATL—left lateral projection.

graphic correlations with angiography were excellent, the true index of significant coronary disease remains unclear. Cases of false positive or false negative scintigrams may in part only reflect our difficulty in assessing the anatomic degree and significance of coronary stenosis. In this respect, scintigraphy may be found helpful in evaluating questionable angiographic findings. Scintigraphic abnormalities have been well correlated with significant coronary lesions measured quantitatively from arteriography.[41]

In several studies, abnormal stress scintigrams supplemented electrocardiographic findings, adding to the over-all sensitivity of stress testing.[14,31] However, both electrocardiographic and scintigraphic methods may be insensitive to subtle ischemic changes and may both appear negative in occasional cases with evident angiographic abnormalities. On the other hand, the exact meaning of the abnormal stress electrocardiogram in the absence of significant coronary lesions remains unclear. It is likely that scintigraphic and electrocardiographic indicators of myocardial ischemia measure different parameters. The stress-induced scintigraphic abnormalities largely reflect segmental perfusion changes, whereas stress-induced electrocardiographic changes most likely reflect hypoxic, metabolic and electrophysiologic alterations, resulting from changes in perfusion. Causes of myocardial ischemia other than coronary disease do not carry the dire prognosis of significant coronary disease and scintigraphy appears more accurate for the diagnosis of large vessel coronary disease than does the stress electrocardiogram.

Technical Considerations

The majority of the studies noted above evaluated the relative sensitivity and specificity of scintigraphy in relation to that of stress electrocardiography for coronary diagnosis using a multiple lead monitoring system. Some studies employed only a single anterior electrocardiographic monitor lead. Although it has been shown that multiple monitor lead systems are advantageous and that the sensitivity of electrocardiographic stress testing may be significantly increased by monitoring inferior as well as anterior leads, this multiple lead system would very likely also decrease the specificity of stress electrocardiography and would probably not help to resolve the equivocal test. Another issue undergoing development is the application of computer techniques to the enhancement of Tl-201 perfusion scintigrams. As yet, there is no totally objective, widely accepted method of such image enhancement. The development of such methods presents significant problems, but promises improved sensitivity, specificity, objectivity and simplicity in image interpretation. However, in spite of the unavailability of such enhancement techniques, results have been impressive and studies to date have revealed a low inter- and intra-observer variability.[32,42]

Summary

The standard for diagnosis of significant coronary narrowing remains the indirect anatomic evidence of selective coronary arteriography. In a rough, imprecise manner, the degree of coronary stenosis is assessed and assumptions are made concerning its effect on myocardial blood supply and its pathologic significance. No effort is made to objectively evaluate myocardial oxygen demands in relation to blood supply.

The stress ECG attempts to assess, in a non-invasive manner, both components of the oxygen supply/demand ratio. Presumably, this test is abnormal when a decrease in this ratio reaches pathologic significance regardless of the observed coronary anatomy. Potentially, this eliminates our need to visually quantitate the coronary lesion involved. However, stress electrocardiography has been shown to be fraught with problems of insensitivity and non-specificity.

Relative myocardial perfusion scintigraphy, using T1-201, is a graphic non-invasive method to diagnose pathologically significant coronary lesions without direct anatomic assessment. As an indicator of relative perfusion, scintigraphy evaluates coronary supply and identifies the heterogeneity of myocardial blood flow evoked by increasing coronary flow demands in vessels with varied and limited abilities to accommodate this demand. Whereas flow through stenotic vessels may be normal at rest, exercise stimulates a less than normal increment in flow through vessels with significant coronary lesions and a diminished flow reserve. The results of such altered reserve among normal, partially stenotic and occluded vessels is stress-induced heterogeneity of coronary flow, appreciated in the scintigram as "hot and cold" regions.

Stress scintigraphy appears to be more sensitive and more specific for coronary diagnosis than stress electrocardiography. The scintigram is of extreme value in assessing the nature of atypical pain and appears to differentiate ischemic syndromes which are related to coronary disease from those related to a non-coronary etiology. Stress scintigraphy maintains its accuracy in the setting of resting baseline electrocardiographic abnormalities in a variety of conditions where interpretation of the stress tracing is hazardous and the results are at best equivocal. The anatomic correlation between T1-201 scintigraphic defects and lesions on angiography is excellent and assumes increased importance in the evaluation of the patient following coronary bypass graft surgery. Although sensitive to coronary diagnosis, scintigraphy is a relative technique and does not always identify all abnormal regions and involved vessels. In cases of multivessel disease, regions of normal flow could not be differentiated from regions of absolutely reduced, yet "best" flow. Nevertheless, scintigraphy may be extremely valuable for the identification of a subgroup of patients with extremely high risk coronary lesions. In association with rest perfusion scintigraphy, stress scintigrams can differentiate reversible ischemia from irreversible infarction.

The clinical evaluation of stress scintigraphy has only just begun. The future of this non-invasive method promises more physiologic and more accurate estimation of coronary stenosis than any method presently available. The technique will very likely aid in the differentiation of ischemia from coronary and non-coronary causes, and will provide a useful objective parameter by which to evaluate therapeutic interventions. In association with rest scintigraphy and other clinical methods, stress scintigraphy promises to provide full appreciation of the extent and distribution of reversibly ischemic and infarcted myocardium. Such evaluation will contribute to improved identification of patients at increased risk, and the more profitable direction of therapy to the maximal preservation and salvation of ischemic myocardium.

REFERENCES

1. Love, W. D., Romney, R. B. and Burch, G. E.: A comparison of the distribution of potassium and exchangeable rubidium in the organs of dogs, using rubidium-86. Circ. Res. 2:112, 1957.
2. Carr, E. E., Jr., Beierwaltes, W. H., Patno, M. E., Bartlett, J. D., Jr. and Wegst, A. V.: The detection of experimental myocardial infarction by photoscanning. Am. Heart J., 64:650, 1962.
3. Carr, E. A., Jr. Gleason, F., Shaw, J. and Krantz, B: The direct diagnosis of myocardial infarction by photoscanning after administration of cesium-131. Am. Heart J., 68:627, 1964.
4. Smith, R. O., Bennett, K. R., Lehan, P. H. and Hellems, H. K.: Myocardial ^{42}K scanning compared with coronary arteriography. J. Nucl. Med. 11:642, 1970.
5. Botti, R. E., MacIntyre, W. J. and Pritchard, W. H.: Identification of ischemic area of left ventricle in visualization of ^{43}K myocardial deposition. Circulation, 47:486, 1973.
6. Yano, Y., Van Dyke, D., Budinger, T. F., Anger, H. O. and Chu, P.: Myocardial uptake studies with ^{129}Cs and the scintillation camera. J. Nucl. Med., 11:663, 1970.
7. Chandra, R., Braunstein, P., Streuli, F. and Hirsch, J.: ^{134}Cs: a new myocardial imaging agent. J. Nucl. Med., 14:243, 1973.
8. Peo, N.: Comparative myocardial uptake and clearance characteristics of potassium and cesium. J. Nucl. Med., 13:557, 1972.
9. Prokop, E. K., Strauss, H. W., Natarajan, J. K., Pitt, B. and Wagner, H. N., Jr.: Comparison of ^{43}K and microsphere methods for detecting myocardial ischemia and infarction. J. Nucl. Med., 14:443, 1973.
10. Botvinick, E. H., Shames, D. M., Gershengorn, K. M., Carlsson, E., Ratshin, R. N. and Parmley, W. W.: Myocardial stress perfusion scintigraphy with rubidium-81 versus stress electrocardiography. Am. J. Cardiol., 39:364, 1977.
11. Harper, P. V., Lathrop, K. A., Frizek, H., Lembares, L., Stark, V. and Hoffer, P. B.: Clinical feasibility of myocardial imaging with ^{13}NH$_3$. J. Nucl. Med., 13:278, 1972.
12. Hoop, B., Jr., Smith, T. W., Burnham, C. A., Correll, J. E., Brownell, G. L. and Sanders, C. A.: Myocardial imaging with ^{13}NH$_4$$^+$ and a multicrystal position camera. J. Nucl. Med. 14:181, 1973.
13. Weich, H. F., Strauss, H. W. and Pitt, B.: Myocardial extraction fraction of thallium-201 (abstr.). Circulation, 53 & 54 (Suppl II):II, 1976.
14. Bailey, I. K., Griffith, L.S.C., Rouleau, J., Strauss, W. and Pitt, B.: Thallium-201 myocardial perfusion imaging at rest and during exercise. Circulation, 55:79, 1977.

15. Zir, L. M., Miller, S. W. and Dinsmore, R. E.: Interobserver variability in coronary angiography. Circulation, *53:*627, 1976.
16. Borer, J. S., Brensiki, J. F. and Redwood, D. R.: Limitations of the electrocardiographic responses to exercise in predicting coronary artery disease. N. Engl. J. Med., *293:*367, 1975.
17. Goldschlager, N., Selzer, A. and Cohn, K.: Treadmill stress tests as indicators of presence and severity of coronary artery disease. Ann. Intern. Med., *85:*277, 1976.
18. Holmgren, A., Johnsson, B. and Lavender, M.: ECG changes in vasoregulatory asthenia and the effects of physical training. Acta Med. Scand. *165:*259, 1959.
19. Harris, C. N., Aronow, W. S. and Parker, D. P.: Treadmill stress test in left ventricular hypertrophy. Chest, *63:*353, 1973.
20. Kawai, C. and Hultgren, H. N.: The effect of digitalis upon the exercise electrocardiogram. Am. Heart J., *68:*409, 1964.
21. Jacobs, W. F., Battle, W. E. and Rowan, J. A.: False-positive ST-T changes secondary to hyperventilation and exercise. Ann. Intern. Med., *81:*479, 1974.
22. Sketch, M. H., Mohiddin, S. M. and Lunch, J. D.: Significance of sex differences in the correlation of electrocardiographic exercise testing and coronary angiograms. Am. J. Cardiol., *36:*169, 1975.
23. Levinson, W. I., Adolph, R. J. and Romhilt, D. W.: Effects of myocardial hypoxia and ischemia on myocardial scintigraphy. Am. J. Cardiol., *35:*251, 1975.
24. Gould, K. L., Lipscomb, K. and Hamilton, G. W.: Physiologic basis for assessing critical coronary stenosis. Am. J. Cardiol., *33:*87, 1974.
25. Roitman, D., Jones, W. B. and Sheffield, L. T.: Comparison of submaximal exercise ECG test with coronary cineangiocardiogram. Ann. Intern. Med., *72:*641, 1970.
26. Pohost, G. M., Zir, L. M., Moore, R. H., McKusick, K. A., Guney, T. E. and Beller, G.: Differentiation of transiently ischemic from infarcted myocardium by serial imaging after a single dose of Thalium-201. Circulation, *55:*294, 1977.
27. Zaret, B. L., Strauss, H. W. and Martin, N. D.: Noninvasive regional myocardial perfusion with radioactive potassium. N. Engl. J. Med., *288:*809, 1973.
28. Zaret, B. L., Stenson, R. E. and Martin, N. D.: Potassium-43 myocardial perfusion scanning for the noninvasive evaluation of patients with false-positive exercise tests. Circulation, *48:*1234, 1973.
29. Berman, D. S., Salel, A. F. and DeNardo, G. L.: Noninvasive detection of regional myocardial ischemia using Rb-81 and the scintillation camera: comparison with stress electrocardiography in patients with arteriographically documented coronary stenosis. Circulation, *52:*619, 1975.
30. McGowan, R. L., Martin, N. D., Zaret, B. L., Hall, R. R., Bryson, A. L., Strauss, H. W. and Flamm, M. D.: Diagnostic accuracy of noninvasive myocardial imaging for coronary artery disease: an electrocardiographic and angiographic correlation. Am. J. Cardiol., *40:*6, 1977.
31. Ritchie, J. L., Zaret, B. L., Strauss, H. W., Pitt, B., Berman, D. S., Schelbert, H. R., Ashburn, W. L. and Hamilton, G. W.: Myocardial imaging with thallium-201 at rest and with exercise—a multicenter study (Abstr.). Am. J. Cardiol., *39:*321, 1977.
32. Botvinick, E. H., Taradash, M. R., Shames, D. M. and Parmley, W. W.: Thallium-210 myocardial perfusion scintigraphy for the clinical clarification of normal, abnormal and equivocal stress tests. Am. J. Cardiol., *41:*43, 1978.
33. Ross, R. S. and Friesinger, G. C.: Coronary arteriography. Am. Heart J., *72:*437, 1966.
34. Weaver, W. D., Lorch, G. S., Alvarez, H. A. and Cobb, L. A.: Angiographic findings and prognostic indications in patients resuscitated from sudden cardiac death. Circulation, *54:*895, 1976.
35. Martin, C. M. and McConahay, D. R.: Maximal treadmill exercise electrocardiography—correlations with coronary arteriography and cardiac hemodynamics. Circulation, *46:*956, 1972.
36. Greenberg, B., Hart, R., Werner, J., Brundage, B., Botvinick, E., Chatterjee, K. and Parmley, W.: Thallium-201 stress imaging in the followup evaluation of coronary bypass patients (Abstr.). Circulation, October, 1977, in press.
37. Dwyer, E. M., Wiener, L. and Cox, J. W.: Angina pectoris in patients with normal and

abnormal coronary arteriograms: hemodynamic and clinical aspects. Am. J. Cardiol., *23*:638, 1969.

38. Massie, B., Botvinick, E., Shames, D., Taradash, M., Werner, J. and Schiller, N.: Myocardial perfusion scintigraphy in patients with mitral valve prolapse: its advantage over stress electrocardiography in diagnosing associated coronary artery disease and its implications for the etiology of chest pain. Circulation, 1978, in press.

39. Botvinick, E. H., Shames, D. M., Ratshin, R. A., Chatterjee, K. and Parmley, W. W.: The physiologic assessment of critical coronary stenosis by relative myocardial perfusion imaging with atrial pacing. Am. J. Cardiol., *37*:122, 1976.

40. Zaret, B. L., Martin, N. D., McGowan, R. L., Strauss, H. W., Wells, N. P., Jr. and Flamm, M. D.: Rest and exercise potassium 43 myocardial perfusion imaging for the noninvasive evaluation of aortocoronary bypass surgery. Circulation, *49*:688, 1974.

41. Massie, B., Morady, E., Botvinick, E., Ratshin, R., Tyberg, J. and Parmley, W.: Quantitative assessment of coronary artery stenosis: Correlation with coronary flow (Abstr.). Circulation, *26* (Suppl. II), 1975.

42. McLaughlin, P. R., Martin, R. P., Doherty, P., Daspit, S., Goris, M., Haskell, W., Lewis, S., Kriss, J. P. and Harrison, D. C.: Reproducibility of thallium-201 myocardial imaging. Circulation, *55*:497, 1977.

15

Value of the Exercise ECG Test for Screening Asymptomatic Subjects for Latent Coronary Artery Disease

James Conklin, M.D. and
V. F. Froelicher, M.D., F.A.C.C.

General Considerations

The most common serious diseases in industrialized countries are the cardiovascular diseases. In the Framingham study, the probability of developing cardiovascular disease by age 65 was 37% for a man and 18% for a woman.[1] One of the greatest scientific accomplishments of the past two decades has been the identification of the risk factors related to the current epidemic of cardiovascular disease. Persons at high risk for cardiovascular disease can be identified from a measurement of their serum cholesterol and blood pressure, a smoking history, an electrocardiogram and a determination of glucose intolerance.[2] The 10% of persons identified at highest risk, using a mathematical equation derived from the Framingham study, account for about one-fifth of the 8 year incidence of coronary atherosclerotic heart disease (CAD) and one-third of the 8 year incidence of stroke, hypertensive heart disease and intermittent claudication. This equation provides a method of identifying persons at high cardiovascular risk who need preventive treatment and those at low risk who need not be alarmed about one elevated risk factor or marker. Blackburn has presented a concise and practical approach to the evaluation and management of cardiovascular risk factors.[3]

In spite of the already declining cardiovascular disease death rate,[4] it will be some time before the primary prevention of these diseases is a reality. Therefore, it is advisable to evaluate screening methods for detecting latent CAD. The relative value of techniques for identifying individuals who have asymptomatic CAD should be assessed in order to optimally and cost-effectively direct preventive efforts to them. Risk factor screening has a limited sensitivity and so other techniques, particularly exercise testing, deserve consideration.

The applications for screening asymptomatic individuals with exercise testing are listed in Table 15-1. An abnormal electrocardiographic response to exercise testing is a demonstrated risk marker for CAD.[5,6] Therefore, one of the established applications of screening asymptomatic men with exercise testing is to identify those at high risk. The exercise test has also been used as an end point for CAD similar to angina, acute myocardial infarction and sudden death in epidemiological studies. Unfortunately, the predictive value of S-T segment depression for CAD is relatively low and it is not as good an end point as these clinical end points.

The exercise test can be used to screen asymptomatic individuals who are detected by other methods to be at high risk for CAD. Those with lipid abnormalities, with hypertension, or with a strong family history of coronary disease can be screened with exercise testing. Asymptomatic individuals in whom sudden incapacitation could compromise public safety have been evaluated with exercise testing. Such individuals include pilots,[7] firemen[8] and policemen.[9] Others who possibly should be screened in this manner include railroad engineers, air traffic controllers and drivers of large commercial vehicles. Because an exercise program does present a risk to sedentary coronary prone middle-aged men,[10, 11] it may be advisable to evaluate such individuals with exercise testing prior to prescribing an exercise program. This is not always practical and if they are properly counseled in a graduated exercise program, an exercise test is not always necessary. There are many research applications for exercise testing asymptomatic individuals. These include establishing normal values for the electrocardiographic response to exercise[12, 13] as well as for physiologic responses.[14] Such values help to determine limits separating categories of patients and to separate healthy individuals from those with specific disease processes. Also, it is important to evaluate the response of women compared to men because the test seems to be less specific in women.[15] Screening asymptomatic individuals also identifies a group of false positives in whom additional techniques such as radionuclides can be assessed for their discriminating power.

In order to evaluate the value of any screening test, sensitivity, specificity, predictive value and relative risk must be calculated.[16] Sensitivity is the

Table 15-1. Applications of Screening Asymptomatic Individuals with Exercise Testing

1. Epidemiological
2. To further screen individuals at high risk for coronary heart disease due to other risk factors or risk markers
3. For public safety reasons
4. To evaluate an individual for an exercise program
5. Research

percentage of times a test gives an abnormal response when those with disease are tested. Specificity is the percentage of times a test gives a normal response when those without disease are tested—a definition quite different from the conventional use of the word "specific". The predictive value of an abnormal test is the percentage of individuals with an abnormal test who have disease. The relative risk of an abnormal test response is the relative chance of having disease if the test is abnormal compared to having disease if the test is normal. As will be demonstrated, the values for these last two terms are dependent upon the prevalence of disease in the population being tested.

Submaximal Exercise Testing with Follow-up

Mattingly[17] and Parmley[18] reported their findings in 300 asymptomatic army officers who were screened with the double Master's test. There were 100 men in each age group of 25–34, 35–44 and 45–60. An abnormal response was considered to be 0.05 mv. or more of horizontal or downward sloping S-T segment depression. There was one abnormal response in the youngest age group, and three in each of the older age groups. After an average follow-up of 15 years, all of the men were re-evaluated. Of the 7 with an abnormal response, 1 had died suddenly and 2 had non-fatal myocardial infarctions. Of the 293 men with normal responses, 5 had died secondary to coronary heart disease, 12 had myocardial infarctions, and 8 had developed angina. Their findings are summarized in Table 15-2. From his extensive experience with the double Master's test, including autopsy results and follow-up of a large asymptomatic group, Mattingly concluded that an abnormal double Master's test did not assure a grave prognosis, nor was it sensitive enough to use as a screening test for early coronary artery disease.

Brody reported his results with the routine clinic use of the double Master's test for evaluating asymptomatic middle-aged businessmen.[19] An abnormal response was considered to be 0.05 mv. or more of horizontal or downward sloping S-T depression. Twenty-three (3%) had an abnormal response. Over the 4 years of follow-up, 6 of these men had myocardial infarctions and 10 developed angina. In a group of 733 with a normal response, 6 developed overt coronary heart disease. Subtle processes working in those being seen in a clinic probably selected a group with a higher prevalence of disease than found in the general population. Such a selection process could explain the relatively high predictive value of the test found by Brody.

Bellet and colleagues studied 795 asymptomatic male Bell Telephone Company employees with the double Master's test.[20] The mean age of this group of men was 51 years. An abnormal response was considered to be 0.1 mv. or more of S-T segment depression or frequent premature ventricular contractions. After 3 years of follow-up, 23 coronary artery disease events

Table 15-2. Studies Reported Screening Asymptomatic Men with Submaximal Exercise Tests and Following Them for End Points of Coronary Artery Disease

Principal Investigator	Number	Years Follow-up	Incidence CAD	Age at Entry	% With Abnormal Test	Sensitivity	Specificity	Predictive Value	Risk Ratio
Mattingly (17)	300	15	9%	25–60	2.3%	10%	99%	43%	5
Brody (19)	756	4	7%	23–74 (Mean 53 yrs.)	3%	34%	99%	70%	14
Bellet (20)	795	3	3%	25–65 (Mean 51 yrs.)	12%	44%	89%	14%	10
Doyle (21)	2003	5	9%	39–54	4%	35%	99%	85%	13
Rumball (22)	660	6	4%	19–54 (Mean 37 yrs.)	10%	62%	92%	23%	15

occurred, including 16 myocardial infarctions, two sudden deaths and the development of angina in 5 men.

A study of asymptomatic men by Doyle and Kinch with follow-up, utilized a submaximal treadmill test comparable in workload to the double Master's test.[21] They used a treadmill walk of 10 minutes at 3 miles/hour with a 5% grade. This was part of a prospective study of New York State employees which began in 1952. The age range of the men was 39–54 years at the study's onset. Flattening or downward sloping of the S-T segment of 0.1 second was considered to be an abnormal response. Of 2,003 men who were tested at least twice over 13 years, 263 men developed angina, a myocardial infarction, or died suddenly. Seventy-five or 30% of the men who developed these coronary artery disease end points had an abnormal exercise test as the first sign of their disease. This study involved multiple examinations, and it is difficult to compare its results to the other studies. Doyle concluded that the submaximal treadmill test used was relatively insensitive but specific for identifying men with clinically silent but far advanced coronary artery disease. The repetition of the tests during the follow-up period probably accounts for the relatively high predictive value reported.

Rumball and Acheson used another type of submaximal step test in evaluating 668 asymptomatic members of the Royal Air Force.[22] Their ages ranged from 19–54 with a mean of 37 years. An S-T segment depression of 0.05 mv. or more was considered an abnormal response. There were no deaths due to coronary artery disease over the 6 years of follow-up and the end point was the clinical finding of "ischemic pain". Only sample groups of those originally studied were re-evaluated. The inadequate sampling and the less definitive end point used could explain the surprisingly high sensitivity of 62% reported in this study.

Maximal or Near Maximal Testing Without Follow-up

An obvious shortcoming of submaximal testing is its low sensitivity. Other shortcomings, specifically of a step test like the double Master's test, are that it cannot be used to evaluate functional capacity and that the ECG is not monitored during exercise. There is a physiologic fallacy in adjusting the number of steps as determined by Master according to body weight. Rowell and colleagues showed that the oxygen consumption per kilogram is much greater for light individuals than heavier individuals when the number of steps performed is in accord with the Master's step tables.[23] The workload can be near maximal for light persons whereas it is minimal for heavy subjects. A danger of the Master's test is that it is usually performed only with the electrocardiogram monitored in the post-exercise period. We have seen a patient who fibrillated during a double Master's test and there is at least one case reported in the literature.[24]

The advantages of a progressive, continuous exercise test with electrocardiographic and blood pressure monitoring during the test have been discussed elsewhere.[25] Numerous studies have been reported screening asymptomatic individuals with such a test without subsequent follow-up data. Only such studies that have evaluated the findings listed in Table 15-3 will be reviewed in this section.

Kattus and colleagues studied 1,013 male volunteers from the Association of Life Insurance Underwriters of Los Angeles County, using a near maximal treadmill test. The subjects ranged in age from 23–82 years with an average of 49 years.[26] A CX5 bipolar lead was monitored. Elevated serum cholesterol, a past history of cardiac symptoms, and an abnormal resting ECG showed a high correlation with an abnormal exercise ECG response. Table 15-4 shows the percentage of abnormal responders per age decade. This study demonstrated that the percentage of abnormal responders is directly related to age. Thirteen of the abnormal responders participated in a supervised physical training program and 4 had a normal response after training.[27] Among those abnormal responders who did not train, 2 had reversion of the abnormal response to normal.

Lester and colleagues compared a submaximal heart rate targeted exercise test and a maximal exercise test.[28] The Bruce treadmill protocol was used for both the maximal and submaximal test: 113 male volunteers ranging in age from 40–75 performed both tests. A CC5 bipolar lead was used, but in the post-exercise period, routine ECG leads were also observed and the subjects were supine rather than sitting. These techniques should have optimized the sensitivity of the tests. The prevalence of abnormal responses to the submaximal exercise test was less than 1% whereas it was 4.5% for the maximal test. Cumming has also evaluated the yield of abnormal exercise-induced S-T segment depression in relation to the exercise intensity in an asymptomatic population.[29] He found that if exercise had been performed to a target heart rate of 85% of expected maximal heart rate, half of the abnormal responses he demonstrated would have been missed. These two studies favor the use of an exercise test to the point of voluntary fatigue if the greatest sensitivity is desired.

Table 15-3. Findings of Near Maximal or Maximal Exercise Test Studies in Asymptomatic Individuals (Without a Follow-up) To Be Reviewed

1. The direct relationship of the prevalence of abnormal S-T segment depression to age
2. Higher prevalence of abnormal responses using maximal testing compared to near maximal exercise testing
3. Higher prevalence of abnormal S-T segment depression in age matched apparently healthy women compared to similar men
4. Relationship of abnormal exercise-induced S-T segment depression to the standard risk factors

Table 15-4. Analysis of the Relationship of the Abnormal Response Rate to Age in an Asymptomatic Male Population Using a Near Maximal Treadmill Test[26]

Age	Number	Number and (%) with Exercise-Induced S-T Segment Depression
23–39	36	0 (0%)
40–49	141	8 (5.7%)
50–59	91	10 (11%)
60–69	39	10 (26%)
70–79	6	2 (33.3%)
Total:	313	30 (9.6%)

Olsson and colleagues reported their results using an exercise test to near maximal heart rate in a hyperlipidemic population.[30] The frequency of abnormal S-T segment depression increased with age, was higher in females than males, and was greater in all types of hyperlipidemia. Invariably, age was the best predictor of S-T segment depression. The lipoprotein fraction giving the highest correlation coefficient was low density lipoprotein cholesterol in both sexes. Allen and colleagues correlated the prevalence of abnormal maximal treadmill tests with coronary risk factors in 1,077 asymptomatic adults.[31] Ten and a half percent of the population had an abnormal exercise test. An abnormal test correlated with male sex, increasing age, a serum cholesterol greater than 200 mg.%, hypertriglyceridemia, cigarette smoking, but not with hypertension, obesity or hyperglycemia.

The four studies listed in Table 15-5 have screened asymptomatic women with exercise testing.[32-35] From these studies it is apparent that even when age-matched, women have 2–3 times the prevalence of abnormal responses as men. This is in spite of their well established lower prevalence of coronary artery disease. The high false positive rate is probably due to the low prevalence of disease in women and also to a lower specificity of the exercise test in them.[15]

Maximal or Near Maximal Testing with Follow-up

Table 15-6 summarizes four follow-up studies that utilized maximal or near maximal exercise testing to screen asymptomatic men for latent CAD.[36-39] The populations in these studies were tested, and followed for end points of CAD, including angina, acute myocardial infarction and sudden death. Angiographic findings were not used as end points in these studies.

Bruce and colleagues studied 221 men in Seattle.[36] A CB$_5$ bipolar lead was used and 0.1 mv. or more of S-T segment depression was the criterion for an abnormal response. The patients were monitored in the sitting

Table 15-5. Results of Four Studies Screening Asymptomatic Women for Latent CAD with Exercise Testing

Investigator	Number	Mean Age	% with Abnormal Exercise Test
Lepeskin (34)	143	41	24%
Astrand (35)	117	50	35%
Profant (32)	144	45	33%
Cumming (33)	357	44	26%

position post-exercise. Ten percent of them had abnormal S-T segment responses to the symptom limited maximal treadmill test. They were followed for 5 years. The relative risk of developing coronary heart disease over the follow-up period was 13.6 times greater for those who had an abnormal S-T segment response to treadmill testing than for those who had a normal response. The probability of developing coronary artery disease with an abnormal treadmill test (the predictive value of an abnormal response) was 13.6%. That is, 13.6% of those who had an abnormal response developed CAD. The sensitivity was 60%; i.e., of those who developed CAD over the follow-up period, 60% had an abnormal treadmill test when they entered the study.

Aronow and colleagues tested 100 men in Los Angeles and followed them for 5 years.[37] A V_5 lead was used and 0.1 mv. or more of S-T segment depression was the criterion for an abnormal response. The patients were monitored in the supine position post-exercise. Thirteen percent of them had an abnormal S-T segment response to near maximal treadmill testing. The risk ratio for an abnormal response was 13.6, the predictive value was 46% and the sensitivity was 67%.

Cumming and colleagues reported their 3 year follow-up of 510 asymptomatic men of whom 12% had an abnormal response to a bicycle exercise test.[38] Maximal or near maximal effort was performed and a CM_5 lead was monitored. The criterion for an abnormal response was 0.2 mv. or more of S-T segment depression and the patients were monitored in the supine position post-exercise. The risk ratio for an abnormal response was 10, the predictive value was 25%, and the sensitivity of the test was 58%.

At the United States School of Aerospace Medicine, maximal treadmill testing has been routinely performed in a consistent fashion on all asymptomatic consultation subjects since 1965. All electrocardiographic records, including the entire exercise test, were microfilmed on 16mm rolls. Selected for testing were 1,390 asymptomatic men who were evaluated from 1965–1968 and who did not have any of the known causes for false positive

Table 15-6. Results of Exercise Testing in Four Prospective Studies Screening Asymptomatic Men for Latent Coronary Artery Disease

Principal Investigator	No.	Incidence CAD	Years Follow-up	% With Abnormal Exercise Test	Sensitivity	Specificity	Predictive Value	Relative Risk
Bruce (36)	221	2.3%	5	11.3%	60%	91%	13.6%	13.6x
Aronow (37)	100	9%	5	16%	67%	92%	46%	13.6x
Cumming (38)	510	4.7%	3	12.8%	58%	90%	25%	10x
Froelicher (39)	1390	3.3%	6.3	10%	61%	92%	20%	14.3x
Average		—	—	12.5%	62%	91%	26%	13x

treadmill tests.[39] They were located after a mean follow-up of 6.3 years. Their exercise tests were re-read; the amount, time occurrence and location of S-T segment depression was carefully coded. Ten percent of these men had abnormal treadmill tests. A CC_5 lead was mainly used but additional leads were obtained in the supine position post-exercise. The criterion for an abnormal response was 0.1 mv. or more horizontal or downsloping S-T segment depression. The risk ratio for an abnormal response was 14.3, the predictive value of an abnormal test was 20%, and the sensitivity of the test was 61%. The results of this study are in remarkable agreement with the other three studies, and the risk ratios obtained with maximal or near maximal exercise testing are relatively high compared to those of other screening techniques.

Some obvious limitations of using maximal or near maximal exercise testing to screen asymptomatic men for latent CAD should be considered. The sensitivity of exercise testing ranged from 58–67%. Only 58–67% of those who developed end points for coronary artery disease had an abnormal response when they were tested. Doyle[21] and Bruce[40] have shown that the sensitivity of exercise testing in a population can be increased if the population is tested serially. Some of those who are going to develop coronary disease will change from normal to an abnormal response when re-tested later. But there are documented cases of individuals with normal maximal treadmill tests and severe coronary artery disease,[41-43] and the exact predictive value of a change from a normal to an abnormal response has not been determined.[44] Another limitation was the predictive value which is the percent of individuals with an abnormal test who will develop coronary disease. It ranged from 13.6–46% with an average of 26% of the abnormal responders developing coronary disease over the follow-up period. Thus, over half of the abnormal responders were "false positives". The possibility exists that some of these individuals have coronary disease that has yet to manifest itself, but angiographic studies have supported this high false positive rate when using the exercise test in asymptomatic populations.

Maximal or Near Maximal Testing with Coronary Angiography

The results of cardiac catheterization have supported the low predictive value found in the follow-up studies. One hundred eleven asymptomatic, apparently healthy men who were found only to have an abnormal treadmill test had coronary angiography performed.[45] Only 30.6% of them had at least one lesion equal to or greater than 50% in a major coronary artery. Thus, the predictive value of an abnormal treadmill test, using coronary angiography as an end point, was 30.6%. Barnard and colleagues have used near maximal treadmill testing to screen randomly selected Los Angeles firefighters.[46] Ten percent showed an abnormal exercise-induced ECG response despite low risk factors for coronary artery disease. Six men with an abnormal exercise test elected to undergo cardiac catheterization.[47] One had severe three-vessel disease and another had a 50% obstruction of the left circumflex coronary artery. The other 4 men had normal coronaries. Borer and colleagues reported their angiographic findings in 11 asymptomatic individuals with hyperlipidemia and an abnormal exercise test.[48] Only 37% of these individuals were found to have angiographic coronary artery disease. Erikssen and colleagues reported their angiographic findings in 105 apparently healthy males aged 40–59 with one or more of the following criteria: 1) a questionnaire for angina pectoris positive on interview; 2) typical angina during a near maximal bicycle test; and 3) a positive exercise ECG during and/or post-exercise.[49] These criteria were combined in their population making it difficult to evaluate the predictive value of any criterion individually. However, it appears that the predictive value ranged from 55–78%. In this selected population, they found an exercise test to have a sensitivity of 84% if a slowly ascending S-T segment pattern was included. The relatively high predictive value in this study might be due to the age of their population. The other angiographic studies dealt with younger individuals.

Biostatistical Considerations

Table 15-7 illustrates how a test with a sensitivity of 70% and a specificity of 90% performs in a population with a 1% prevalence of disease. As previously demonstrated, these values approximate the sensitivity and specificity of maximal or near maximal exercise testing. Since 1% of the 10,000 men have disease, 100 men have disease. In the middle column are the number of men with abnormal tests and in the far right column are the number with normal tests. Since the test is 70% sensitive, 70 of those with disease will have abnormal tests and are true positives. The remaining 30 have normal tests and are false negatives. Since the test is 90% specific, 90% of the 9,900 without disease are true negatives, whereas the remainder are

Table 15-7. Performance of a Test with a 70 % Sensitivity and a 90 % Specificity in a Population with a 1 % Prevalence of Disease

	No. with Abnormal Test		No. with Normal Test	
100 Diseased	70	(TP) (Sensitivity)	30	(FN)
9,900 Non-diseased	990	(FP) (Specificity)	8,910	(TN)
Total	1,060		8,940	

$$\text{Predictive value of an abnormal test} = \frac{TP}{TP + FP} = \frac{70}{1,060} = 6.6\%$$

$$\text{False positive rate} = 100 - 6.6 = 93.4\%$$

$$\text{Relative risk} = 19.4 \text{ x}$$

Table 15-8. Performance of a Test with a 70 % Sensitivity and a 90 % Specificity in a Population with a 50 % Prevalence of Disease.

	No. with Abnormal Test		No. with Normal Test	
5,000Diseased	3,500	(TP) (Sensitivity)	1,500	(FN)
5,000 Non-diseased	500	(FP) (Specificity)	4,500	(TN)
Total	4,000		6,000	

Predictive value of an abnormal test	$= \dfrac{TP}{TP + FP}$	$= \dfrac{3,500}{4,000}$	$=$	87.5%
False positive rate	$=$	$100 - 87.5$	$=$	12.5%
Relative risk	$=$	$3.5\ x$		

false positives. To calculate the predictive value, the true positives are divided by all of those with an abnormal test. Table 15-8 shows the performance of a test with the same 70% sensitivity and 90% specificity in a population with a 50% prevalence of disease. After performing the same calculations as in Table 15-7, it is obvious that using the test in a population with a greater disease prevalence reduces the false positive rate.

There are more false positive responses when exercise testing is used in a population with a low prevalence of disease than there are in a population with a high prevalence of disease. This explains the greater number of false positives found when using the test as a screening procedure compared to when using it as a diagnostic procedure in patients with symptoms that most likely are due to coronary artery disease.

No matter what techniques are used, there is a reciprocal relationship between sensitivity and specificity. The more specific a test is (i.e., the more able it is to determine who is disease free), the less sensitive it is. The values for sensitivity and specificity can be altered by adjusting the criterion for abnormal responses. For instance, when the criterion for an abnormal exercise-induced S-T segment response is altered to 0.2 mv. depression to make it more specific for coronary artery disease, the sensitivity of the test can be cut in half.[16] For unknown reasons, the specificity of the S-T response is decreased when the test is used in patients with S-T segment depression at rest[50] or when it is used in women.[15]

The information most important to the clinician is the likelihood of a patient having the disease once his test result is known. Such a likelihood cannot be estimated just from the test result and the diagnostic characteristics of the test. It also requires knowledge of the prior probability of the patient having the disease before the test was administered. The probability of an individual having the disease after a test depends upon the probability before the test and on the test's sensitivity and specificity.

Table 15-9 consists of four 2 × 2 tables demonstrating the impact of prior probability on exercise test results. The test is considered to have a 70% sensitivity and a 90% specificity. The probability of CAD was obtained from angiographic studies which investigated the prevalence of significant CAD in patients with different chest pain syndromes.[51-54] Approximately 90% of the patients with true angina pectoris and 50% of the patients presenting with atypical angina pectoris were found to have significant angiographic coronary disease. By atypical is meant that the pain had an unusual location, prolonged duration, inconstant precipitating factors or did not respond to nitroglycerin. Thus, the patient with typical angina pectoris has a 90% chance of having significant CAD. An abnormal exercise test increases the probability to 98%. Because such a patient still has a 75% probability of disease after a negative test, angiography may still be required to definitely rule out coronary disease. The greatest diagnostic impact would be in patients with atypical angina. An abnormal test result would increase the probability from 50-88%, and for practical purposes, establish the diagnosis. With a normal test, the probability of coronary disease would be reduced to 25%.

The patient with non-anginal chest pain has a 10% probability of having coronary disease. An abnormal exercise test increases this to approximately 44% whereas a negative test decreases it to 3.5%. An angiographic study by Gensini in patients undergoing catheterization for reasons other than symptoms of coronary disease suggests that the probability of an asymptomatic person having angiographic coronary disease would be about 5%.[55] An abnormal exercise test would increase this probability to 27%. This probability or predictive value is amazingly similar to the 20% reported in a follow-up study[39] and the 30% reported in an angiographic study.[45] A negative test would decrease the probability to 2%.

A recent study used extensive risk factor screening in addition to exercise testing and found that the exercise test added little predictive information in their middle-aged population.[56] This finding is controversial and another careful study using standard risk factors and exercise testing should be performed in order to compare their prognostic value. Such a study would help to demonstrate the most cost effective way to screeen for latent coronary disease. An interesting consideration is that the major end point reported in most prospective studies has been angina pectoris. One wonders if those with an abnormal exercise test were biased to report angina pectoris sooner than those with a negative test who were not made anxious about symptoms of coronary artery disease.

Table 15-10 lists some of the causes for false positive exercise tests. These have been reviewed in detail in a previous publication.[16] Table 15-11 lists some of the causes for false negatives. The studies of Cumming and Lester have shown that maximal testing is more sensitive than submaximal testing. Although 70-80% of the abnormal responders will be abnormal in V_5 alone

Table 15-9. 2×2 Tables Showing the Principles of the Predictive Model Using Exercise Testing in Different Populations*

$$**p(B|A) = \frac{p(A|B)\,p(B)}{p(A)} \quad \text{or} \quad p(A|B) = \frac{p(B|A)\,p(A)}{p(B)}$$

CLASSIC ANGINA SYMPTOMS → p(A) = 0.9

	A (disease)	Ā (no disease)	Total
B (+ test)	AB^{63}	$\bar{A}B^{1}$	B^{64}
B̄ (− test)	$A\bar{B}^{27}$	$\bar{A}\bar{B}^{9}$	$\bar{B}^{36}$
Total	A^{90}	$\bar{A}^{10}$	100

Sensitivity = $p(B|A) = AB/A = 63/90 = 0.7$
Specificity = $p(\bar{B}|\bar{A}) = \bar{A}\bar{B}/\bar{A} = 9/10 = 0.9$
p(disease | + test) = $p(A|B) = AB/B = 63/64 = 98\%$
p(disease | − test) = $p(A|\bar{B}) = A\bar{B}/\bar{B} = 27/36 = 75\%$

NON-ANGINAL PAIN → p(A) = 0.1

	A (disease)	Ā (no disease)	Total
B (+ test)	AB^{7}	$\bar{A}B^{9}$	B^{16}
B̄ (− test)	$A\bar{B}^{3}$	$\bar{A}\bar{B}^{81}$	$\bar{B}^{84}$
Total	A^{10}	$\bar{A}^{90}$	100

Sensitivity = $p(B|A) = AB/A = 7/10 = 0.7$
Specificity = $p(\bar{B}|\bar{A}) = \bar{A}\bar{B}/\bar{A} = 81/90 = 0.9$
p(disease + test) = $p(A|B) = AB/B = 7/16 = 43.75\%$
p(disease − test) = $p(A|\bar{B}) = A\bar{B}/\bar{B} = 3/84 = 3.5\%$

ATYPICAL ANGINA PECTORIS → p(A) = 0.5

	A (disease)	Ā (no disease)	Total
B (+ test)	AB^{35}	$\bar{A}B^{5}$	B^{40}
B̄ (− test)	$A\bar{B}^{15}$	$\bar{A}\bar{B}^{45}$	$\bar{B}^{60}$
Total	A^{50}	$\bar{A}^{50}$	100

Sensitivity = $p(B|A) = AB/A = 35/50 = 0.7$
Specificity = $p(\bar{B}|\bar{A}) = \bar{A}\bar{B}/\bar{A} = 45/50 = 0.9$
p(disease | + test) = $p(A|B) = AB/B = 35/40 = 87.5\%$
p(disease | − test) = $p(A|\bar{B}) = A\bar{B}/\bar{B} = 15/60 = 25\%$

ASYMPTOMATIC PERSON → p(A) = 0.05

	A (disease)	Ā (no disease)	Total
B (+ test)	$AB^{3.5}$	$\bar{A}B^{9.5}$	B^{13}
B̄ (− test)	$A\bar{B}^{1.5}$	$\bar{A}\bar{B}^{85.5}$	$\bar{B}^{87}$
Total	A^{5}	$\bar{A}^{95}$	100

Sensitivity = $p(B|A) = AB/A = 3.5/5 = 0.7$
Specificity = $p(\bar{B}|\bar{A}) = \bar{A}\bar{B}/\bar{A} = 85.5/95 = 0.9$
p(disease | + test) = $p(A|B) = AB/B = 3.5/13 = 27\%$
p(disease | − test) = $p(A|\bar{B}) = A\bar{B}/\bar{B} = 1.5/87 = 2\%$

* Courtesy of Dr. Michael Criqui, Division of Epidemiology, Department of Community Medicine, University of California, San Diego.
** Note that p(B|A) means the probability of event B occurring given the pre-existing condition of A. Thus p(B|A) = AB/A.

Table 15-10. Conditions That Can Possibly Result in an Exercise-induced Abnormal S-T Segment Depression Without the Presence of Coronary Artery Disease (False Positive Exercise Test)

Valvular heart disease	Left ventricular hypertrophy
Congenital heart disease	WPW syndrome
Cardiomyopathies	Pre-excitation variants
Pericardial disorders	Mitral valve prolapse syndrome
Drugs	Vasoregulatory abnormality
Electrolyte abnormalities	Hyperventilation repolarization ab-
Non-fasting state	normalities
Anemia	Hypertension
Sudden excessive exercise	Excessive double product
Inadequate recording equipment	Improper lead systems
Bundle branch block	Incorrect criteria
Improper interpretation	

Table 15-11. Causes of False Negative Exercise ECG Test

1. Inadequate exercise stress
2. Too few leads monitored
3. Beta-blocking agents
4. Cancelling S-T segment vectors
5. Improper recording equipment
6. Failure to consider other abnormal end points
7. Coronary lesions not causing ischemia

or in addition to other leads, an additional 20–30% will be abnormal only in other leads.[25, 57] Therefore, unless these other leads are monitored, the exercise test will have a decreased sensitivity. Beta-blocking drugs such as propranolol lower the heart rate response to exercise and can normalize exercise-induced S-T segment depression.[58] Multiple ischemic areas can generate cancelling S-T segment vectors which can result in no S-T segment changes on the surface electrocardiogram in individuals with severe coronary artery disease.[59] The prevalence of this occurrence is uncertain but it is probably rare in asymptomatic individuals since it usually indicates that severe left ventricular dysfunction is present. If the frequency response of the monitoring equipment is improper, S-T segment depression can be altered. It has been shown that there are other end points of exercise testing that can be as predictive for coronary disease as S-T segment depression. These include anginal chest pain during exercise,[60] S-T segment elevation,[61] an inadequate heart rate response[62] and exercise-induced hypotension.[63] Another cause for false negatives is coronary lesions that do not cause ischemia but can still be life threatening.

Summary

When screening asymptomatic men, an abnormal response to an exercise test identifies a group at high risk for having coronary heart disease. The prevalence of exercise-induced S-T segment depression increases with age. Maximal exercise testing has an increased sensitivity compared to submaximal exercise testing. An abnormal response to exercise testing correlates with standard risk factors.

As demonstrated in the biostatistical section, the predictive value of an abnormal exercise test response is directly related to the prevalence of disease in the population tested. Thus, the usefulness of the test is enhanced in populations with increased risk factors or markers for coronary heart disease. Another group of asymptomatic individuals that deserve consideration for exercise testing are those in whom sudden incapacitation has a high probability of endangering many people. These include pilots, firemen, policemen, railroad engineers and drivers of large commercial vehicles. In certain situations, middle-aged sedentary individuals who are planning to begin intensive physical training programs should undergo exercise testing.

Maximal exercise testing has a sensitivity of approximately 70% and a specificity of nearly 90% for coronary artery disease. An abnormal test does not absolutely predict the presence of coronary artery disease or its future development, and a normal test does not rule out coronary artery disease or the future occurrence of coronary events. Good clinical judgment and risk factor analysis must be utilized to avoid the iatrogenic complication of "cardiac cripples." At the present time, there is no secondary line of non-invasive studies that can provide the same information nor absolutely separate a false positive exercise test response from a true positive exercise test response.

Exercise testing has a number of valid applications for screening asymptomatic individuals but it should not be used indiscriminately. In a population with a relatively low prevalence of coronary artery disease, such as asymptomatic young people, the test will have a predictive value of only about 25%. Thus, 75% of the abnormal responders will be false positives. Considering the detrimental impact of the test on the false positive responders and the cost of the test, it may not be the most cost effective way to screen for latent coronary artery disease. Many important studies have been performed with asymptomatic individuals that have led to a better understanding of exercise testing. Exercise testing asymptomatic individuals has a place in the health care system but it should not be a frequent precursor to coronary artery bypass surgery.

REFERENCES

1. Kannel, W. B., McGee, D. and Gordon, T.: A general cardiovascular risk profile: The Framingham study. Am. J. Cardiol., 38:46, 1976.

2. Kannel, W. B.: Some lessons in cardiovascular epidemiology from Framingham. Am. J. Cardiol., *37:*269, 1976.
3. Blackburn, H.: Coronary risk factors. How to evaluate and manage them. Eur. J. Cardiol. *2/3:*249, 1975.
4. Kuller, L. H.: Epidemiology of cardiovascular diseases: Current perspectives. Am. J. Epidemiol., *104:*425, 1976.
5. Froelicher, V. F.: The application of electrocardiographic screening and exercise testing to preventive cardiology. Prev. Med., *2:*592, 1973.
6. Froelicher, V. F.: Review of epidemiology in clinical cardiology. Aviat. Space Environ. Med., *48(7):*659, 1977.
7. Froelicher, V. F., Thompson, A. J., Yanowitz, F. and Lancaster, M. C.: Treadmill exercise testing at the USAFSAM: Physiological responses in aircrewmen and the detection of latent coronary artery disease. AGARDOGRAPH No. 210, 1975, NTIS, Springfield, V.
8. Barnard, R. J. and Duncan, H. W.: Heart rate and ECG responses of fire fighters. J. Occup. Med. *17(4):*247, 1975.
9. Faris, J. V., McHenry, P. L. and Jordan, J. W.: The prevalence and reproducibility of exercise-induced PVCs during maximal exercise in normal men. Am. J. Cardiol., *37:*617, 1976.
10. Shephard, R. J.: Do risks of exercise justify costly caution? Physician and Sports Medicine *5:*58, 1977.
11. Froelicher, V. F.: Does exercise conditioning delay progression of myocardial ischemia in coronary disease? *in* Controversies in Cardiology, edited by E. Corday and A. Brest, Cardiovasc. Clin., *8/1,* Philadelphia, F. A. Davis, 1977.
12. Simoons, M. L. and Hugenholtz, P. G.: Gradual changes of ECG and waveform during and after exercise in normal subjects. Circulation, *52:*570, 1975.
13. Rautaharju, P. M., Punsar, S., Blackburn, H., Warren, J. and Menotti, A.: Waveform patterns in Frank-lead rest and exercise electrocardiograms of healthy elderly men. Circulation, *48:*541, 1973.
14. Wolthuis, R. A., Froelicher, V. F., Fischer, J. et al.: The response of healthy men to treadmill exercise. Circulation, *55:*153, 1977.
15. Sketch, M. H., Mohinddin, S. M., Lynch, J. D. et al.: Significant sex differences in the correlation of electrocardiographic exercise testing and coronary arteriograms. Am. J. Cardiol., *36:*169, 1975.
16. Froelicher, V. F., Thompson, A. J., Longo, M. R. et al.: Value of exercise testing for screening asymptomatic men for latent coronary artery disease. Prog. Cardiovasc. Dis., *43:*265, 1976.
17. Mattingly, T. W.: The postexercise electrocardiogram. Its value in the diagnosis and prognosis of coronary arterial disease. A. J. Cardiol., *9:*395, 1962.
18. Parmley, L. F.: Personal communication.
19. Brody, A. J.: Master two-step exercise test in clinically unselected patients. J. A. M. A., *171:*1195, 1959.
20. Bellet, S., Roman, L., Nichols, G. and Muller, O.: Detection of coronary-prone subjects in a normal population by radio-electrocardiographic exercise test-follow-up studies. A. J. Cardiol., *19:*783, 1967.
21. Doyle, J. T. and Kinch, S. H.: The prognosis of an abnormal electrocardiographic stress test. Circulation, *41:*545, 1970.
22. Rumball, A. and Acheson, E. D.: Latent coronary heart disease detected by electrocardiogram before and after exercise. B. Med. J., *1:*423, 1965.
23. Rowell, L. B., Taylor, H. L., Simonson, E. and Carlson, W.: The physiologic fallacy of adjusting for body weight in performance of the Master two-step test. Am. Heart J., *70:*461, 1965.
24. Yigitbasi, O., Nalbantigil, I. and Kiliccioglu, B.: Ventricular fibrillation after exercise test. Communications to the Editor, Chest, *68:*747, 1975.
25. Koppes, G., Bassan, M., McKiernan, T. and Froelicher, V.: Treadmill exercise testing, *in* Current Problems in Cardiology, Chicago, Year Book Medical Publishers, Nov. & Dec., 1977.
26. Kattus, A. A., Jorgensen, C., Worden, R. and Alvaro, A.: S-T segment depression with near-maximal exercise in detection of preclinical coronary heart disease. Circulation, *44:*585, 1971.

27. Kattus, A. A., Jorgensen, C., Worden, R. and Alvaro, A.: S-T segment depression with near-maximal exercise; Its modification by physical conditioning. Chest, 62:678, 1972.
28. Lester, F. M., Sheffield, L. T. and Reeves, T. J.: Electrocardiographic changes in clinically normal older men following near maximal and maximal exercise. Circulation, 36:5, 1967.
29. Cumming, G. R.: Yield of ischaemic exercise electrocardiograms in relation to exercise intensity in a normal population. Br. Heart J., 34:919, 1972.
30 Olsson, A., Ekelund, L. and Carlson, L.: Studies in asymptomatic primary hyperlipidaemia. Acta Med. Scand., 198:187, 1975.
31. Allen, W. H., Aronow, W. S. and DeCristofaro, D.: Treadmill exercise testing in mass screening for coronary risk factors. Catheterization and Cardiovascular Diagnosis, 2:39, 1976.
32. Cumming, G. R., Dufresne, C. and Samm, J.: Exercise ECG changes in normal women. CMA Journal, 109:108, 1973.
33. Profant, G. R., Early, R. G., Nilson, K. L. et al.: Responses to maximal exercise in healthy middle-aged women. J. Appl. Physiol., 33:595, 1972.
34. Lepeshkin, E. and Surzwicz, B.: Characteristics of true positive and false positive results of electrocardiographic Master-two-step exercise test. New Engl. J. Med., 258:511, 1958.
35. Astrand, I.: Exercise electrocardiograms recorded twice with an 8-year interval in a group of 204 women and men 48–63 years old. Acta Med. Scand., 178:27, 1965.
36. Bruce, R. A. and McDonough, J. R.: Stress testing in screening for cardiovascular disease. Bull. N.Y. Acad. Med., 45:1288, 1969.
37. Aronow, W. S. and Cassidy, J.: Five year follow-up of double Master's test, maximal treadmill stress test, and resting and postexercise apexcardiogram in asymptomatic persons. Circulation, 52:616, 1975.
38. Cumming, G. R., Samm, J., Borysyk, L. et al.: Electrocardiographic changes during exercise in asymptomatic men: 3-year follow-up. Can. Med. Assoc. J., 112:578, 1975.
39. Froelicher, V. F., Thomas, M., Pillow, C. et al.: An epidemiological study of asymptomatic men screened with exercise testing for latent coronary heart disease. Am. J. Cardiol., 34:770, 1974.
40. Bruce, R. A.: Exercise electrocardiography, in Heart, edited by W. B. Hurst, New York, McGraw-Hill, 1974.
41. Sweet, R. L. and Sheffield, L. T.: Myocardial infarction after exercise induced ECG changes in a patient with variant angina pectoris. Am. J. Cardiol., 33:813, 1974.
42. Gradman, A. H., Bell, P. A. and DeBusk, R. F.: Sudden death during ambulatory monitoring: Clinical and electrocardiographic correlations—Report of a case. Circulation, 55:210, 1977.
43. Lintgen, A. B.: Death from myocardial infarction after exercise test with normal result. J.A.M.A., 235:837, 1976.
44. Thompson, A. J., Froelicher, V. F., Longo, M. R. et al.: Normal coronary angiography in an aircrewman with serial exercise test changes. Aviat. Space Environ. Med., 46:69, 1975.
45. Froelicher, V. F., Thompson, A. J., Wolthuis, R., Fuchs, Balusek, R. et al.: Angiographic findings in asymptomatic aircrewmen with electrocardiographic abnormalities. Am. J. Cardiol., 39:32, 1977.
46. Barnard, R. J., Gardner, G. W., Diaco, N. V. and Kattus, A. A.: Near-maximal ECG stress testing and coronary artery disease risk factor analysis in Los Angeles City fire fighters. J. Occup. Med. 17(11):693, 1975.
47. Barnard, R. J., Gardner, G. W. and Diaco, N. V.: "Ischemic" heart disease in fire fighters with normal coronary arteries. J. Occup. Med., 18(12):818, 1976.
48. Borer, J. S. Brensike, J. F., Redwood, D. R., Itscoitz, S. B. et al.: Limitations of the electrocardiographic response to exercise in predicting coronary-artery disease. New Engl. J. Med., 293:367, 1975.
49. Erikssen, J., Enge, I., Forfang, K. and Storstein, O.: False positive diagnostic tests and coronary angiographic findings in 105 presumably healthy males. Circulation, 54:371, 1976.
50. Kansal, S., Roitman, D.and Sheffield, L. T.: Stress testing with S-T segment depression at rest: An angiographic correlation. Circulation, 54:636, 1976.
51. Proudfit, W. L., Shirey, E. K. and Sones, F. M.: Selective cine coronary angiography: correlation with clinical findings in 1000 patients. Circulation, 33:901, 1966.

52. Friesinger, G. C. and Smith, R. F.: Correlation of electrocardiographic studies and arteriographic findings with angina pectoris. Circulation 46:1173, 1972.
53. McConahay, D. R., McCallister, B. D. and Smith, R. E.: Post-exercise electrocardiography: correlation with coronary arteriography and left ventricular hemodynamics. Am. J. Cardiol., 28:1, 1972.
54. Campeau, L., Bourassa, M. G., Bois, M. A. et al.: Clinical significance of selective coronary cinearteriography. Can. Med. Assoc. J., 99:1063, 1968.
55. Gensini, G. G. and Kelly, A. E.: Incidence and progression of coronary artery disease. An angiographic correlation in 1,263 patients. Arch. Intern. Med., 129:814, 1972.
56. Wilhemson, L.: Multivariate risk prediction in a 15 year follow-up using risk factors and exercise testing (Abstr.). Labax and Univ. of Bordeau Exercise Testing Symposium, Bordeau, France, June, 1977.
57. Mason, R. E., Likar, I., Biern, R. O. and Ross, R. S.: Multiple-lead exercise electrocardiography. Experience in 107 normal subjects and 67 patients with angina pectoris, and comparison with coronary cinearteriography in 84 patients. Circulation 36:517, 1967.
58. Reybrouch, T., Amery, A. and Billiet, L.: Hemodynamic response to graded exercise after chronic beta-adrenergic blockade. J. Appl. Physiol., 42:133, 1977.
59. Manvi, K. N. and Ellestad, M. H.: Elevated S-T segment with exercise in ventricular aneurysm. J. Electrocardiol., 5:317, 1972.
60. Weiner, D. A., McCabe, C., Hueter, D., Hood, B. and Ryan, T.: The predictive value of chest pain as an indicator of coronary disease during exercise testing (Abstr.). Circulation, 53/54(Supp. II): 10, 1976.
61. Fortuin, N. J. and Friesinger, G. C.: Exercise induced S-T segment elevation. Am. J. Med., 49:459, 1970.
62. Ellestad, M. H. and Wan, M. K.: Predictive implications of stress testing. Follow-up of 2700 subjects after maximum treadmill stress testing. Circulation, 51:363, 1975.
63. Morris, S. N. and McHenry, P. L.: The incidence and significance of decreases in systolic blood pressure during graded treadmill exercise testing. Am. J. Cardiol., 41:221, 1978.

16

Circulatory Adjustments to Exercise

Jan Praetorius Clausen, M.D.

General Considerations

This chapter presents physiologic background information on circulatory regulation during exercise that can be useful in the interpretation of exercise ECG tests. The material utilized is derived mainly from experiments that include invasive techniques, which are not applicable as a routine in clinical exercise ECG tests. However, with basic knowledge of the response and interdependence of the different circulatory variables, it is possible from easily obtainable measures like the heart rate and the arterial blood pressure, together with the clinical reaction, to make deductions about a number of other central and peripheral circulatory parameters. This can be illustrated by a few examples. Since the oxygen costs of simple forms of exercise such as bicycling and walking vary only slightly in different subjects (about 5%), the capacity for increased oxygen transport, i.e., for augmenting the cardiac output, can be grossly assessed from the workload the subject can sustain during 3- to 6-minute periods. The increase in heart rate and the rise in systolic blood pressure reflect the concomitant increase in myocardial oxygen uptake and blood flow. The increase in arterial blood pressure also provides information about the total peripheral vascular resistance. Moreover, the increase in heart rate is an indicator of sympathetic activation which can be used to predict the degree of peripheral vasoconstriction. The color and the temperature of the skin as well as the degree of filling of cutaneous veins indicate something about the contribution of thermal stress to the sympathetic activation. By putting together such pieces of information it is, for instance, possible in a given patient to decide whether his entire circulatory system is severely challenged at the moment when precordial pain and/or ECG changes occur or whether local ischemia in a small part of his myocardium limits his performance. If the reading of this chapter inspires the reader in the context of understanding and interpreting exercise ECG tests, it has served its purpose.

Muscle Metabolism and Blood Flow

Although interest focuses on circulatory and ventilatory variables in clinical exercise ECG tests, it should not be forgotten that the primary events during muscle activity take place at the level of the skeletal muscle fibers. Figure 16-1 gives a synopsis of the metabolic processes which cover the energy expenditure in the contracting skeletal muscle cell. The mechanical energy created by the sliding movement of the actin and myosin filaments is provided by splitting of the energy-rich phosphate compounds adenosine triphosphate (ATP) and creatinine phosphate (CP). The stores of ATP and CP in the muscle cell are small and only sufficient for very short periods of activity. Thus, continuous or repeated contractions require that ATP and CP are resynthesized pari passu with the rate of splitting. This is obtained by the breakdown of glucose and free fatty acids and the metabolic systems involved are activated by the presence of splitting products from ATP. The substrates are available as intracellular stores of glycogen grains and fat droplets, but can also be taken up from the blood perfusing the muscle. The fastest way to generate ATP is the anaerobic glycolysis, i.e., the breakdown of glycogen to pyruvate, which is subsequently converted to lactate or alanine. Whereas this anaerobic process ensures rapid ATP supply without oxygen consumption, in a quantitative sense the ATP yield obtained in this way is modest and the cumulation of lactate

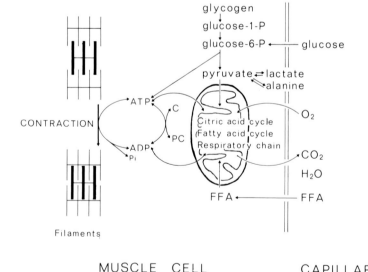

MUSCLE   CELL   CAPILLARY

Fig. 16-1 Schematic presentation of the most important metabolic events in contracting muscle cell. For explanation, see text.

leads to a deterioration of the internal cellular milieu, especially by reducing the pH, which, after a short time, may prevent further function. If muscle contractions are to be continued for minutes or longer, the main part of the ATP production must derive from aerobic intramitochondrial complete breakdown to CO_2 and H_2O of pyruvate and free fatty acids. Hereby 34 mol. of ATP are generated/mol. of glucose compared to 2 mol. ATP by anaerobic glycolysis.[20]

The ensuing augmented oxygen demand is covered by increased oxygen extraction as well as by increased perfusion of the muscle. The increase in blood flow is adjusted to the actual oxygen demands by graded vasodilation caused by local release of vasodilator metabolites.[27] The exact nature of these metabolites is not yet established.

The muscle blood flow does not depend solely on the degree of metabolic vasodilation, however. The local vasodilator mechanism acts in competition with a neurogenic sympathetic vasoconstrictor influence on the resistance vessels, which tends to limit the increase in blood flow.[27] Furthermore, muscle contractions interfere mechanically with the blood flow. During static or isometric muscle contractions during which the muscle tension increases, but no shortening of the muscle takes place, an impediment of blood flow due to compression of the vessels becomes appreciable at about 15% of the maximal contraction force and at 60–70% the blood flow is virtually arrested.[12] This explains, at least in part, an inverse relationship between the force of a muscle contraction and the time it can be maintained. If the contraction is sustained for several minutes the contraction force must constitute less than 15–25% of the maximal contraction force, i.e., be at a level at which the blood flow is still not seriously hampered.[12] However, other factors contribute to explain the shorter endurance time with increasing force of contraction. Skeletal muscle, unlike the myocardium, is composed of various types of fibers with different enzymatic and functional characteristics. Some fibers are like the myocardial fibers rich in oxidative intramitochondrial enzymes connected to the citric acid cycle, the fatty acid cycle and the respiratory chain. These are the classical "red" muscle fibers. At the other end of a continuous spectrum is the typical "white" muscle fiber with a high content of enzymes necessary for anaerobic glycolysis, but containing few mitochondria. Due to their great capability for aerobic metabolism, red fibers sustain contractions for long periods of time, whereas the anaerobic white fibers require longer aerobic restitution phases even after short periods of activity. At lower levels of force development only red fibers are activated, but with increasing force an augmented number of motor units with anaerobic enzymatic profile and short function time is recruited.[19, 19]

During rhythmic or dynamic contractions the muscle shortens and produces external work. In this situation the working time is also an inverse function of the force of each contraction and, in addition, of the frequency of contractions. The oxygen uptake is a linear function of the external work produced. As in the case with static exercise, during dynamic exercise continued for several minutes or more, only about 15–25% of a muscle's maximal force of contraction can be utilized.

Nevertheless, much higher values for muscle blood flow and local oxygen consumption can be measured during dynamic exercise: The maximal muscle blood flow during dynamic exercise is 70–100 ml. $\times$ 100 g.$^{-1}$ $\times$ min.$^{-1}$ compared to about 30–40 ml. $\times$ 100 g.$^{-1}$ $\times$ min.$^{-1}$ at the end of a prolonged static contraction.[5, 12] The difference in blood flow can be related to the fact that the alternating contraction and relaxation phases during dynamic exercise make the muscle function as an efficient pump. During heavy physical exercise the vascular bed in muscles fills and empties in a way very similar to the events in the heart ventricles. During the contraction (systolic) phase there is virtually no inflow of blood, but a vigorous ejection takes place. In between contractions (in the diastole) there is little or no venous outflow from the muscle, the evacuated vascular bed being filled up by a maximal inflow.[15]

It takes from 2–3 minutes before the oxygen uptake reaches a steady level during dynamic exercise. Since the muscle blood flow attains its final value within less than a minute[5] (Figure 16-2), this delay must be due to tardiness of the metabolic reactions. During this initial period, lactate is released from the muscle even at light work intensities showing that part of the ATP expenditure is covered by anaerobic glycolysis. During heavy physical exercise the lactate production may continue throughout the exercise period.[25]

Systemic Circulatory Adjustments

A. Variations in Response to Different types of Exercise

The increase in oxygen demands caused by weak contractions of small muscle groups probably may be covered exclusively by the local metabolically controlled vasodilation. However, almost any form of muscle activity elicits nervous cardiovascular reflexes, causing, first and foremost, an increased sympathetic and reduced parasympathetic nervous stimulation of the heart, together with an increased sympathetic stimulation of the peripheral vessels.[14] Apart from an increase in cardiac output, muscle activity therefore normally results in an augmentation of the heart rate and the arterial blood pressure which is proportional to the work intensity. However, the relative affection of the different variables depends on the type of exercise performed. If the major part of the active skeletal muscles contracts rhythmically in young healthy subjects during walking, running, swimming, bicycling and rowing, a large increase in cardiac output (4–6 times the resting value) and in the heart rate (up to 200 beats/minute at maximal work intensity) is accompanied by a relatively modest increase in mean

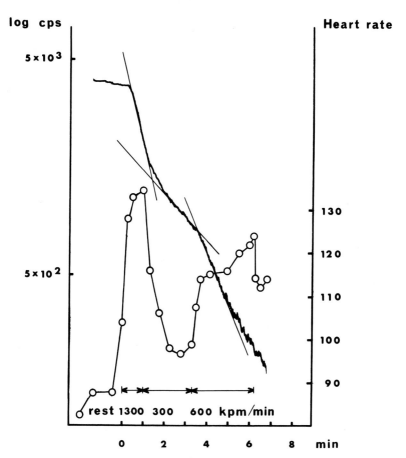

Fig. 16-2   Muscle blood flow assessed from the elimination rate of [133] Xenon in the vastus lateralis muscle during exercise on bicycle ergometer at three successive workloads. The rapid changes in blood flow with the transition from rest to exercise and with a decrease or an increase in workload should be noted. The corresponding heart rate is shown by the open circles. (From Clausen & Lassen: Cardiovasc. Res., 5:245, 1971.)

arterial blood pressure (MBP) up to about 110–120 mm. Hg. By contrast during isometric effects, e.g., handgrip, the mean arterial blood pressure may attain 150–160 mm. Hg concomitant to a heart rate of only 120–130 beats/minute. Although, in this situation, cardiac output increases more in relation to the oxygen uptake than during dynamic exercise, the absolute augmentation is modest (about 2 times the value at rest). It is noteworthy that the increase in MBP during isometric exercise is a function of the force of contraction in percent of the maximal force of contraction of the muscle group in question, but widely independent of the size of the active muscle mass.[12] The same pressure response is elicited by a handgrip as by leg extension when the relative force of contraction is the same.

The pressure response to isometric contractions is added to that of ongoing dynamic exercise. If a person carries a weight or performs a handgrip during walking or bicycling, an extra increase in MBP is seen and, in essence, it corresponds to that expected from the isometric effort alone.[12] Similarly, dynamic exercise which involves a strong component of static muscle activity for maintenance of the body position, e.g., arm cranking or wood sawing, causes a much steeper rise in MBP for a given oxygen uptake than does walking or running.[6] It is important to recall this fact when choosing the type of exercise for the exercise ECG test and when recommending leisure time activity to cardiac patients and elderly individuals. It is the "volume load" on the heart and on the peripheral circulatory system inherent in dynamic muscle activity and the central and peripheral circulatory adaptive changes resulting from this kind of exercise that are supposed to be of prophylactic value against coronary artery disease and beneficial in patients with known coronary heart disease. The "pressure load" on the circulatory system imposed by isometric exercise is not thought to be of any value in this context. On the contrary, many cardiologists have the opinion that the abrupt pressure response related to static efforts is hazardous in cardiac patients and elderly subjects. This point of view does not agree with the common attitude among laymen. Normally, people are willing to accept that they are too old to perform vigorous dynamic activities such as running, bicycling and ball games, but they do not often hesitate to demonstrate their muscle power in isometric efforts. We shall return to the possible risks of isometric exercise in cardiac patients later on.

B. Variations in Response to Increasing Workloads

(1) Cardiac Output and Its Distribution

Figure 16-3 gives a comprehensive picture of the changes in some important circulatory variables during 2 types of dynamic exercise valid for a young healthy subject. Both ordinary bicycling and arm cranking are shown in order to demonstrate differences and similarities in circulatory adjustments in 2 types of exercise. In one form of exercise great muscle groups perform the external dynamic work with only a small component of static work, and in another form of exercise, the muscle groups engaged in dynamic exercise are smaller and the concomitant isometric effort is greater.

From the diagram, cardiac output, its regional distribution, the heart rate, the cardiac stroke volume and the arterial blood pressure can be read for any oxygen uptake from the resting condition through the entire range of submaximal workloads up to maximal exercise. Maximal exercise is defined as the work intensity which elicits the highest attainable oxygen uptake for the given type of exercise. Beyond this level, further increase of

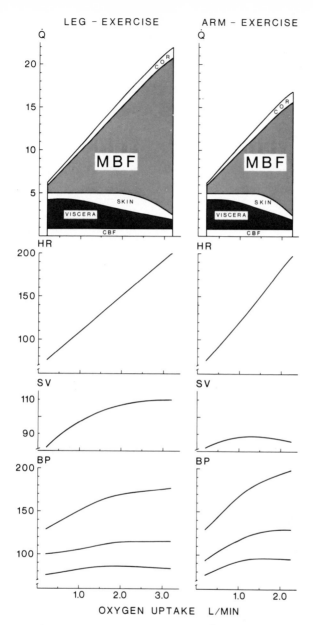

Fig. 16-3 Cardiac output (Q) in $1 \times min^{-1}$ and estimates of its regional distribution to the exercising muscles (MBF), to the myocardium (COR), to the skin, to the abdominal viscera and to the brain (CBF), together with corresponding values for heart rate (HR), stroke volume (SV) in ml., systolic, diastolic and mean arterial blood pressure in mm. Hg, all related to the oxygen uptake at rest and during exercise with the legs (left panel) or with the arms (right panel). At any oxygen uptake the values apply to the situation after 5–7 minutes of exercise when oxygen uptake and cardiac output have reached a steady state. (Modified from Clausen, 1976.)

the workload does not lead to further augmentation of the oxygen uptake (Figure 16-4). Normally, exercise of this intensity leads to exhaustion within 5–10 minutes.

It appears from Figure 16-3 that the cardiac output is a linear function of the oxygen uptake during both types of work. The increase in total flow is essentially the same for a given increase in oxygen uptake during arm and leg exercise, namely about 6 liters/liter extra oxygen uptake. The main part of the increase in cardiac output is directed to the exercising muscles, and the difference between arm and leg exercise with respect to the maximal cardiac output is explained by the difference in the mass of skeletal muscles performing dynamic exercise.

Part of the increase in cardiac output is directed to the respiratory muscles and the myocardium. The fraction allotted to the respiratory muscles is proportional to the ventilatory effort and the pulmonary oxygen

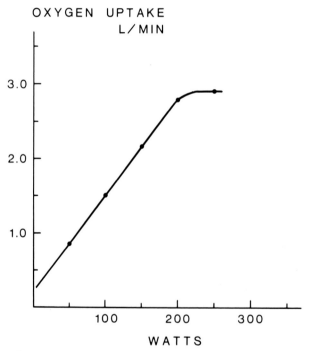

Fig. 16-4 The oxygen uptake at different workloads during exercise on bicycle ergometer measured after 5–7 minutes of exercise in a young healthy subject. At submaximal levels oxygen uptake is a linear function of the workload. In this subject maximal oxygen uptake (2.91 × min^{-1}) was reached at 220 watts and further increase of the workload did not result in augmented oxygen uptake.

uptake. Normally, it is assumed that the respiratory muscles account for 10–20% of the increase in pulmonary oxygen uptake and a corresponding fraction of the increase in cardiac output goes to these muscles.[7] Myocardial blood flow is adapted to local oxygen demands through metabolically controlled vasodilation. Myocardial oxygen consumption is analogous to that of skeletal muscles, determined by the force and the frequency of contractions. The force of contraction or the tension development depends on the intraventricular pressure in systole, the initial length of myocardial fibers (end-diastolic volume), the ventricular wall thickness and the contractile state of the myocardium.[35] A close relationship has been demonstrated in man between coronary blood flow and oxygen uptake and the product of the heart rate and systolic blood pressure or the heart rate alone.[22] The correlation of myocardial blood flow with the heart rate and systolic blood pressure means that myocardial blood flow is a function of total body oxygen uptake in percent of the maximal oxygen uptake rather than the external workload the subject performs. Thus, at a given pulmonary oxygen uptake, the lower the myocardial blood flow, the higher the maximal oxygen uptake. The fraction of cardiac output assigned to the heart is probably below 4% even at maximal exercise.

Skin blood flow in response to exercise is complicated, because 2 different mechanisms tend to change flow in opposite directions.[32] Skin is supplied by vasoconstrictor nerves mediating flow reduction during exercise. On the other hand, reflexes related to body thermoregulation tend to cause vasodilation to facilitate heat dissipation. As a net result, during exercise in thermal neutral environments, skin flow decreases during the first 5 minutes, but subsequently increases above resting values provided the workload requires less than about 60% of the maximal oxygen uptake. At still high workloads, skin flow again decreases, and at maximal levels working time is normally too short to allow development of pronounced hyperthermia and skin remains vasoconstricted. This will be discussed in detail later in this chapter.

Blood flow to most other non-exercising tissues, with the blood flow to the brain as an important exception, is reduced due to the increased sympathetic vasoconstrictor influence. Quantitatively most important in this context are the blood flows to the abdominal viscera (splanchnic-hepatic and renal blood flows), and the blood flow to non-working muscles. As far as the abdominal viscera are concerned, it has been shown that the decrease in perfusion during exercise is a linear function of the relative severity of exercise expressed as the actual oxygen uptake in percent of the maximal oxygen uptake for the given type of exercise. Thus as seen in Figure 16-3, a given oxygen uptake causes a greater reduction in the visceral flow during arm exercise than during leg exercise, whereas during maximal exercise the flow is reduced to about 20% of the resting value in both situations.[6, 32]

(2) Heart Rate, Stroke Volume and Arterial Blood Pressure

The heart rate is, like the peripheral vasoconstriction, a linear function of the oxygen uptake in percent of the maximal oxygen uptake. Thus, when related to the absolute oxygen uptake as shown in Figure 16-3, the increase is steeper during arm exercise than during leg exercise, but at a workload requiring maximal oxygen uptake for the respective types of exercise, approximately the same maximal heart rate value is attained.

During exercise performed in the upright position, cardiac stroke volume normally increases until about 50% of the maximal oxygen uptake is attained. Thereafter it remains essentially unchanged. The final value is often the same as that measured at rest in the supine position. Due to the fact that cardiac output increases by the same number of liters per liter as the increase in oxygen uptake during the two types of exercise, and the fact that heart rate is a function of the oxygen uptake in percent of the maximal oxygen uptake, stroke volume becomes considerably lower during arm exercise compared to leg exercise (Figure 16-3).

The arterial blood pressure increases with increasing workload, reflecting that the cardiac output increases relatively more than the total peripheral resistance decreases. As previously stated, the increase is steeper during arm exercise than during leg exercise. The augmentation in arterial blood pressure during exercise and the large difference in this respect between arm and leg exercise may seem surprising in view of the fact that the systemic circulation is provided with a control system aimed at preventing major fluctuations in arterial pressure. It seems, however, that during exercise the baroreceptor response to increased pressure is modified at the level of the vasomotor center[30] so that the arterial pressure becomes a more or less passive function of the actual cardiac output and the peripheral resistance.

C. Integrated Cardiovascular Response to Exercise

The above described normal response to exercise depends on a multiplicity of regulatory changes involving virtually every circulatory component. Furthermore, most of the changes interact: a change in one factor regularly necessitates readjustments of the other.[14, 34] In order to get a comprehensive view we will attempt to reduce the multiplicity of interacting processes to some basic patterns by an acceptable simplification.

The reduction in vascular resistance in the contracting muscles caused by locally controlled vasodilation is directly responsible for the increased oxygen supply in proportion to the increased demands. However, vasodilation in greater muscle groups would lead to a marked fall in arterial blood pressure and insufficient filling of the heart without the compensatory interventions mediated especially through the sympathetic division of the autonomic nervous system. These nervous interventions are directed toward maintaining the arterial blood pressure and ensuring optimal conditions for an increased venous return. The sympathetic effects can be divided in peripheral and cardiac effects and the peripheral effects further divided into arterial and venous, i.e., in influences on the resistance and the capacitance vessels.[14, 34]

The sympathetic activation causes reinforced arterial vasoconstriction in almost any tissue of the body, with the brain as an important exception. The vasoconstrictor influence even includes the resistance vessels in the working muscles, but here it is more or less completely overridden by the metabolic vasodilation.[7, 27]

The sympathetic venoconstriction facilitates the venous return by pressing tighter on the blood stream and makes a main contribution to increase the driving force tending to return the blood to the heart. At the same time the arterial and venous constriction diminish the volume of blood in the non-exercising tissues, causing a release of blood volume into the main stream, which further improves the filling conditions of the heart.

The importance of the sympathetic peripheral vasoconstriction is disclosed by the effects of deficient function. If peripheral vasoconstriction can not occur during exercise due either to lesions of the sympathetic nervous system or to administration of drugs with antagonistic effects, exercise elicits an abrupt fall in arterial blood pressure even when performed in the supine position.[26]

The sympathetic stimulation of the heart enables it to forward a 4- to 6-fold greater output with virtually unchanged filling pressures, reduced diastolic volume and a stroke volume which does not exceed that seen at rest in the supine position. This improvement in pump function is achieved by the combined effects of the increase in heart rate and the increased myocardial contractility. The systolic heart volume is also reduced and the heart does thus contribute an additional volume of blood to the peripheral vascular bed.[28, 34]

Whereas the absence of the peripheral vasoconstriction results in a serious limitation of the ability to perform exercise, the lack of sympathetic stimulation of the heart has much less influence on the physical performance capacity. Administration of a beta-receptor blocking agent like propranolol (Inderal) reduces markedly the heart rate and the contractility during exercise; maximal heart rate may be reduced by 40–50 beats/minute. Nevertheless, through a compensatory increase in the stroke volume young healthy subjects provide a sufficient cardiac output to maintain a normal oxygen uptake up to the maximal level.[13] Likewise, subjects with congenital atrioventricular (A-V) block show a normal increase in cardiac output in relation to the oxygen uptake during exercise.[21] However, during beta-receptor blockade at least this maintained capacity for oxygen transport, despite the lack of cardiac sympathetic stimulation, is not achieved exclusively by the Frank-Starling mechanism. It requires, at the same time, an exaggerated peripheral vasoconstriction at a given oxygen uptake,[6] which certainly reduces the adaptability to the further stress associated with prolonged effort or additional thermal stress. Although an almost normal circulatory oxygen transport can be attained for the short period of time required to obtain maximal oxygen uptake, the time during which severe exercise can be sustained is clearly reduced.[13]

The vasodilation in skeletal muscle and the concomitant activation of the sympathetic nervous system may be considered an obligatory response to exercise which always is seen independent of the duration of exercise. Exercise continued for more than about 5 minutes makes further major circulatory adjustments necessary because of the need for elimination of large quantities of heat to keep body temperature at acceptable levels.[32]

This is accomplished by selective vasodilation of the skin vessels. Variations in the state of contraction of these vessels may have important consequences for the total peripheral vascular resistance and the distribution of the total blood volume. With maximal cutaneous vasodilation as much as 7–8 liters of blood/minute can be directed to this regional bed, and an important amount of blood volume can be pooled in the capacious cutaneous veins. Although skin is never allowed to vasodilate completely during exercise, the fall in vascular resistance and the displacement of blood volume which occurs especially in hot environments do require marked compensatory adjustments to prevent a fall in arterial blood pressure. During very mild prolonged exercise in the heat the increase in skin blood flow causes an augmentation in cardiac output as it is seen also at rest. During heavier but still moderate submaximal exercise the cardiac output does not increase and the cutaneous vasodilation is compensated by further sympathetic activation, causing additional reduction in visceral perfusion and further augmentation of the heart rate. The compensation is not complete. Even in thermal neutral environments prolonged exercise is characterized by a cardiovascular drift, i.e., a progressive decline in arterial blood pressure and in stroke volume. Near the maximal work intensity, at which there is no further possibility for visceral vasoconstriction (or increase in heart rate), skeletal muscles and the skin compete for cardiac output. As far as short-lasting maximal efforts are concerned, heat accumulation does not reach pronounced degrees; skin remains vasoconstricted and maximal muscle blood flow and maximal oxygen uptake can be obtained even in the heat. During prolonged severe exercise, however, cutaneous vasodilatation may induce a reduction in muscle blood flow and set the limitation for the duration of exercise especially in hot environments. A fall in arterial blood pressure as well as increased sympathetic vasocontrictor activity may contribute to the decrement in muscle blood flow in this situation.

Even during the short-lasting maximal efforts, during which cutaneous vasodilatation does not interfere with the muscle blood flow, the sympathetic vasoconstrictor tones in the muscle resistance vessels apparently set the upper limit for muscle blood flow and thus for cardiac output and the maximal oxygen uptake. This has at least been shown to apply to exercise with great muscle groups (bicycling, combined arm and leg exercise).[7] The greater the active muscle mass, the more pronounced is the vasoconstriction. Therefore, a given muscle group has a greater maximal blood flow when it is working alone, than when other muscle groups are active at the same time. Thus, the addition of further muscle groups (e.g., arm exercise to

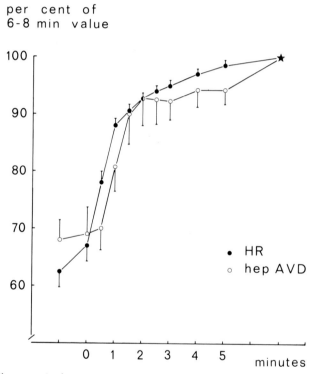

Fig. 16-5 Changes in heart rate (HR) and in splanchnic-hepatic blood flow assessed from variations in the arterio hepatic venous oxygen difference (hep AVD) immediately before and during the first 6–8 minutes of exercise. Both variables are expressed in percent of the 6–8 minute value. As can be seen the reduction in splanchnic blood flow (= increase in hep AVD) has the same time course as the increase in heart rate. The delay of the hep AVD values of about 30 seconds during the first 1.5 minutes is due to the transit time for blood in the splanchnic-hepatic circuit. (From Clausen and Trap-Jensen: J. Appl. Physiol., 37:716, 1974.)

ongoing leg exercise) does not increase the maximal oxygen uptake in proportion to the metabolic capacity of the extra muscle mass.

Although the increased sympathetic nervous activity plays a dominant role for the circulatory regulation during exercise, the mechanism behind this increased activation remains to be clarified. It seems reasonable to assume that the sympathetic outflow to the heart and the peripheral vascular bed is controlled by the same mechanism: there is a close correlation between the change in the heart rate and the change in perfusion of the abdominal viscera,[6, 32] and these two variables have a common time course during the initial phases of exercise (Figure 16-5). It is a characteristic feature that the sympathetic outflow to the heart and to the abdominal viscera occurs in proportion to the relative severity of exercise rather than to the absolute external work produced.[6, 32] In other words, the degree of activation depends on how close the exercising muscles are to their maximal capacity for aerobic metabolism. This suggests that the sympathetic activation is controlled by a feedback mechanism involving muscle afferents connected to metabolic receptors. The existence of such reflex mechanism has been demonstrated in animal experiments.[10] However, at the same time it is known, that an autonomic activation pattern similar to that seen during exercise can also be elicited from centers in the brain, and that this "central command" does play a role for the increase in heart rate and peripheral vasoconstriction at least at the onset of exercise.[14, 17] The relative importance of the feedback information from the muscles and of the central command in matching the sympathetic activity so precisely to both muscle metabolism and thermoregulatory needs remains to be established and represents a major unsolved problem within exercise physiology.

Long-term Cardiovascular Adaptations

A. Effects of Physical Conditioning

Physical conditioning performed as dynamic exercise increases the maximal circulatory capacity for oxygen transport and thereby the maximal oxygen uptake, and reduces the circulatory stress imposed by a given submaximal workload. Both local adaptations in the trained muscles and improved cardiac function contribute to this change.[7]

The peripheral changes include oxidative enzymatic adaptations, i.e., increased number and/or greater and more enzyme rich mitochondria,[20] together with increased maximal muscle blood flow.[7] The cardiac adaptations make the heart a more powerful pump and enable it to produce a greater maximal cardiac output.[33] These two kinds of circulatory adaptations occur in proportion to the relative stress imposed on the heart and on the peripheral circulation, respectively. To obtain marked improvement of the cardiac function, exercise with great muscle groups is required which elicits high values for cardiac output and stroke volume. In contrast, peripheral effects can be obtained to the same extent using exercise with smaller muscle groups as during exercise with great muscle groups.[7] Due to the increase in maximal oxygen uptake, a given submaximal oxygen uptake constitutes a smaller relative workload. Therefore, after training at a given submaximal oxygen uptake, the sympathetic activation is less pronounced and the heart rate as well as the peripheral vasoconstriction is less augmented. This means that the same workload imposes less strain on the heart and that the perfusion of the abdominal viscera is closer to that seen at rest.

B. Long-term Adaptation to Exercise in Heat

Also, the circulatory response to exercise in heat is modified by chronic exposure to this type of stress.[32] Acclimatization to work in heat brings about an earlier onset of sweating and an increment in sweat-rate and evaporative cooling. Thus, the need for sympathetic activation at a given oxygen uptake and external temperature is reduced, and the heart rate and the vascular resistance in visceral organs increase less.

Circulatory Adjustments to Exercise in Patients with Coronary Heart Disease

Most patients who are subjected to the exercise ECG test are between 35 and 65 years of age. Both the aging process and myocardial lesions contribute to the modification of the circulatory response to exercise in this age group compared to healthy young individuals.

In advanced age, especially after 60 years, the circulation tends to become hypokinetic, i.e., the cardiac output is low in relation to the oxygen uptake. However, the reduction in cardiac output also applies to the condition at rest, and the increase in cardiac output with a given increase in oxygen uptake is essentially the same in older as in younger subjects. The cardiac stroke volume is normally lower in older subjects, whereas the arterial blood pressure as well as the peripheral vascular resistance are higher. The maximal heart rate and probably also the maximal degree of sympathetic vasoconstriction decline with age. Both the maximal cardiac output and the maximal oxygen uptake diminish with aging.[23, 36]

In general, the presence of coronary heart disease subtracts further from physical performance capacity, but depending on the premorbid level and the severity of the disease, a wide range of impairment in cardiovascular adjustment to exercise may be encountered among patients with coronary heart disease.[3] Some coronary patients can hardly be distinguished from healthy subjects, but the majority of patients are likely to have a lower than normal maximal cardiac output and maximal oxygen uptake. The patients with angina pectoris tend to have a lower "symptom-limited" maximal oxygen uptake than the patients with uncomplicated healed myocardial infarction.

The reduced maximal oxygen uptake in coronary patients is associated with subnormal values for stroke volume and heart rate during maximal exercise. The arterial blood pressure during maximal exercise may be elevated, normal, or reduced; the latter is most often seen in patients with more advanced impairment of left ventricular function and/or angina pectoris. The increase in cardiac output in proportion to the oxygen uptake is often the same as in healthy subjects of the same age, but it tends to decline with increasing severity of coronary heart disease. With very severe impairment, very little or no increase in cardiac output is seen at the transition from rest to exercise, and the increase in heart rate only results in a fall in stroke volume.[8] However, for obvious reasons, such patients are seldom candidates for the exercise ECG test.

In most patients with coronary artery disease, an abnormal response of the stroke volume is observed during exercise. Not only is the stroke volume lower than normal and the heart rate higher during submaximal exercise, but the stroke volume decreases markedly at workloads requiring more than about 60–70% of the maximal oxygen uptake (Figure 16-6). This probably reflects impaired left ventricular function at higher relative workloads due to reversible myocardial ischemia. Other such signs are reduced left ventricular contractility, as judged from a slower rate of rise of left ventricular pressure and a reduced mean systolic ejection rate and an increased left ventricular end-diastolic pressure and volume during exercise.[6]

The peripheral circulatory regulation in patients with coronary artery disease corresponds in principle to that described for young healthy subjects.[6] Peripheral vasoconstriction is related to the increase in heart rate and the oxygen uptake in percent of the maximal oxygen uptake just as in healthy subjects, but the extent of change in both variables is reduced mainly due to aging. The maximal muscle blood flow is lower in proportion to the reduction in the maximal cardiac output.

A. Angina Pectoris

Although patients with angina pectoris often have a more profound impairment of left ventricular function and physical working capacity than patients with coronary artery disease without angina, there does not seem to be any specific differences in their central and peripheral circulatory regulation which separate them from other cardiac patients. However, from the exercise physiologist's viewpoint, the patient with angina pectoris is peculiar in that his capacity for dynamic exercise is not primarily limited by his ability to transport oxygen to the exercising muscles, but rather by the maximal oxygen supply to myocardial regions supplied by narrowed coro-

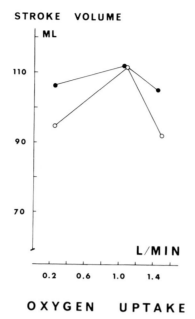

STROKE   VOLUME

Fig. 16-6 Mean values from 6 patients with coronary heart disease for stroke volume measured at rest, supine, and during exercise in the sitting position at a moderate and heavy submaximal workload before and after a period of physical conditioning. Both before and after training, stroke volume was higher during moderate submaximal exercise than during heavy submaximal exercise. In normal subjects stroke volume is maintained unchanged up to maximal levels of exercise (cf. Figure 16-3). (Modified from Clausen and Trap-Jensen, 1970.)

nary arteries. If pain is prevented by prophylactic administration of nitroglycerin, a patient with angina pectoris can exercise longer at a given workload or achieve higher workloads, and thus a higher maximal oxygen uptake.[11]

As previously mentioned, the myocardial oxygen demands are, among other factors, related to the heart rate and the arterial blood pressure. When chest pain is provoked in patients with angina pectoris, this occurs at an individually fairly constant threshold value for the product of the heart rate and the systolic blood pressure, the so-called rate pressure product (RPP).[31] Expressed by the coefficient of variation the reproducibility of this pain threshold value is on an average about 6%.[9] The constancy of the individual RPP pain threshold value also applies to situations which facilitate provocation of chest pain, as exercise in reduced or elevated environmental temperature, in the post-prandial period, after smoking or under influence of emotional stress.[16] It appears that the extra increase in heart rate and/or systolic blood pressure under these conditions is added to that caused by exercise. Thus, a smaller amount of exercise can be produced before the critical threshold value for RPP is reached.

The close relationship between the onset of angina and the RPP or the heart rate indicates that other determinants of myocardial oxygen demands, such as the contractile state or the diastolic ventricular volume, vary in proportion to the heart rate or are unchanged during upright exercise. However, the significance of an increased end-diastolic volume in augmenting the myocardial oxygen consumption is probably demonstrated during exercise performed in the supine position. In this situation the diastolic filling of the heart is greater and angina pectoris is provoked at a lower heart rate and RPP compared to the threshold value determined in the upright position.[4]

Conversely, during exercise with smaller muscle groups like, e.g., arm exercise, most patients tolerate a higher heart rate and RPP before chest pain is provoked,[6] despite the fact that there is a steeper increase in systolic pressure with increasing workload (Figure 16-3). Two differences between the circulatory adjustment to arm and leg exercise may help to explain this. The first is that the left ventricular end-diastolic volume, like the stroke volume, is smaller during arm exercise than during leg exercise. The other is that arm exercise, in variance with leg exercise, causes a significant increase not only in the systolic blood pressure, but also in the diastolic blood pressure (Figure 16-3). Since the myocardial perfusion mainly takes place during diastole, the increase in diastolic pressure means an increased effective perfusion pressure and an improved myocardial blood supply.

The additon of an isometric effort to dynamic exercise does not lead to earlier precipitation of chest pain, despite the resulting extra augmentation in RPP. On the contrary, some patients are able to exercise longer at a given workload on a bicycle ergometer when performing with a handgrip at the same time.[18, 24] These observations raise the question of whether the practice of isometric exercise really presents a particular risk in patients with coronary artery disease as it is generally believed. As assessed from the fact that it is rather difficult to provoke anginal pain and ECG changes using isometric efforts alone,[18, 24] myocardial ischemia is not especially easily provoked by this type of exercise. However, the problem needs further systematic study. Since the long-term adaptive changes resulting from isometrics are hardly of specific value for the patients, there seems to be no reason to directly recommend isometric exercise to patients with coronary artery disease.

Effect of Training on Patients with Coronary Heart Disease

Patients with coronary artery disease, with or without angina pectoris, who are able to participate in a physical training program obtain an increased exercise tolerance just as healthy individuals do. Like healthy subjects, they show an increase in maximal oxygen uptake and a reduced sympathetic activation during the submaximal exercise, with the ensuing decrement in heart rate and peripheral vasoconstriction at a given submaximal workload.[6] Although both cardiac and peripheral adaptations contribute to augment the working capacity in healthy subjects, most cardiac patients are probably not able to improve their cardiac function directly. The improved exercise tolerance they obtain from training is predominantly due to adaptive changes in the trained muscles. Nonetheless, these adaptations in the skeletal muscles are of great value for the cardiac functional conditions in these patients, because they reduce the need for sympathetic stimulation of the heart, and thus the myocardial oxygen demands during exercise. This is of specific significance for the patient with angina pectoris, because it enables him to achieve a greater amount of work before his critical RPP threshold value is reached.[9]

Effect of Drugs

The sympathetic stimulation of the heart during exercise can also be reduced by administration of beta-receptor blocking agents, and the resulting impaired heart rate and blood pressure response lead to an increased exercise tolerance in many patients because more work can be performed before the RPP threshold is attained. However, at the same time the RPP threshold is reduced[2] probably because maximal myocardial blood flow is diminished.[22] This effect can be explained either by the fact that the left ventricular end-diastolic volume is augmented during beta-receptor blockade or as the effect of a changed relation between the sympathetic vasoconstrictor activity on coronary resistance vessels and the local metabolic vasodilator influence.[1] It is probably due to these effects that some patients do not show increased exercise tolerance after beta-receptor blockade. Futhermore, beta-receptor blockade has adverse effects on peripheral circulatory regulation. In contrast to training, which diminishes both the sympathetic stimulation of the heart and the peripheral vasoconstrictor activity, causing a more ample perfusion of visceral organs during exercise, beta-receptor blockade reflexly mediates an exaggerated visceral vasoconstriction as a compensation for the reduction in cardiac output and in arterial blood pressure.[6]

Nitroglycerin has a well established ability to alleviate chest pain in patients with angina pectoris and to increase their working capacity when administered prophylactically.[9, 11, 16] During a period of 30–60 minutes, the drug produces an improvement in exercise capacity which is equal to that obtained by an effective training program.[9] The mechanism behind the effect of nitroglycerin is, however, quite different. Nitroglycerin acts by causing a general peripheral vasodilatation including both resistance and capacitance vessel. Due to the lower vascular resistance and the peripheral pooling of blood, the cardiac diastolic filling and the arterial blood pressure decrease. The reduction in myocardial oxygen demands obtained in this way is sufficient to override the extra energy costs induced by a concomitant compensatory increase in heart rate mediated by the arterial baroreceptors.[16] It is conceivable that nitroglycerin, at the same time, has a direct vasodilator action on coronary vessels. It can be doubted, however, that this effect includes the vessels with obliterative arteriosclerotic lesions and can cause an increased perfusion of myocardial regions, which suffer ischemia with increased demands for oxygen.

Summary

During muscular exercise several minutes in duration the main part of the energy expenditure in the active muscles must be covered by aerobic metabolic processes and the most important problem is to ensure sufficient oxygen supply to contracting skeletal muscles. The vasodilatation in muscle is adjusted to the metabolic demands by release of vasodilator metabolites. This local mechanism for flow regulation competes with a concomitant increased sympathetic vasoconstrictor activity. In addition, muscle contractions interfere mechanically with blood flow. During isometric contractions (static exercise), impediment of blood flow is appreciable at 15% of the maximal contraction force and complete at about 65%. During rhythmic contractions (dynamic exercise), in contrast, muscle blood flow is facilitated by alternating emptying and filling of the vascular bed caused by the contractions. Much higher values for muscle blood flow are thus seen during dynamic exercise.

Both isometric and dynamic exercise result in major central circulatory adjustments. During *isometric exercise* a modest increase in cardiac output (2 times the resting value) and in heart rate (up to 120–130 beats/minute) is accompanied by a marked increase in arterial mean blood pressure (up to 150–160 mm. Hg). During maximal *dynamic exercise* cardiac output can increase 4–6 times the resting level and heart rate attain 200 beats/minute, but the arterial mean blood pressure seldom exceeds 110–120 mm. Hg. However, if the dynamic exercise involves a concomitant isometric effort, the mean arterial pressure may increase in proportion hereto.

The augmentation in cardiac output during dynamic exercise amounts to 6 liters/minute/extra liter of oxygen uptake/minute and is directed to the active skeletal muscles (the respiratory muscles included), the myocardium, and, if exercise is continued for more than about 5 minutes, also to the skin to facilitate heat dissipation. The perfusion of most other non-exercising tissues is reduced due to increased activation of the sympathetic vasoconstrictor system. As far as the splanchnic-hepatic blood flow and the renal blood flow are concerned, the reduction in flow during exercise is closely related to the increase in heart rate. Both manifestations of increased sympathetic nervous activity occur in proportion to the relative severity of exercise expressed as the actual oxygen uptake in percent of the maximal oxygen uptake for the given type of exercise. Thus, at a given oxygen uptake, the degree of sympathetic activation is greater during exercise with smaller muscle groups (e.g., the arms) than during exercise with great muscle groups (e.g., the legs). The arterial mean blood pressure has also a steeper rise with increasing oxygen uptake during arm exercise due to the more pronounced peripheral vasoconstriction in proportion to the increase in cardiac output, which in turn is explained by a higher relative workload, and a greater component of isometric effort.

The integrated circulatory regulation during exercise depends mainly on 2 events: (a) the locally regulated vasodilatation in skeletal muscle which is the prime determinant of the cardiac output, and (b) the autonomic cardiovascular nervous reflexes, which make the heart a more efficient pump and ensure maintenance of arterial blood pressure and optimal conditions for venous return through peripheral vasoconstriction. During prolonged exercise, heat dissipation necessitates vasodilatation in skin, which is compensated by additional sympathetic activation causing further increase in heart rate, reinforced vasoconstriction in abdominal viscera and, at strenuous loads, probably also vasocontriction in active muscles.

The circulatory adjustments to exercise and thermal stress undergo adaptive changes with chronic exposure. Physical training results in a greater maximal cardiac output and maximal oxygen uptake and a modified response to submaximal exercise, many variables being less changed from the condition at rest at a given oxygen uptake. Both local adaptations in the trained muscles and improved cardiac function contribute to the changed circulatory response after training. The circulatory response to exercise in heat is modified by chronic exposure in such a way that the subjects rely more on sweating and evaporative cooling for heat dissipation so that vasodilatation in the skin can be less pronounced at a given heat load.

The circulatory adjustment to exercise in patients with coronary artery disease typically differs from that of normal subjects in that the maximal values for cardiac output, oxygen uptake, heart rate and arterial blood pressure are lower and the relation between cardiac output and oxygen uptake during submaximal exercise tends to be reduced. Most patients exhibit signs of left ventricular failure during exercise: the stroke volume declines at higher workloads, myocardial contractility is reduced and the end-diastolic left ventricular pressure and volume are increased.

In patients with angina pectoris, the exercise capacity is limited by a subnormal maximal myocardial oxygen supply. A given patient has a reproducible pain threshold value for easily obtainable indices of myocardial oxygen requirements, such as the heart rate and the product of heart rate and arterial systolic blood pressure. Training can increase the exercise capacity in the patients by reducing the heart rate and the blood pressure at a given workload, and thus enable a greater amount of exercise to be done before the critical level is attained at which myocardial ischemia occurs. A similar effect on the heart rate and blood pressure can be obtained by beta-receptor blocking agents. However, this intervention has adverse effects on the peripheral circulatory regulation, causing an increased vasoconstriction in visceral organs. Nitroglycerin dilates both resistance and capacitance vessels and the resulting reduced pressure and volume load on the heart diminish myocardial oxygen requirements and thereby the exercise capacity is increased.

REFERENCES

1. Abboud, F. M., Heistad, D. D., Mark, A. L. and Schmid, P. G.: Reflex control of the peripheral circulation. Prog. Cardiovasc. Dis., *18:*371, 1976.
2. Areskog, N. H. and Adolfsson, L.: Effects of a cardio-selective beta-adrenergic blocker (ICI 50172) at exercise in angina pectoris. Br. Med. J., *2:*601, 1969.
3. Bruce, R. A., Kusumi, F., Niederberger, M. and Petersen, J. L.: Cardiovascular mechanisms of functional aerobic impairment in patients with coronary heart disease. Circulation, *49:*696, 1974.
4. Bygdeman, S. and Wahren, J.: Influence of body position on the anginal threshold during leg-exercise. Eur. J. Clin. Invest., *4:*201, 1974.
5. Clausen, J. P.: Muscle blood flow during exercise and its significance for maximal performance, *in* Limiting Factors of Physical Performance, edited by J. Keul, pp. 253–266, Stuttgart, Georg Thieme, 1973.
6. Clausen, J. P.: Circulatory adjustments to dynamic exercise and effect of physical training in normal subjects and in patients with coronary artery disease. Prog. Cardiovasc. Dis., *18:*459, 1976.
7. Clausen, J. P.: The effect of physical training on cardiovascular adjustments to exercise in man. Physiol. Rev., *4557:*779, 1977.
8. Clausen, J. P. and Trap-Jensen, J.: Effects of training on the distribution of cardiac output in patients with coronary artery disease. Circulation, *42:*611, 1970.
9. Clausen, J. P. and Trap-Jensen, J.: Heart rate and arterial blood pressure during exercise in patients with angina pectoris. Effect of training and of nitroglycerin. Circulation, *53:*436, 1976.
10. Coote, J. H., Hilton, S. M. and Perez-Gonzales, J. F.: The reflex nature of the pressor response to muscular exercise. J. Physiol. (London), *215:*789, 1972.
11. Detry, J. M. R. and Bruce, R. A.: Effects of nitroglycerin on "maximal" oxygen intake and exercise electrocardiogram in coronary heart disease. Circulation, *43:*155, 1971.
12. Donald, K. W., Lind, A. R., McNicol, G. W., Humphreys, R. W., Taylor, S. H. and Staunton, H. P.: Cardiovascular responses to sustained (static) contractions. Circ. Res., 21 (Suppl.) *I:*15, 1967.
13. Ekblom, B., Goldbarg, A. N., Kilbom, A. and Åstrand, P. O.: Effects of atropine and propranolol on the oxygen transport system during exercise in man. Scand. J. Clin. Lab. Invest., *30:*35, 1972.
14. Folkow, B. and Neil, E.: Circulation, New York, Oxford University Press, 1971.
15. Folkow, B., Haglund, U., Jobal, M. and Lundgren, O.: Bood flow in the calf muscle of man during heavy rhythmic exercise. Acta Physiol. Scand., *81:*157, 1971.
16. Goldstein, R. E. and Epstein, S. E.: Medical management of patients with angina pectoris. Prog. Cardiovasc. Dis., *14:*360, 1972.
17. Goodwin, G. M., McCloskey, D. I. and Mitchell, J. H.: Cardiovascular and respiratory responses to changes in central command during isometric exercise at constant muscle tension. J. Physiol. (London), *226:*173, 1972.

18. Haissly, J. C., Messin, R., Degre, S., Vandermoten, P., Demaret, B. and Denolin, H.: Comparative response to isometric (static) and dynamic exercise tests in coronary disease. Am. J. Cardiol., 33:791, 1974.
19. Hennemann, E. and Olson, C. B.: Relations between structure and function in the design of skeletal muscle. J. Neurophysiol., 28:581, 1965.
20. Holloszy, J. O.: Biochemical adaptations to exercise: Aerobic metabolism, in Reviews In Exercise and Sports Sciences, edited by J. H. Willmore, pp. 45–71, New York, Academic Press, 1973.
21. Holmgren, A., Karlberg, P. and Pernow, B.: Circulatory adaptation at rest and during muscular work in patients with complete heart block. Acta Med. Scand., 164:119, 1959.
22. Jorgensen, C. R., Wang, K., Wang, Y., Gobel, F. L., Nelson, R. R. and Taylor, H.: Effect of propranolol on myocardial oxygen consumption and its hemodynamic correlates during upright exercise. Circulation, 48:1173, 1973.
23. Julius, S., Amery, A., Whitlock, L. S. and Conway, J.: Influence of age on the hemodynamic response to exercise. Circulation, 36:222, 1967.
24. Kerber, R. E., Miller, R. A. and Najjar, S. M.: Myocardial ischemic effects of isometric, dynamic and combined exercise in coronary artery disease. Chest, 67:388, 1975.
25. Klausen, K., Rasmussen, B., Clausen, J. P. and Trap-Jensen, J.: Blood lactate from exercising extremities before and after arm or leg training. Am. J. Physiol., 227:67, 1974.
26. Marshall, R. J. and Sphepherd, J. T.: Cardiac Function in Health and Disease. Philadelphia, W. B. Saunders, 1968.
27. Mellander, S. and Johansson, B.: Control of resistance, exchange, and capacitance functions in the peripheral circulation. Pharmacol. Rev., 20:117, 1968.
28. Mitchell, J. H. and Wildenthal, K.: Left ventricular function during exercise, in Coronary Heart Disease and Physical Fitness, edited by O. A. Larsen and O. Malmborg, pp. 93–96, Copenhagen, Munksgaard, 1971.
29. Pette, D. and Staudte, H. W.: Differences between red and white muscles, in Limiting Factors of Physical Performance, edited by J. Keul, pp. 23–35, Stuttgart, Georg Thieme, 1973.
30. Pickering, T. G., Gribbin, B., Petersen, E. S., Cunningham, D. H. C. and Sleight, P.: Effects of autonomic blockade on the baro-reflex in man at rest and during exercise. Circ. Res., 30:177, 1972.
31. Robinson, B. F.: Relation of heart rate and systolic blood pressure to the onset of pain in angina pectoris. Circulation, 35:1073, 1967.
32. Rowell, L. B.: Human cardiovascular adjustments to exercise and thermal stress. Physiol. Rev., 54:75, 1974.
33. Scheuer, J.: Physical training and intrinsic cardiac adaptations. Circulation, 47:677, 1973.
34. Smith, E. E., Guyton, A. C., Manning, R. D. and White, R. J.: Integrated mechanisms of cardiovascular response and control during exercise in the normal human. Prog. Cardiovasc. Dis., 18:421, 1976.
35. Sonnenblick, E. H., Ross, J. and Braunwald, E.: Oxygen consumption of the heart. Newer concepts of its multifactoral determination. Am. J. Cardiol., 22:328, 1968.
36. Strandell, T.: Circulatory studies on healthy old men. Acta Med. Scand (Suppl.), 414:1, 1964.

17

Complications of the Exercise ECG Test and Some Aspects of Medicolegal Problems

Lewis W. Gray, M.D. and
Edward K. Chung, M.D., F.A.C.P., F.A.C.C.

General Considerations

The submaximal or maximal exercise (stress) ECG test is designed to obtain diagnostic and functional data concerning the cardiovascular system. Various exercise ECG test protocols have been developed in order to obtain information not available at rest. Intuitively, then, it is expected that the exercise ECG test is not without inherent risks, and that complications can and do occur. To quote a report of the American Heart Association's Committee on Stress, Strain and Heart Disease:[1] "A single episode of stress in individuals rendered susceptible because of underlying heart disease, if of sufficient intensity and duration appears capable of eliciting adverse responses which may trigger or hasten certain cardiac lesions and dysfunctions. These may include angina pectoris, a cardiac dysrhythmia, acute congestive failure, or possibly a myocardial infarction."

The incidence of various complications is greatly influenced by many factors, including the method of the exercise ECG test, selection of the patients, facilities of the exercise ECG laboratory, etc. Fortunately, the incidence of complications is low,[2] and with careful precautions, the incidence can be kept low even in a risky population subgroup.[3, 4] Rochmis and Blackburn reported on the safety of exercise ECG test in 1971, using the combined center experience of 170,000 tests. The mortality rate was about 1:10,000; the combined mortality and morbidity rate was only 4:10,000.[2] Ellestad's experience confirms this data, and he has noted no mortality in his experience by using his own protocol.[3] Similarly, no major complications have been encountered and no death has been observed in the past 6 years at the Exercise ECG Laboratory of the Thomas Jefferson University Hospital by utilizing Chung's exercise ECG test protocol (see Chapter 9).

The law has become a necessary component of the medical curriculum, largely because the practice of medicine involves the weighing of competing personal values of the patient that the physician is not equipped to deal with alone.[5]

Various complications which may be observed during and after the exercise ECG test are summarized in Table 17-1. The criteria used at Thomas Jefferson University Hospital for terminating the exercise ECG test are described in Chapter 9.

Cardiac Complications

1. Cardiac Arrhythmias

(a) Tachyarrhythmias

Various cardiac arrhythmias are the most common complications of the exercise ECG test. It is not unusual to observe atrial arrhythmias, mostly

Table 17-1. Complications of Exercise ECG Test

Cardiac complications:
  Cardiac arrhythmias
    Tachyarrhythmias
      Atrial
      A-V junctional
      Ventricular
    Bradyarrhythmias
      Sinus
      A-V junctional
      Ventricular
      A-V block
      Asystole
    Brady-tachyarrhythmia syndrome
  Sudden death
  Angina pectoris
  Myocardial infarction
  Congestive heart failure
  Hypertension
  Hypotension and shock
Non-cardiac complications:
  Musculoskeletal trauma
  Peripheral claudication
  Cerebrovascular accidents
  Phlebitis
  Retinal separation
Ill-defined and miscellaneous complications:
  Severe fatigue, dizziness, fainting, general malaise,
  ill-defined body ache, etc., due to various causes.

atrial premature beats, during and immediately after exercise. Transient atrial arrhythmias, however, are considered clinically insignificant. Similarly, occasional ventricular premature beats are relatively common even in healthy individuals, especially when they are unifocal in origin. In general, most of these premature beats disappear at higher heart rates, perhaps returning during the resting period after the exercise ECG test. The clinical significance of these ventricular premature beats is not clearly known, although some investigators proposed that ventricular premature beats may have an association with coronary artery disease.[6] In general, ventricular premature contractions which become more frequent during higher degrees of exercise are considered clinically significant and these appear to have a more definite association with coronary artery disease.[7]

Needless to say, ventricular tachycardia, fibrillation and flutter during and after exercise are the worst cardiac rhythm problems which may lead to sudden death (will be discussed later). These ventricular tachyarrhythmias are often initiated by multifocal ventricular premature contractions, the R-on-T phenomenon and grouped ventricular beats.

(b) Bradyarrhythmias

Various bradyarrhythmias may occur during and after exercise but they are extremely uncommon. The occurrence of bradyarrhythmias, by and large, indicates a serious outcome, although the fundamental mechanism involved in the production of a given arrhythmia significantly influences the true clinical implication.

(c) Brady-tachyarrhythmia Syndrome

The term, brady-tachyarrhythmia syndrome is used when the cardiac rhythm disturbance consists of a component of bradyarrhythmias and a component of tachyarrhythmias. When brady-tachyarrhythmia syndrome is observed during and after exercise, it is a very serious problem, but its presence does not necessarily indicate coronary heart disease. In fact, sick sinus syndrome is the usual underlying process for brady-tachyarrhythmia syndrome. Cardiac arrhythmias during and after exercise will be discussed in detail in Chapter 13.

2. Sudden Death

Without a doubt, the most feared complication is sudden death, probably occurring as a result of ventricular tachyarrhythmias in the majority of instances. The incidence of ventricular tachycardia and ventricular fibrillation is said to be about 1 in 5,000 cases in Bruce's study,[8] but cardioversion was not required for cardiac arrhythmias in 12,000 exercise tests in another study by McHenry.[4]

As McHenry[4] points out, the key aspect is the ability to recognize a subgroup at increased risk for exercise-induced sudden death. In fact, there was a readily recognized subgroup with both proven coronary artery disease and exercise-induced hypotension which has an apparent 2.2% incidence of exercise-induced ventricular fibrillation.[4]

It is apparent that the classic diagnostic criteria of the S-T segment changes for interpreting the exercise ECG test are not sensitive enough to recognize every case of coronary heart disease and that there are other parameters useful in recognizing those individuals with coronary artery disease. Data generated by the Seattle Heart Watch[9] has shown that the variation in systolic blood pressure during exercise is highly correlated with the risk of subsequent death related to coronary artery disease. The annual sudden death rate decreased as the maximal attained systolic blood pressure increased among groups of men as follows:

Systolic blood pressure (mm. Hg):	Below 140	140–199	Above 200
Death Rate:	98/1,000	25/1,000	6.6/1,000.

In another study,[10] Bruce described the data on 6 men requiring electrical cardioversion after performing an exercise ECG test. In each case, there was the finding of a decrease or limited increase (less than 10 mm. Hg) in the systolic blood pressure with exercise. In all cases, the arrhythmia developed at the end of or after exercise. The author presumed that the failure of the cardiac output to rise with the peripheral demand for flow leads to regional myocardial ischemia with its attendant electrical instability. Of course, ventricular premature beats by themselves can lead to transient reduction in coronary arterial perfusion pressure, causing further ischemia and instability.

There is an interesting case report describing a post-exercise death from myocardial infarction in a patient with a negative exercise ECG test.[11] This 56-year-old male was exercised to 88% of maximal predicted heart rate using a 2-lead monitoring system. The test was entirely negative and the 10-minute post-exercise ECG was likewise normal. Thirty minutes later he complained of chest pain and suddenly collapsed; he was found to be in ventricular fibrillation. Autopsy revealed an aorta and coronary artery system free of atherosclerosis except for a left anterior descending coronary artery which was completely occluded by a fresh hemorrhage into an intimal plaque.

3. Angina Pectoris and Myocardial Infarction

One of the main purposes of the exercise ECG test is, of course, to elucidate and partially quantitate the cause of a patient's chest pain. One of the most important points in diagnosing angina pectoris is the association of chest discomfort with the S-T segment depression (rarely elevation) during and/or after exercise. It can be said that the diagnostic S-T segment change with or without angina pectoris is a signal of an imbalance between oxygen demand and supply in the heart. The possibility of myocardial damage is real under such circumstances, and as such the test must be monitored assiduously for possible development of acute myocardial infarction.

It should be noted that there is a possible risk of inducing acute myocardial infarction by exercise in every case with coronary heart disease, although its incidence is fortunately low. There has not been a single case of a patient developing acute myocardial infarction as a result of the exercise ECG test at the Exercise ECG Laboratory of Thomas Jefferson University Hospital in the past 6 years.

4. Congestive Heart Failure

It is well recognized that left ventricular compliance is reduced in the presence of myocardial ischemia. This is seen in the catheterization laboratory as an elevated mean pulmonary capillary wedge pressure and as a prominent atrial "kick" on the left ventricular pressure tracing. In the face of a reduced myocardial reserve, the strain of exercise can raise pulmonary venous pressure into the transudative pressure range, and hence cause the manifestation of congestive heart failure. Studies being conducted in the Exercise ECG Laboratory at Thomas Jefferson University Hospital have supported this finding. In preliminary studies, there has been a close correlation between a decline in post-exercise vital capacity and the presence of either a pre-existing compensated state of left ventricular failure, or severe coronary artery disease causing global ischemia with marked rises in left ventricular filling pressure during angina.[12] These results and methods are supported, also, by a study by Parker and Gorlin.[13]

5. Hypertension and Hypotension

Systolic blood pressure above 220 mm. Hg during exercise is considered an abnormal response. A more serious problem is the actual development of hypotension or no significant rise in blood pressure by exercise. Blood pressure change of physiologic versus abnormal response during exercise is described in detail in Chapter 11.

Non-cardiac Complications

1. Musculoskeletal Trauma

A variety of musculoskeletal trauma may be observed during the exercise ECG test. This is particularly true in elderly individuals who lose their balance during exercise. Furthermore, the incidence of trauma will increase when proper instructions regarding the test are not given to the patient. Musculoskeletal trauma in connection with the exercise ECG test is extremely important from a medico-legal viewpoint. It should be avoided with extreme care.

2. Peripheral Claudication

Atherosclerosis is a systemic disease. Thus, the stressing of skeletal muscle with a residual vascular reserve may produce as much symptomatology as stressing cardiac muscle. The only major problem as a result of exercise-induced claudication is that the exercise ECG test has to be terminated prematurely in these individuals. Peripheral claudication usually improves upon resting.

3. Cerebrovascular Accidents and Phlebitis

Cerebrovascular accidents and phlebitis in connection with the exercise ECG test have been reported [14] but their relationship to the exercise itself is not as direct as most of the other complications. These complications are generally very rare, and there has been no case of a patient developing a cerebrovascular accident during or after exercise at the Exercise Laboratory of Thomas Jefferson University Hospital in the past 6 years.

4. Retinal Separation

As a rare complication, retinal separation has been described and it is a real danger.[14] This complication is more likely to be seen in patients with a history of retinal separation or in those patients who have had previous cataract surgery.

Ill-defined and Miscellaneous Complications

Other than the above-mentioned complications, any possible untoward event may occur in connection with the exercise ECG test. These may include severe fatigue, dizziness, near-fainting or actual fainting, general malaise, ill-defined body ache, etc., due to various organic as well as functional causes. Every symptom should be evaluated carefully for possible serious complications when the symptom is severe enough.

Medico-legal Problems

Despite careful precautions and rigidly applied criteria for the exercise ECG test, complications can, and do, occur. This is unfortunate, particularly in light of our current medico-legal climate. Some definitions of legal terminology will be discussed first.

A suit against a physician or exercise laboratory can involve charges of negligence and/or battery. "Battery" may be defined simply as the "unconsented touching" of a patient.

Defining "negligence" is more complicated. In determining negligence, there are four criteria:

(1) Interests that are sacrificed if the activity is not undertaken.
(2) The likelihood of harm.
(3) The safety measures available to reduce the likelihood of harm. This is largely covered in the foregoing discussion. In regard to the safety measures, it is the usual practice of all exercise ECG laboratories to have full resuscitative equipment available to handle any emergency. This would include a defibrillator, a full complement of cardiovascular medications, materials for starting an intravenous line and for endotracheal intubation and respiratory support.
(4) Whether or not harm actually results.

Whereas negligence requires some "bad" outcome, battery incurs liability regardless of outcome, and, interestingly, is often excluded in malpractice insurance policies.

The exercise ECG test is an elective diagnostic procedure. In dealing with elective diagnostic procedures, the physician has 2 basic responsibilities:[15]

(1) That the patient must be made aware of foreseeable risks of that procedure, and that with such knowledge he consents to it.
(2) That the procedure be carefully performed and that all steps to minimize the risks to the patient be taken.

We have already presented most of the knowledge necessary to discharge the second responsibility. A few words on the term "carefully performed" are appropriate. This term indicates that the procedure should be administered only by a physician trained in its administration, and trained in dealing with the problems which may arise. Medico-legal risks may arise whenever a physician seeks to define a patient's condition. "In the physician-patient relationship, the physician has the responsibility of providing proper care and applying his skill, learning and judgement in accordance with the standards of his specialty and the generally accepted practice of the community."[16] It is the responsibility of the physician to select the technique most likely to provide the required data at the least risk to the patient. The test must be properly administered with adequate medical staff and equipment.

The first responsibility is the so-called "informed consent," legally defined as "a reasonable disclosure to the patient of the nature of his disease, of the treatment, and of the probable consequences of the treatment".[17] The exercise ECG test should not be performed without first obtaining a document of informed consent, signed by the patient and witnessed by the physician who will supervise the test (see Chapter 3). The consent form may not be absolutely required in many European or Asian countries, but it is mandatory in the United States of America at present because various medico-legal problems may be minimized or even avoided by obtaining the consent form.

As expected, after reading the consent form, some patients may refuse to undergo the exercise ECG test. This has led to an argument among physicians that the consent form may needlessly frighten the patient away from a diagnostically useful and safe test. A Cleveland Clinic study[18] seems to argue for a written and complete consent form. The authors concluded that the more detailed the explanatory forms, the more likely the patients were to sign for the test. This is because the patient may appreciate being included in the decision making process and may react favorably to having complete foreknowledge.

However, there is agreement among jurists that fully informed consent is not always necessary or desirable. Some patients often request that detailed explanation be avoided. For example, some patients may feel: "I came here for this test, let's get on with it. Don't scare me." Legal precedent has determined that:

(1) A patient's expressed desire not to be told about risks should be honored, and
(2) If the physician can document that risk disclosure will make the patient so distraught as to preclude a rational discussion, no such disclosure need be made.[19]

The exercise ECG test requires sophisticated equipment, and, consequently, one or more technical assistants may be required along with the physician. The roles of nurses and paramedical personnel are not clear from the medico-legal viewpoint.[20] It is a general agreement that only a physician may diagnose, treat, assess the progress of disease, or perform complex procedures on a human body. Some exercise ECG laboratories assign control of the exercise ECG test and aftercare to paramedical staff, nevertheless. Even though they may be fully familiar with the entire procedure, the physician is fully responsible for selecting trained and competent assistants. Depending upon the circumstances, he may be liable legally for malpractice along with them for breach of duty or negligence on their part.[16] It is safe to say, however, that a technician, no matter how well trained, may not and should not be the sole administrator of the exercise ECG test. The physician who supervised the exercise ECG test and/or the physician-in-charge of the exercise ECG laboratory will be totally responsible for the entire procedure, including the interpretation of the test, from the medico-legal viewpoint.

Summary

This chapter has reviewed the known complications of the exercise ECG test and the medico-legal aspects resulting from these complications. It is not possible to create a cookbook guide for the performance of an exercise ECG test that will avoid all complications in all patients and will guarantee the complete absence of court subpoena. Each patient must be tested and treated individually; each test may be modified in order to insure safety. The exercise ECG test should be avoided in high-risk patients. Possible contraindication for the exercise ECG test should be carefully considered (see Chapter 8).

Obtaining the consent from (see Chapter 3) is a mandatory procedure before the exercise ECG test, particularly in the United States of America. In addition, the entire procedure of the test must be supervised by a physician who is fully familiar with the exercise ECG test.

"The patient is best served by rendition of the best medical care available. Even if the end results are not as desired, there will be no basis for blame, since medicine is not an exact science which is capable of achieving a specific planned benefit."[16]

Preparations and precautions for the exercise ECG test are described in detail in Chapter 3.

REFERENCES

1. A report of the Committee on Stress, Strain and Heart Disease. American Heart Association. Circulation, 55:825A, 1977.
2. Rochmis, P. and Blackburn, H.: Exercise tests: A survey of procedures, safety, and litigation experience in 170,000 tests. J.A.M.A., 217:1061, 1971.
3. Ellestad, M. H.: Stress Testing. Philadelphia. F. A. Davis, 1975.
4. McHenry, P. L.: Risks of graded exercise testing. Am. J. Cardiol., 39:935, 1977.
5. Informed consent and the dying patient. Yale Law J., 83:1632, 1974.
6. Anderson, M. T., Lee, G. B., Champion, B. C. et al.: Cardiac dysrhythmias associated with exercise stress testing. Am. J. Cardiol., 30:763, 1972.
7. Goldschlager, N., Cake, D. and Cohn, K.: Exercise-induced ventricular arrhythmias in patients with coronary artery disease: Their relation to angiographic findings. Am. J. Cardiol., 31:434, 1973.
8. Bruce, R. A.: Progress in exercise cardiology, in Progress in Cardiology, edited by P. N. Yu and J. F. Goodwin, Vol. 3, pp. 113–169, Philadelphia, Lea & Febiger, 1974.
9. Irving, T. B., Bruce, R. A. and DeRouen, T. A.: Variations in and significance of systolic pressure during maximal exercise (treadmill) testing. Am. J. Cardiol., 39:841, 1977.
10. Irving, T. B. and Bruce, R. A.: Exertional hypotension and post-exertional ventricular fibrillation in stress testing. Am. J. Cardiol., 39:849, 1977.
11. Lintgen, A. B.: Death from myocardial infarction after exercise testing with normal result. J.A.M.A., 235:837, 1976.
12. Gray, L. W. and Chung, E. K.: Unpublished data.
13. Parker, G..W. and Gorlin, R.: Immediate post exercise vital capacity: A measure of increased pulmonary capillary pressure. Am. J. Med. Sci., 257:365, 1969.
14. Hamrell, B. B., Blackburn, H. and Taylor, H. L.: Disabling complications of physical exercise training in middle-age, coronary-prone American men, in Exercise and the Heart: Guidelines for Exercise Programs, edited by R. L. Morse, p. 188, Springfield, Ill., Charles C Thomas, 1972.
15. Siegel, G. H.: Legal aspects of informed consent, stress testing and exercise programs (the law and cardiac rehabilitation), in Exercise Testing and Exercise Training in Coronary Heart Disease, edited by J. P. Naughton, H. K. Hellerstein and I. C. Mohler, p. 387, London, Academic Press, 1973.

16. Ladimer, I.: Professional liability in exercise testing for cardiac performance. Am. J. Cardiol., *30:*753, 1972.
17. McNiece, H. F.: Legal aspects of exercise testing. N. Y. State J. Med., p. 1822, July, 1972.
18. Alfidi, R. J.: Informed consent—a study of patient reaction. J.A.M.A., *216:*1325, 1971.
19. Annas, G. J.: Legal aspects of informed consent. New Engl. J. Med., *297:*228, 1977.
20. Bacon, R.: Legal aspects of exercise stress testing and exercise therapy, *in* Medical Aspects of Exercise Testing and Training, edited by L. Zohman and B. Phillips, p. 156, New York, Intercontinental Medical Book Corp., 1973.

INDEX*

* Italics indicate major discussion.